International and Cultural Psychology

Series Editor

Anthony J. Marsella

More information about this series at http://www.springer.com/series/6089

Farah A. Ibrahim • Jianna R. Heuer

Cultural and Social Justice Counseling

Client-Specific Interventions

Springer

Farah A. Ibrahim
University of Colorado Denver
Denver, CO, USA

Jianna R. Heuer
LaGuardia Community College
Long Island City, NY, USA

ISSN 1574-0455 ISSN 2197-7984 (electronic)
International and Cultural Psychology
ISBN 978-3-319-35799-7 ISBN 978-3-319-18057-1 (eBook)
DOI 10.1007/978-3-319-18057-1

Springer Cham Heidelberg New York Dordrecht London

Softcover re-print of the Hardcover 1st edition 2016

Printed on acid-free paper

Springer International Publishing AG Switzerland is part of Springer Science+Business Media (www.springer.com)

It is with deep gratefulness and sincere
appreciation that I acknowledge the support
and encouragement I have received
from my family, especially my mother,
Iffat Almas, my brother, Naeem Khan,
and my children, Jianna and Aaron,
my mentors, Drs. Edwin L. Herr,
Allen E. Ivey, and Clemmont Vontress,
and my students and clients over
the last 37 years. The gifts I have received
from all these sources have facilitated
my research endeavors, and my work
on cultural competence, cultural
responsiveness, and social justice
in counseling interventions.

Farah A. Ibrahim

I want to thank my mother for inviting
me to participate in writing this book;
it has enhanced my knowledge and skills.
Your love and support throughout my life
has empowered me to be who I am today.
To my brother, Aaron Schroeder, thank you
for making me believe in second chances,
I love you. To my partner, Jason Heuer,
this book would not exist without

your love and support—you are my rock and inspiration. To my mentors, grateful thanks to Diana Gasperoni, for always believing in me and for sharing your invaluable knowledge and skills with me, and Gina Barreca, for helping me believe I really could be a writer. To the students, staff, and interns I have worked with at LaGuardia Community College, thank you for teaching me patience, acceptance, and tolerance and allowing me to be a part of your journey. To my friends and therapist, thank you for your support and care.

Jianna R. Heuer

Disclaimer

The cases in this text are developed on hypothetical clients, designed to demonstrate using the cultural assessments to make the interventions client specific. Any resemblance to any specific client, or situation is coincidental, and the profiles are not specific to any specific person or situation.

Introduction

What Does This Book Offer You, the Professional, and Our Profession?

A new book, at its best, offers new, challenging, and important insight leading us to the future. This is a book that can and will make a difference for your daily practice and/or teaching. In addition, it is a book that leads to increasing competence and understanding for counselors, psychologists, social workers, and human service professionals.

You will soon start reading the work of Farah A. Ibrahim and Jianna R. Heuer, so I'll be brief with bullet points. I suggest special attention to the following issues:

- We talk about multiculturalism with awareness that diversity is complex and multifaceted. Rather than just sharing broad differences in culture, this book shows how to assess the individual client and then establish appropriate interventions that make sense to the client and lead to change.
- The above tall order is achieved through presenting specific steps for operationalizing treatment plans based on acculturation status within one's own culture, as well as acculturation to the dominant culture within which the client lives.
- We now all agree that William Cross' cultural identify theory (CIT) is an essential part of counseling and clinical practice. The authors show how concepts of worldview may be assessed in conjunction with CIT leading to individually unique understandings and actions.
- I am impressed with the authors' discussion of acculturation. The practical and useful balance for assessing acculturation is essential for us all. Too much of our multicultural thought is focused on cultural "difference." Of course, this is central, but the authors move us forward with innovative insights—particularly, interventions need to be in accord with the acculturation of the client. For example, clients of Mexican descent may be recent immigrants or they could have been in the USA for generations. They have in common discrimination and other cultural traits, but their level of acculturation and accompanying counseling needs varies extensively.

- Social justice action has become increasingly central to our profession, and its focus on community and social change is critical, but insufficient attention has been given to the social justice implications of psychotherapy—and the authors show how profoundly important it is to include ideas of social justice in the individual interview.
- Understanding immigrants and refugees become the focus of two separate chapters—definitive in nature. Trauma is a feature of both experiences and here the discussion will again be most helpful.
- Fascinating, relevant, and highly useful case studies provide the conclusion of this book. Here, we see how the concepts presented earlier are implemented in counseling and clinical practice.

In short, there is a lot here to absorb, as several concepts will be practice changing. Each of us will take something unique from this book that will make a difference. We are all lucky to have the wisdom of Farah A. Ibrahim and Jianna R. Heuer. Enjoy your time with them.

University of Massachusetts Amherst
Amherst, MA, USA
University of South Florida
Tampa, FL, USA

Allen E. Ivey, Ed.D., A.B.P.P.

Preface

This text addresses a void in the literature on diverse counseling encounters by providing tools and approaches for cultural assessment. It also presents social justice variables of privilege and oppression to help make the counseling intervention (process and goals) relevant and meaningful to the client. Several texts have addressed the issue of counseling the "other" or counseling within-group, and counseling clients from other cultural contexts than the helper's, i.e., culture (ethnicity, nationality), disability, gender, and sexual orientation, and these include books on theories, strategies, and skills, along with guidelines and competency statements issued by professional associations to increase efficacy in counseling across cultures, genders, sexual orientations, spirituality or religions, developmental stages, and ability/disability levels. In addition, researchers have addressed the importance of social class, and contexts that clients come from, cultural and geographic.

However, no text has addressed how the counselor or clinician can formulate a counseling intervention plan, by providing specific information for addressing all the cultural and social justice variables that are contextual for a client. As Marsella (2015) notes "How can successful counseling ignore or be indifferent to the cultural context of a person's life? How can the personal history of being a racial or ethnocultural minority be avoided or denied with all of its consequences for accumulated injustices, oppression, and abuses? When this occurs, it is no longer counseling as a healing art and science that is present, rather it is simply a re-socialization" (p. vii). Although texts exist that address these variables individually, this leaves the average counselor/therapist wondering how they can attend to so many factors, while also focusing on the client, the presenting problem, and building a therapeutic relationship.

This text helps mental health professionals in (a) identifying the cultural and contextual variables significant for a client by getting the information from the client, (b) building a therapeutic relationship during this process, and (c) incorporating client-specific cultural information in developing the goals for counseling, and making the intervention culture specific. We continue to hear about early terminations, and disappointing counseling encounters for culturally different clients (Sue, Zane, Hall, & Berger, 2009). These negative outcomes are the result of an inability to incorporate the client-specific cultural variables, client values, beliefs and assumptions, and contextual variables, such as social class and place in a hierarchical society, into the counseling intervention. When we are presented with broad guidelines either about a cultural group, or counseling competency statements, without any guidance on how to operationalize the information and make it relevant to a client's situation, it results in confusion for the helping professional, and frustration for the client. Shin (2015) notes that "a common criticism of racial/ethnic identity stage theories, offered previously by several scholars, is the fact that the models fail to capture the vast intra-group differences in identity development within all racial and ethnic groups" (p. 13). This stance can be generalized to most of the information one finds in the multicultural counseling domain, ergo the need to "decolonize" the field of cross-cultural, multicultural, transcultural counseling, by taking away the generalities common to psychology to describe cultural groups, without providing the tools to make information applied to counseling settings client specific. The primary goal in providing therapeutic services is to initially develop a therapeutic relationship. However, focusing on what the profession wants, recommendations from the research literature, and the training that professionals undergo, and requirements for ethical practice create a dilemma for a therapist.

Making the intervention meaningful to a client is the goal of this text, using specific cultural assessment tools, and providing case studies to highlight how the assessments were helpful in making the intervention client specific. The purpose of counseling is to help the client in making his or her life more manageable; by providing knowledge and skills that will provide insights, and enhance the client's ability to negotiate the personal, cultural, social, and occupational world successfully. Given this goal, it is evident that a text is needed to address the issue of how to manage the body of literature available in a meaningful manner, and to incorporate the knowledge, skills, and competencies into each specific counseling intervention, and to meet the client in his or her cultural, familial, social, and occupational world, along with recognizing the personal variables, such as personal style, and attitudes, that are commonly addressed in counseling encounters.

This text addresses critical information needed to conduct appropriate cultural assessments and incorporate the results into the counseling interventions, i.e., development of goals and process. As counseling and psychology goes international due to impact of globalization, it is critical that theory, practice, and research consider meaningfulness of theories, competency and ethical guidelines, and assessment models for a global audience (Friedman, 1999; Leach & Gauthier, 2012; Leong, Pickren, Leach, & Marsella, 2012). This is especially critical as many developing and developed nations look to American Psychology as the standard for theory, practice, and research. The chapters present information on the rationale and research for using cultural assessments; the information is grounded in professional, and ethical guidelines for assessment, and counseling interventions. Not only does the text identify the key cultural domains that need assessment to understand the client's cultural identity and context, it also includes cases (Chap. 8) to show how the information is incorporated into the counseling process.

The cases utilize assessment strategies needed for each case to develop interventions that are culturally sensitive, and tailored to address the client's presenting problem, incorporating culturally relevant strategies and goals for a positive outcome. The strategies and tools presented are not the only the ones in the research literature, several instruments and tools exist, we encourage you to consider cultural assessment strategies that would be specific and useful for the client you are working with, and to develop your interventions incorporating the domains identified in this text, i.e., incorporating cultural identity, worldview, acculturation, privilege and oppression, and other client-specific issues that may be relevant. Good luck with your interventions and may you be highly successful in your chosen profession and provide culturally sensitive, and responsive counseling and psychotherapy in all your settings.

Denver, CO Farah A. Ibrahim, Ph.D., L.P. (CO)

References

Friedman, T. L. (1999). *The lexus and the olive tree: Understanding globalization*. New York: Farrar, Straus, & Giroux.

Leach, M. M., & Gauthier, J. (2012). Internationalizing the professional ethics curriculum. In F. T. L. Leong, M. M. Leach, & M. Malikiosi-Loizos (Eds.), *Internationalizing the psychology curriculum in the US* (pp. 201–224). New York: Springer.

Leong, F. T. L., Pickren, W. E., Leach, M. M., & Marsella, A. J. (Eds.). (2012). *Internationalizing the psychology curriculum in the US*. New York: Springer.

Marsella, A. J. (2015). Foreword. In R. D. Goodman & P. C. Gorski (Eds.), *Decolonizing "multicultural" counseling through social justice* (pp. vii–x). New York: Springer.

Shin, R. Q. (2015). The application of critical consciousness and intersectionality as tools for decolonizing racial/ethnic identity development models in the fields of counseling and psychology. In R. D. Goodman & P. C. Gorski (Eds.), *Decolonizing "multicultural" counseling through social justice* (pp. 11–22). New York: Springer.

Sue, S., Zane, N., Hall, G. C. N., & Berger, L. K. (2009). The case for cultural competency in psychotherapeutic interventions. *Annual Review of Psychology, 60*, 525–548. doi: 10.1146/annurev.psych.60.110707.163651

Contents

1 Social Justice and Cultural Responsiveness in Counseling Interventions: Using Cultural Assessments 1
Introduction and Overview 1
Cultural Identity 2
Worldview 3
Why Focus on Worldview and Cultural Identity? 4
Privilege and Oppression 5
Acculturation 6
Identifying Healing Systems in the Client's Cultural World 7
Scope of This Text 9
Summary 10
References 10

2 Cultural Identity: Components and Assessment 15
Ethnicity 16
Age and Developmental Stage 19
Gender 20
Gender Identity 22
Transgender Identity 23
Sexual Orientation 24
Cultural Background 25
Migration Status 25
Languages 27
Religion and Spirituality 28
Ability/Disability Status 30
Composition of the Family 31
Birth Order 32
Geographical Environment 33
Social Class 34

Three Key Domains of Identity That Feature in the Presenting Problem.... 35
Conclusion 37
References.... 37

3 **Worldview: Implications for Culturally Responsive and Ethical Practice**.... 51
Worldview Defined 51
Worldview and Counseling.... 54
Conducting Worldview Assessment 56
Establishing a Positive Therapeutic Relationship.... 57
Using Worldview Information to Facilitate Counseling Interventions.... 59
Optimistic Worldview 61
Traditional Worldview 62
Here-and-Now/Spontaneous Worldview.... 65
Pessimistic Worldview.... 66
Research Overview: The Scale to Assess Worldview.... 67
Research on Worldview 67
Conclusion 69
References.... 70

4 **Understanding Acculturation and Its Use in Counseling and Psychotherapy**.... 77
Introduction.... 77
Rationale for Incorporating Assessment of Acculturation.... 78
Acculturation.... 79
Acculturation: Conceptual Approaches 81
Changing Assumptions.... 84
Psychological Well-Being and Acculturation.... 85
Psychological Assessment: Conceptual and Methodological Issues.... 86
Assessment of Acculturation 87
Counseling Implications 90
Conclusion 91
References.... 91

5 **Incorporating Social Justice and Advocacy in Counseling and Psychotherapy**.... 99
Introduction.... 99
Social Justice: Meaning and Implications.... 99
Demographics of the United States.... 103
Social Justice Concerns and Advocacy in Counseling 104
Social Justice Principles and Advocacy Competencies 105
Operationalization of Social Justice Principles.... 108
Counseling Modalities and Social Justice.... 109
The Individual Level.... 109
Group Level 110

Societal and Global Contexts ... 111
Therapist Characteristics for Effective Social Justice Work ... 112
Assessment of Social Justice Concerns ... 114
References ... 116

6 **Immigrants: Identity Development and Counseling Issues** ... 123
Introduction ... 123
Identity Development ... 123
Role of Ethnic or Personal Identity ... 124
Integration in Host Culture ... 125
Phases of Development ... 128
Counseling Strategies and Psychotherapy ... 132
Challenges for Immigrant Populations ... 136
Recommendations for Interventions for Positive Immigrant Identity Development ... 138
Conclusion ... 140
References ... 141

7 **Refugees: Adaptation and Psychological Interventions** ... 151
Who Are Refugees? ... 151
Identity Development of Refugees ... 154
Trauma and Its Impact on Refugees ... 158
Implications for Counseling Refugees ... 160
Treatment Modalities ... 162
Summary ... 163
References ... 164

8 **Application of Social Justice and Cultural Responsiveness Strategies: Using Cultural Assessments in Counseling and Psychotherapy** ... 169
Introduction ... 169
Process for Conducting Cultural Assessments ... 169
Cultural Information: Application in Counseling ... 170
Implications for Psychological Interventions ... 171
Being Authentic ... 171
Connecting with the Client with Empathy ... 172
Mutual Relationship and Co-construction ... 172
The Not-Knowing Perspective ... 173
Identify and Affirm the Client Strengths ... 173
Dynamics of a Dyadic Relationship and Collaborative Goal Setting ... 173
Evaluate the Effectiveness of the Intervention ... 174
Recognize Limits of Cultural Competence ... 175
Case 1: Counseling a Native American Client ... 176
Aimee Aron-Reno
Introduction ... 176
Client Information ... 176

Presenting Problem 176
Social/Educational Background 177
Assessments 178
Other Relevant Assessments 179
Counselor Biases 180
Intervention Strategies 180
Evaluation of the Assessments and the Intervention 183
Summary 185
Case 2: Counseling a Cross-Racial African American Adoptee 186
Kimberly Berkey
Introduction 186
Client Information 187
Assessments 188
Counselor Biases 190
Intervention 190
Evaluation of the Assessments and the Intervention 191
Summary 192
Case 3: Counseling a Bicultural Native American Client 193
Jennifer Anne Blair
Client Information 193
Presenting Problem 193
Social/Educational Background 194
Assessments 195
Counselor Biases 198
Client Goals 199
Intervention 199
Evaluation of the Assessments and Interventions 202
Summary 204
Case 4: Counseling a Colombian Immigrant Client 204
Carlo A. Caballero
Client Information 204
Cultural Background 204
Presenting Problem 204
Social/Educational Background 205
Assessments 205
Other Assessments 207
Overall Intervention Plan 208
Summary 209
Case 5: Counseling a Lesbian Latina Client 210
Bryce Carithers
Client Information 210
Background Information 210
History of Presenting Problem 210
Family Structure 211
Client Strengths 211

Assessments 212
Intervention 214
Summary 217
Case 6: Counseling a Transgender Client 217
Jianna R. Heuer
Client Information 217
Presenting Problem 218
Assessments 219
Behavioral Observations 221
Risk Assessment 221
DSM-5 Diagnosis 221
Counselor Biases 222
Client Goals 222
Intervention 222
Evaluation of the Assessments and Interventions 224
Intervention Evaluation 224
Summary 224
Case 7: Counseling an Iranian Immigrant Client 225
Lisa Taggart
Client Information 225
Cultural Background 225
Presenting Problem 225
Assessments 227
Counselor Biases 228
Intervention 229
Evaluation of Assessments and Intervention 230
Summary 231
References 232

Appendix A Cultural Identity Check-List-Revised© 239

Appendix B Scale to Assess World View© 241

Appendix C United States Acculturation Index© 247

Index 249

List of Figures

Fig. 1.1 Factors influencing cultural identity and worldview. *Key*: *CI* cultural identity, *WV* worldview, *AC* acculturation, *EI* ethnic identity, *GI* gender identity, *PO* privilege and oppression, *R/S* religion/spirituality, *SI* sexual identity, *SPH* sociopolitical history 2

Fig. 7.1 The multidimensionality of cultural identity. *AC* acculturation, *CI* cultural identity, *EI* ethnic identity, *GI* gender identity, *PO* privilege and oppression, *R/S* religion/spirituality, *SI* sexual identity, *SPH* sociopolitical history, *WV* world view 156

Fig. 7.2 Refugee cultural identity 157

List of Tables

Table 3.1 Comparison of Kluckhohn's existential value orientations and Schwartz's empirically derived universal values 53
Table 3.2 Four worldviews derived for the US sample 56

Contributors

Aimee Aron-Reno, M.A., N.C.C., L.P.C. University of Colorado Denver, Denver, CO, USA

Kimberly Berkey BMGI International Consulting, Denver, CO, USA

Jennifer Anne Blair, M.A., L.P.C.C. Jennifer Blair Counseling, Denver, CO, USA

University of Colorado Denver, Denver, CO, USA

Carlo A. Caballero University of Colorado Denver, Denver, CO, USA

Bryce Carithers University of Colorado Denver, Denver, CO, USA

Lisa Taggart, M.B.A., M.A., N.C.C. Four Directions Counseling LLC, Denver, CO, USA

University of Colorado Denver, Denver, CO, USA

About the Authors

Farah A. Ibrahim, Ph.D., L.P. (CO) is a fellow of the American Psychological Association (Society for Counseling Psychology) and a licensed psychologist (CT, DC, CO). She is past president of Counselors for Social Justice (2002–2003), a division of the American Counseling Association. She has served at the University of Connecticut, Howard University, and as Chair of Teacher and Counselor Education at Oregon State University as a tenured full professor. She is currently serving as full professor in the School of Education and Human Development at the University of Colorado Denver. She is the author of the Existential Worldview theory and is the developer of the following instruments: *Scale to Assess Worldview*© with Harris Kahn, the "Cultural Identity Check List©" (Ibrahim, 1990, 2007), the "Cultural Competence Survey©" (Ibrahim, 2005), and the United States Acculturation Index© (Ibrahim, 2008). She has conducted research on worldview and training for cultural effectiveness, gender and worldview, organizational culture and worldview, identity development, South Asian identity issues, trauma and posttraumatic stress disorder (PTSD) due to oppression, and infusion of social justice and cultural competencies in counseling curricula. Her latest research has focused on counseling Muslims in the West. She has a video on "Counseling Muslims" marketed by Microtraining Associates. She has assisted with several grant projects as a consultant or as co-principal investigator focusing on cultural competence training, effect of domestic violence on children and adolescents, and intergenerational trauma and its impact and health and mental health. Her current research interests are cultural competence and social justice training, cross-cultural research on worldviews, assessment in cross-cultural settings, identity development in a diverse society, Counseling South Asian immigrants and international students, and alleviation, and elimination of trauma and violence in society, social justice, and cultural competence in group work.

Jianna R. Heuer, M.A., L.C.S.W., Ph.D. has a Master's degree in Social Work from New York University. She currently serves as a part-time counselor for students with disabilities at LaGuardia Community College. Her research interests focus on cultural responsiveness and social justice concerns. She also maintains a private practice in New York City where she focuses on college coaching as well as relationship issues, trauma, disability issues, anxiety, and depression.

Chapter 1
Social Justice and Cultural Responsiveness in Counseling Interventions: Using Cultural Assessments

Introduction and Overview

This chapter provides an overview of the variables necessary for conducting a cultural assessment for counseling and psychotherapy to provide services with competency in both social justice interventions and cultural responsiveness. Guidelines and competency statements of all mental health professional organizations require attention to these issues, i.e., American Counseling Association (ACA, 1992, 2014), American Psychological Association (APA, 2002, 2010), American Psychiatric Association (APA 2013a, 2013b), American Association for Marriage and Family Therapists, (AAMFT, 2012), and the National Association of Social Workers (NASW), 2008). The key variables identified by the various professional associations and current research on cultural responsiveness, indicate an understanding of cultural identity (cultural/racial/ethnic identity), cultural context, and other relevant cultural issues, and the meaning of these issues in the client's culture, and context (Marsella, 2015). Mental health service providers are also mandated to have knowledge of possible resolutions based on the client's culture, client philosophy of life, social class, educational level, and other significant variables such as gender identity, sexual orientation, age and the meaning ascribed to life stages, spiritual and/or religious affiliation, languages spoken, social class, etc. (Conwill, 2015; Goodman, 2015; Reyes Cruz & Sonn, 2015; Smith & Chamber, 2015). A brief overview of key variables follows determined to be useful in cultural competence and responsiveness. Figure 1.1 shows all the variables that influence an individual's cultural identity and worldview.

F.A. Ibrahim, J.R. Heuer, *Cultural and Social Justice Counseling*,
International and Cultural Psychology, DOI 10.1007/978-3-319-18057-1_1

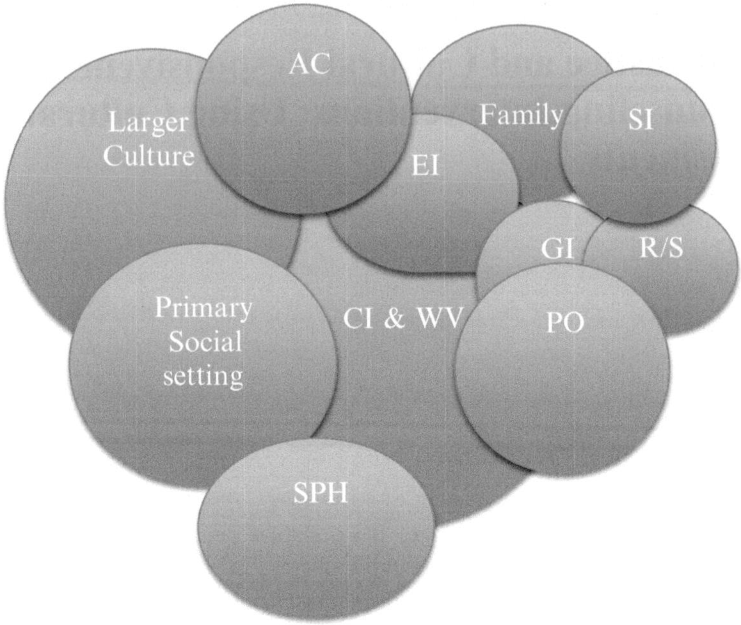

Fig. 1.1 Factors influencing cultural identity and worldview. *Key*: *CI* cultural identity, *WV* worldview, *AC* acculturation, *EI* ethnic identity, *GI* gender identity, *PO* privilege and oppression, *R/S* religion/spirituality, *SI* sexual identity, *SPH* sociopolitical history

Cultural Identity

Cultural identity is a person's sense of self, developed within a familial, social, cultural, and political world and is influenced by several variables. Psychological theories have evolved significantly in the last 40 years to recognize that identity, which was considered a unitary model known as self-identity (Burke, 1980; McCall & Simmons, 1978; Stryker, 1968, 1987), to recognizing that identity can have several aspects such as racial identity (Cross, 1978, 1991; Helms, 1990; Shin, 2015), gender identity (Downing & Roush, 1985; Money, 1973; Stewart & McDermott, 2004), ethnic identity (Phinney, 1990; Shin, 2015), sexual identity (Cass, 1979; McCarn & Fassinger, 1996; Smith & Geroski, 2015), and social class identity (Liu, 2001; Smith & Chamber, 2015). Ibrahim (1991, 2007) recommended that cultural identity should be viewed as a multidimensional construct, with personal, cultural/ethnic, familial, social, historical, ability/disability perspectives and provided a Cultural Identity Check List© to identify variables important to a client. Over time, these identity dimensions have emerged as significant in terms of understanding clients to provide counseling and psychotherapy in a diverse society (Hipolito-Delgado, 2009).

The social construction of identity as noted in psychological reports that describe a client as "John is a Black male…" places the emphasis on color and considers a client only from the perspective of race or ethnicity and gender. This stance is limited in identifying all the influences that form identity. Ibrahim (1999, 2003) notes that various aspects of identity may be significant to the specific presenting problem, as context changes and how people relate to an issue. This text focuses on helping counselors and therapists in identifying all the relevant variables that will affect goals and processes for counseling to make the intervention culturally relevant, sensitive, and meaningful to a client.

The issue of cultural identity and context was formalized in the Diagnostic and Statistical Manual-IV (DSM-IV, APA 1994, 2000). It was recommended by the American Psychiatric Association that a diagnosis could not be made without understanding the client's culture, and socialization. The recent revision of the DSM-5 (APA, 2013a, 2013b) requires a "Cultural formulation interview" to understand a client's cultural world, identity, and context. The variables to consider in a formal formulation of cultural identity for diagnosis focus on the intersections of a person's multidimensional identity and include: Cultural and racial identity, including ethnicity or ethnicities; gender identity and sexual orientation; partnering status, i.e., single, divorced, widowed, coupled, original partnership or blended family, nuclear family or extended family living arrangement, single career or dual career couple; age and life stage; ability and disability status; spirituality and/or religion; socioeconomic status (SES); educational level of immediate family members, and client's educational level; native to the culture in which they are being evaluated, or immigrant, generation in the United States, region of the world they came from, and the culture of origin versus the culture they are in now, enculturation to primary culture, and acculturation to host culture. Subsumed, in this analysis is the client's cultural group, how it was received and integrated in the host culture, leading to an assessment of acculturation; privilege and oppression analysis; and the geographical environment, (urban, suburban, or rural) that clients come from, and where they are living now. All these variables may not be salient to the presenting problem or the focus of the intervention, however, knowing the client's cultural, personal, familial, historical, and social world helps in clarifying how many variables will need to be addressed, or incorporated into the specific intervention. Chapter 2 will elaborate on these variables.

Worldview

Initially cultural efficacy was linked with understanding the client's worldview (Ibrahim, 1984, 1985; Ibrahim & Arredondo, 1986). Sue (1978) was the original proponent of the importance of worldview in cross-cultural counseling; he noted that worldview could be linked to two psychological theories, i.e., Locus of Control (Rotter, 1966, 1975) and Attribution Theory (Weiner, 1974). Both these theories address issues of collectivism and individualism, and the influence of the socialization process, based on cultural context. In the social sciences, the concept of worldview was considered important in sociological and anthropological theories and research.

Focusing on identifying the differences between people socialized in collectivistic or individualistic cultural systems. Historically, societies of Asian, African, Middle Eastern origin were and still tend to be closer to the collectivism end of the continuum, and Western Europe and Europe in general, tends to be toward the individualism end of the continuum with variations based on locale, sociopolitical history, religion, and culture. Locus of Control theory posits that socialization in a collectivistic system leads to an external locus of control, whereas socialization within individualistic cultural systems leads to an internal locus of control. Similarly Attribution Theory posits that attribution of control over assumptions, ways of decision-making and problem-solving, is influenced by the social system (collectivistic), or the assumption is that responsibility for attribution of control, assumptions, ways of decision-making, etc., rests with an individual, even when people do not have control over their world (individualism).

Ibrahim (1984, 1985, 2003) defines worldview as the core of cultural identity, pertaining to beliefs, values, and assumptions that are derived from the socialization process, in a specific cultural, familial, social, and historical context. Placing worldview at the core of cultural identity is based on data collected on the Scale to Assess World View (Ibrahim, 1987; Ibrahim & Kahn, 1984; Ibrahim & Owen, 1994). The data shows that several individuals with very different cultural identities tended to have similar beliefs, values, and perspectives. It became clear that value congruence among people with very different cultural backgrounds was influenced by several variables usually not considered to be culture, such as privilege, oppression, social class, educational level, professional identity, etc. This finding led to a review of demographic data on respondents to the SAWV, to identify specific variables that may have influenced values, beliefs, and assumptions of people who appeared to be culturally different entities, yet had similarity of core assumptions. It stimulated the development of the original Cultural Identity Check List© (Ibrahim, 1990). The data derived from the SAWV also revealed that theorists and researchers in the domain of cultural psychology were making some grave errors simply collecting data by race, instead of considering additional demographic variables that should include other mediating factors in understanding identity (Ibrahim, 2003). The key to accurately understanding worldview within a person's multidimensional identity lies in considering variables that a person considers primary to their cultural identity, and the congruence between their core values and cultural identity variables. The concept of worldview, and how to use it in counseling and psychotherapy is discussed in detail in Chap. 3.

Why Focus on Worldview and Cultural Identity?

Understanding the importance of core values and cultural identity in all its complexity will help clinicians when counseling in a culturally sensitive and relevant manner in a diverse society. However, other critical variables that pertain to issues of social justice and equity need to be incorporated to understand the client's reality in social systems where there are dominant and nondominant cultural groups based on race, ethnicity, gender, sexual orientation, social class, religion, age, life stage, ability/disability. In hierarchical social systems, the issue of privilege (opportunities available on the basis of race/ethnicity, gender, sexual orientation, etc.) helps in identifying issues of privilege and oppression (Gorski & Goodman, 2015; Hage & Kenny, 2009). The variables used to access the client perception of his or her place in the system can be done using the Miami Family Therapy Institute's (n.d.), *Privilege Oppression Continuum*, or the *Privilege Oppression Inventory* (Hays, Chang, & Decker, 2007).

Privilege and Oppression

Clients' perceptions of their place in social systems, and what they believe they can and cannot do, can be immensely helpful in counseling and psychotherapy. This analysis will help us in determining if the privilege and oppression identified by the client is based on societal conditions, published reports in the psychological literature, newspaper stories, statistics on poverty, racism and sexism, occupational accident and absentee reports, etc. Or does the client have the means to do more with his or her life, than he or she believes. Clients who lack access to opportunities to achieve the "good life" have been treated negatively in counseling and psychotherapy on the basis of race, gender identity, sexual orientation, culture, age, religion, social class, and disability due to the inability of mental health professionals to understand their challenges and limitations, given that the education and training of clinicians and educators does not specifically focus on understanding these dimensions (Dana, 1997; Goodman et al., 2004).

The lack of emphasis on social justice and equity issues in training is responsible for this oversight by professionals. In addition Nagayama Hall, Lopez, and Bansal (2001) identified a training issue that influences the perspectives of clinicians from underprivileged backgrounds once they are in graduate training programs. Graduate schools initiated recruiting students from nondominant, and lower social class, after reports were circulated that clients from nondominant and lower social classes were terminating counseling services within the first three sessions (Sue & Zane, 1987; US Department of Health & Human Services, 2001). Graduate programs hoped that recruiting students from underserved groups would facilitate effective culturally meaningful services to their own cultural and economic groups. However, Nagayama Hall et al. note that the graduate schools culture and the socialization of faculty were not taken into account. Students from nondominant cultural groups and lower social class feel they must acculturate to the values of the dominant system to survive, and graduate from the training programs and an implicit process took place, which resulted in changing the students. They ended up buying into the assumptions and values of the graduate schools they attended, and emerged with their degrees with the same attitudes as the faculty that trained them, resulting in not taking the client's issues seriously, and blaming them for lack of progress in counseling by "choosing to not change" or showing "resistance." Our perspective on resistance is that it is not something that we can attribute to the client, it is the result of setting goals and using a communication process for counseling that may have no meaning for the client. We recommend going back to the drawing board to identify what the client wants to work on in counseling, what issues or conditions the client thinks led to the presenting problem, what the client believes will bring homeostasis to his or her world, and help resolve the problem (Castillo, 1997).

The emphasis in training programs needs to go beyond cultural competence, to helping students understand, and have the ability to identify privilege and oppression issues in society, which are external factors that induce mental illness, and many physical ailments, and psychological problems such as race-related trauma, PTSD as a result of being a member of a lower social class, or being a minority in a dominant culture (Dohrenwend, 2006; Evans, Jacobs, Dooley, & Catalano, 1987; Goodman, 2015). The experiences of people within these social contexts have attributed to drug and alcohol addiction, diabetes, obesity, heart disease, and several major life-threatening health conditions (Dyrbye et al., 2007; Epel et al., 2006).

The stress associated with not being a "valued" gender, or from a lower social class, or different nationality, or cultural group is always much higher than for others with the same credentials, because other factors attributed to "difference" can result in reducing their credibility as social equals, workers, partners, etc. (Conwill, 2015; Ensher, Grant-Vallone, & Donaldson, 2001; Ibrahim & Ohnishi, 2001). We encourage mental health professionals to identify their own privilege and oppressions, and review the effect on their lives. We also encourage learning more about how different cultural groups are treated, and valued or devalued in society, to increase their ability to understand the circumstances, and stressors diverse clients may face (Reyes Cruz, 2002). Too long we have relied on our ability as helpers to simply be empathic and caring. Unfortunately, training in psychological principles and applied psychology or any of the helping professions focuses to a large extent on theoretical knowledge, research and counseling skills, without addressing the person of the therapist who is expected to be a positive, caring, therapeutic agent (Goodman et al., 2004, 2015). Good intentions do not always translate into efficacy in working with oppressed populations. We encourage professionals to take every opportunity they can to learn more about themselves, and the biases they may have acquired from their own socialization process, their educational environments, and to confront their attitude and lack of empathy for a client they do not understand (Kiselica, 1999; Leong, Leach, & Malikiosi-Loizos, 2012). Privilege and oppression, along with other training prerequisites for effective counseling for social justice and equity in will be addressed in Chap. 5.

Acculturation

Acculturation and adaptation processes can help or hinder successful integration into a cultural system (Berry, 1980; Poston, 1990; Van De Vijver & Phalet, 2004). This construct has been used mostly to understand the adaptation of culturally different clients who are new to a host culture, such as immigrants, refugees, sojourners, foreign workers, etc. However, we posit that cultural hierarchies within a social system create socializing environments that result in cultural identities that may not be similar to the dominant cultural group. People born in a specific country, regardless of their positional status (dominant or nondominant cultural group of identification) will share some larger national assumptions based on national philosophy, education, and other national socializing aspects of their larger social system (Ibrahim, Roysircar-Sodowsky, & Ohnishi, 2001). Being identified as a racial-cultural minority also creates a cultural context, not just for race and ethnicity but also for gender, sexual orientation, age/life stage, ability/disability, religion, educational level, and type of training (science, humanities, etc.). We argue that being members of several cultural subgroups, and a member of a larger social system requires acculturation to the larger system which can be facilitated, or retarded by positive or negative experiences through childhood to adulthood, generally, during the most formative years of a person's life. Reyes Cruz and Sonn (2015), note that the concept of acculturation to the dominant culture, implies that diversity and dissent will not be tolerated, which can be very oppressive for nondominant populations coming from cultural systems that may be very different.

Acculturation or lack of it, to the larger social system, or identification, with or rejection of primary cultural group can provide very important insights into how comfortable the client is with his or her world, and how much stress is experienced, as the client negotiates everyday life (Ibrahim & Ohnishi, 2001). This is another variable that can effectively facilitate cross-cultural and within culture therapeutic encounters. Psychology views human development from neurological, biological, familial, and social perspectives (Rosenberg & Kosslyn, 2011). Understanding acculturation status or a client's adaptation to the world he or she lives in, can help us in understanding the environmental stressors that may be the cause of the presenting problem, or exacerbating it. Addressing problems from these specific perspectives and recognizing that that social conditions may have contributed to the presenting problem has a much higher chance of developing a successful client-specific intervention. It helps the client in negotiating his or her world, changing behavior, or identifying the opportunity to teach specific skills that a client may need to develop, to negotiate his or her world as a resilient, purposeful individual. Acculturation will be addressed in Chap. 4.

Identifying Healing Systems in the Client's Cultural World

Another important variable to consider is the client as a collaborator in the counseling or problem-resolution process. Castillo (1997) notes that beyond identifying cultural identity and cultural context, we need to also review with the client what his/her/zir perception is of the cause and the remedy for the presenting problem. This focuses on identifying healing systems within the client's cultural, social, and spiritual world. The solutions that the client identifies should be incorporated into the intervention in a culturally meaningful manner, e.g., when I worked with Puerto Rican clients in the North East of the United States, some of the clients wanted a "Spiritist" involved in the therapeutic process, and I made arrangements for their personal spiritual leader to be involved with the identification of goals, and possible solutions for achieving homeostasis for the client. This involved having the Spiritist conduct some aspects of the healing process, specifically focused on spiritual healing, or resolution of some issues for the client (Ibrahim, 1992). In other cases, some Jewish clients wanted the Rabbi involved, I made this accommodation and it resulted in the client resolving the presenting problem with the peace of mind that he or she was not violating any religious tenets (Ibrahim, 1987). Religion or spirituality, and culture of origin seems to be the strongest variables that influence cultural identity and exploration of these assumptions can be very helpful for the client in assuring them that they would not be moving into unknown territory with the psychological intervention, it also helps in creating safety for a client, and increases the helper's trustworthiness and credibility.

In other situations where we are dealing with transsexual concerns (gender identity), gay or lesbian issues, and bisexuality (sexual orientation), it is important to find out what others may have done to resolve similar crisis or psychological issues, and to clarify what worked for whom, under what conditions, with the specific clientele. Actions taken by individuals in the same cultural group may also be predicated by their attributes, such as gender, and gender identity, race-ethnicity, age, geographical location, spirituality/religion, etc. Resolutions that did work must be explored keeping all dimensions of privilege, and oppression in view, so that decisions to pursue a similar course of action is well thought out and tested in vivo prior to putting it to a real-world test.

Keeping the client involved in the decision-making process in identifying goals for counseling, theoretical perspectives, and strategies that can help to get the needed outcome for a specific client, must be explored in depth before taking any action (Tate, Torres Rivera, & Edwards, 2015; Smith & Chamber, 2015). Culturally, and philosophically, most cultures of the world value an individual's right to self-determination. This is evident in the literature and poetry of first-, second-, and third-world cultures. Humans are innately opposed to having personal decisions being made by another, and the process of arriving at solving very personal, psychological, or cultural problems that are presented in therapy must primarily honor the client's decisions in counseling. In cases where there is some argument if the client is able to make these decisions, the most effective therapies tend to be ones that engage the client and then work with them to help identify how the path they are on could be destructive such as Dialectical Behavior Therapy for Borderline and suicidal clients (Linehan, 1993) and for addictions, e.g., Motivational Interviewing (Miller & Rollnick, 2002).

It is apparent from successful therapeutic endeavors, such as Dialectical Behavior Therapy and Motivational Interviewing for alcohol abuse (Linehan, 1993; Miller & Rollnick, 2002) and from the last 45 years of research on counseling and psychotherapy that the most important variable is the therapeutic relationship that is genuine, warm, and caring (Rogers, 1959). The second variable that these approaches employ is the therapists' ability to create dissonance in self-perceptions (Bem, 1967; Festinger, 1957; Miller & Rose, 2009). These are important considerations in developing a positive and trusting relationship with the client. In cross-cultural encounters, as well as in within-group encounters, it is critical that mental health professionals have the ability to develop warm, caring, and empathic relationships with clients. This is exemplified in Torrey's (1986) review of healing systems in several cultures of the world. Essentially, the therapist must also be trustworthy and have credibility for the client.

Scope of This Text

This text attempts to help therapists understand effective cultural assessments that will help in facilitating counseling in diverse cultural systems. The diversity within a culture is reported to be higher than the much-highlighted diversity between cultures (Sundberg, 1982). The focus is on the assessment components that will facilitate counseling and psychotherapy within and across cultures. The goal is not to cover therapeutic theories and strategies as we are relying on mostly evidence-based interventions and matching them to client variables in a culturally sensitive manner (APA, 2005; Zane, Sue, Young, Nunez, & Hall, 2004). In spite of over 30 years of rhetoric about cultural sensitivity, Caplan and Ford (2014) report that the experiences of ethnic/racial nondominant populations, on campuses show widespread psychological abuse through racism, sexism, and microaggressions. Further, they show that institutions fail to include active opposition to exclusion and prejudice, or a comprehensive agenda to change the campus environment. Cultural sensitivity comes from understanding the client from multiple perspectives, which include cultural identity, worldview, acculturation, along with privilege and privilege and oppression analysis, and recognizing how one's socialization and life experiences may have affected one's ability to be sensitive, and caring to culturally marginalized clients. Cultural identity covers several personal, familial, cultural, historical, and social variables, and these will be described in detail in Chap. 2.

The case studies that are presented using the assessment perspectives outlined in this text will address counseling interventions that are accepted and meaningful in our professional literature. However, the text will not cover the usefulness of the various therapeutic approaches as we are attempting to use the assessment component to identify what would be useful, and therapeutic in a specific case, considering the client and his or her context. Each case study will identify the salient factors that were significant in developing the intervention and will also evaluate the success or failure of an intervention and discuss the reasons for it. These will be presented in Chap. 8.

Summary

This chapter identified the scope of this text and highlighted the specific components that will require assessment, and the ability to apply the information in a meaningful manner. It highlights the importance of identifying the client's cultural identity, worldview, recognizing the importance of privilege and oppression, and assessing acculturation to mainstream society before planning a counseling intervention. It also identifies all the variables that must be considered prior to setting goals, and process for an intervention, and emphasizes the importance of evaluating the effectiveness of an intervention. The case studies provide information on how the assessments influenced the development of the counseling interventions, and will provide a useful template for interventions with diverse clients.

References

American Association of Marriage and Family Therapy (AAMFT). (2012). *Code of ethics*. Alexandria, VA: Author.

American Counseling Association (ACA). (1992). *Multicultural competencies*. Alexandria, VA: Author.

American Counseling Association (ACA). (2014). *Code of ethics*. Alexandria, VA: Author.

American Psychiatric Association. (1994). *The diagnostic and statistical manual of mental illness-IV (DSM-IV)*. Washington, DC: American Psychiatric Association.

American Psychiatric Association (APA). (2000). *Diagnostic and statistical manual of mental disorders-IV-TR*. Washington, DC: Author.

American Psychiatric Association. (2013a). *Diagnostic and statistical manual of mental disorders* (5th ed.). Washington, DC: Author.

American Psychiatric Association. (2013b). *The principles of medical ethics with annotations especially applicable to psychiatry*. Washington, DC: Author.

American Psychological Association (APA). (2002). *Guidelines on multicultural education, training, research, practice, and organizational change for psychologists*. Washington, DC: Author.

American Psychological Association (APA). (2005). *Report of the 2005 presidential task force on evidence-based practice*. Washington, DC: Author.

American Psychological Association (APA). (2010). *Ethical principles of psychologists and code of conduct: With 2010 amendments*. Washington, DC: Author (Original work published 2002).

Bem, D. J. (1967). Self-perception: An alternative interpretation of cognitive dissonance phenomena. *Psychological Review, 74*, 183–200.

Berry, J. W. (1980). Acculturation as varieties of adaptation. In A. Padilla (Ed.), *Acculturation: Theory, models and some new findings* (pp. 9–25). Boulder, CO: Westview.

Burke, P. J. (1980). The self: Measurement requirements from an interactionist perspective. *Social Psychology Quarterly, 44*, 18–29.

Caplan, P. J., & Ford, J. C. (2014). The voices of diversity: What students of diverse races/ethnicities and both sexes tell us about their college experiences and their perceptions about their institutions' progress toward diversity. *Aporia, 6*(3), 30–69.

Cass, V. C. (1979). Homosexual identity formation: A theoretical model. *Journal of Homosexuality, 4*, 219–235.

Castillo, R. (1997). *Culture and mental illness*. Pacific Grove, CA: Brooks/Cole.

Conwill, W. L. (2015). De-colonizing multicultural counseling and psychology: Addressing race through intersectionality. In R. D. Goodman & P. C. Gorski (Eds.), *Decolonizing "multicultural" counseling through social justice* (pp. 117–126). New York: Springer.

Cross, W. E., Jr. (1978). The Thomas and Cross models of psychological nigrescence: A review. *Journal of Black Psychology, 5*, 13–31.
Cross, W. E., Jr. (1991). *Shades of black: Diversity in African-American identity*. Philadelphia, PA: Temple University Press.
Dana, R. H. (1997). *Understanding cultural identity in intervention and assessment*. Thousand Oaks, CA: Sage.
Dohrenwend, B. P. (2006). Inventorying stressful life events as risk factors for psychopathology: Toward resolution of the problem of intracategory variability. *Psychological Bulletin, 132*(3), 477–495. doi:10.1037/0033-2909.132.3.477.
Downing, N. E., & Roush, K. L. (1985). From passive acceptance to active commitment: A model of feminist identity development for women. *The Counseling Psychologist, 13*, 695–709.
Dyrbye, L. N., Thomas, M. R., Eacker, A., Harper, W., Massie, F. S. J., Power, D. V., et al. (2007). Race, ethnicity, and medical student wellbeing in the United States. *Archives of Internal Medicine, 167*(19), 210321. doi:10.1001/archinte.167.19.2103.
Ensher, E. A., Grant-Vallone, E. J., & Donaldson, S. I. (2001). Effects of perceived discrimination on job satisfaction, organizational commitment, organizational citizenship behavior, and grievances. *Human Resource Development Quarterly, 12*(1), 53–72.
Epel, E., Lin, J., Wilhelm, F., Wolkowitz, O., Cawthon, R., Adler, N., et al. (2006). Cell aging in relation to stress arousal and cardiovascular diseases risk factors. *Psychoneuroendocrinology, 31*(3), 277–287. doi:10.1016/j.psyneuen.2005.08.011.
Evans, G. W., Jacobs, S. V., Dooley, D., & Catalano, R. (1987). The interaction of stressful life events and chronic strains on community mental health. *American Journal of Community Psychology, 15*(1), 23–34. doi:10.1007/BF00919755.
Festinger, L. (1957). *A theory of cognitive dissonance*. Stanford, CA: Stanford University Press.
Goodman, R. D. (2015). A liberatory approach to trauma counseling proposes a liberatory approach to trauma counseling. In R. D. Goodman & P. C. Gorski (Eds.), *Decolonizing "multicultural" counseling through social justice* (pp. 55–72). New York: Springer.
Goodman, L. A., Liang, B., Helms, J. E., Latta, R. E., Sparks, E., & Weintraub, S. R. (2004). Training counseling psychologists as social justice agents: Feminist and multicultural principles in action. *The Counseling Psychologist, 32*(6), 793–837. doi:10.1177/0011000004268802.
Goodman, R. D., Williams, J. M., Chung, R. C.-Y., Talleyrand, R. M., Douglas, A. M., McMahon, H. G., et al. (2015). Decolonizing traditional pedagogies and practices in counseling and psychology education: A move towards social justice and action. In R. D. Goodman & P. C. Gorski (Eds.), *Decolonizing "multicultural" counseling through social justice* (pp. 147–164). New York: Springer.
Gorski, P. C., & Goodman, R. D. (2015). Introduction: Toward a decolonized multicultural counseling and psychology. In R. D. Goodman & P. C. Gorski (Eds.), *Decolonizing "multicultural" counseling through social justice* (pp. 1–10). New York: Springer.
Hage, S. M., & Kenny, M. E. (2009). Promoting a social justice approach to prevention: Future directions for training, practice, and research. *Journal of Primary Prevention, 30*(1), 75–87.
Hays, D. G., Chang, C. Y., & Decker, S. L. (2007). Initial development and psychometric data for the privilege and oppression inventory. *Measurement and Evaluation in Counseling and Development, 40*(2), 66–72. doi:10.1002/j.1556-6678.2007.tb00480.x.
Helms, J. (1990). *Black and White racial identity: Theory, research, and practice*. Westport, CT: Greenwood Press.
Hipolito-Delgado, C. P. (2009). Cultural identity: Understanding development and integration of multiple identities. In C. C. Lee, D. A. Burnhill, A. L. Butler, C. P. Hipolito-Delgado, M. Humphrey, O. Munoz, & H. Shin (Eds.), *Elements of culture in counseling*. Columbus, OH: Pearson.
Ibrahim, F. A. (1984). Cross-cultural counseling and psychotherapy: An existential-psychological perspective. *International Journal for the Advancement of Counseling, 7*, 159–169.
Ibrahim, F. A. (1985). Effectiveness in cross-cultural counseling and psychotherapy: A framework. *Psychotherapy, 22*, 321–323.
Ibrahim, F. A. (1987). *Case notes: Sarah Ann, Jewish-American female client*, Storrs, CT. Unpublished document.

Ibrahim, F. A. (1990). *Cultural identity check list©*, Storrs, CT. Unpublished document.
Ibrahim, F. A. (1991). Contribution of cultural worldview to generic counseling and development. *Journal of Counseling and Development, 70*, 13–19.
Ibrahim, F. A. (1992). *Case notes: Jose, Puerto Rican client*, Storrs, CT. Unpublished document.
Ibrahim, F. A. (1999). Transcultural counseling: Existential world view theory and cultural identity: Transcultural applications. In J. McFadden (Ed.), *Transcultural counseling* (2nd ed., pp. 23–57). Alexandria, VA: ACA Press.
Ibrahim, F. A. (2003). Existential worldview theory: From inception to applications. In F. D. Harper & J. McFadden (Eds.), *Culture and counseling: New approaches* (pp. 196–208). Boston: Allyn & Bacon.
Ibrahim, F. A. (2007). *United States acculturation index©*, Denver, CO. Unpublished document.
Ibrahim, F. A., & Arredondo, P. M. (1986). Ethical standards for cross-cultural counseling: Preparation, practice, assessment and research. *Journal of Counseling and Development, 64*, 349–351.
Ibrahim, F. A., & Kahn, H. (1984). *Scale to assess world view©* (SAWV), Storrs, CT. Unpublished document.
Ibrahim, F. A., & Ohnishi, H. (2001). Posttraumatic stress disorder and the minority experience. In D. R. Pope-Davis & H. L. K. Coleman (Eds.), *The intersection of race, class, and gender in multicultural counseling* (pp. 89–119). Thousand Oaks, CA: Sage Publications.
Ibrahim, F. A., & Owen, S. V. (1994). Factor-analytic structure of the scale to assess World view. *Current Psychology, 13*, 201–209.
Ibrahim, F. A., Roysircar-Sodowsky, G. R., & Ohnishi, H. (2001). Worldview: Recent developments and needed directions. In J. G. Ponterotto, M. J. Casas, L. A. Suzuki, & C. M. Alexander (Eds.), *Handbook of multicultural counseling* (p. 430). Thousand Oaks, CA: Sage Publications.
Kiselica, M. (Ed.). (1999). *Confronting prejudice and racism during multicultural training*. Alexandria, VA: American Counseling Association.
Leong, F. T. L., Leach, M. M., & Malikiosi-Loizos, M. (2012). Internationalizing the field of counseling psychology. In F. T. L. Leong, W. E. Pickren, M. M. Leach, & A. J. Marsella (Eds.), *Internationalizing the psychology curriculum in the United States* (pp. 201–224). New York: Springer.
Linehan, M. M. (1993). *Cognitive-behavioral treatment of borderline personality disorder*. New York: Guilford Press.
Liu, W. M. (2001). Expanding our understanding of multiculturalism: Developing a social class worldview model. In D. B. Pope-Davis & H. L. K. Coleman (Eds.), *The intersection of race, class, and gender in counseling psychology* (pp. 127–170). Thousand Oaks, CA: Sage.
Marsella, A. J. (2015). Foreword. In R. D. Goodman & P. C. Gorski (Eds.), *Decolonizing "multicultural" counseling through social justice* (pp. vii–x). New York: Springer.
McCall, G. J., & Simmons, J. L. (1978). *Identities and interactions*. New York: Free Press.
McCarn, S. R., & Fassinger, R. E. (1996). Revisioning sexual minority identity formation: A new model of lesbian identity and its implications for counseling and research. *The Counseling Psychologist, 24*, 508–534. doi:10.1177/0011000096243011.
Miami Family Therapy Institute. (n.d.). *Privilege-oppression continuum*. Miami, FL: Miami Family Therapy Institute.
Miller, W. R., & Rollnick, S. (2002). *Motivational interviewing: Preparing people for change* (2nd ed.). New York: Guilford Press.
Miller, W. R., & Rose, G. S. (2009). Toward a theory of motivational interviewing. *American Psychologist, 64*(6), 527–537.
Money, J. (1973). Gender role, gender identity, core gender identity: Usage and definition of terms. *Journal of the American Academy of Psychoanalysis, 1*, 397–403.
Nagayama Hall, G. C., Lopez, I., & Bansal, A. (2001). Academic acculturation. In D. Pope-Davis & H. Coleman (Eds.), *The intersection of race, class, and gender in multicultural counseling* (pp. 171–188). Thousand Oaks, CA: Sage.
National Association of Social Workers (NASW). (2008). *Code of ethics*. Washington, DC: National Association of Social Workers.
Phinney, J. S. (1990). Ethnic identity in adolescents and adults: Review of research. *Psychological Bulletin, 10*(3), 499–514.

Poston, W. A. C. (1990). The biracial identity development model: A needed addition. *Journal of Counseling and Development, 69*, 152–155.

Reyes Cruz, M. (2002). *Multiple contexts, multiple identities: Puerto Rican women's Perspectives on race, ethnicity, discrimination and identity*. Unpublished masters' thesis, University of Illinois, Urbana-Champaign.

Reyes Cruz, M., & Sonn, C. C. (2015). (De)colonizing culture in community psychology: Reflections from critical social science. In R. D. Goodman & P. C. Gorski (Eds.), *Decolonizing "multicultural" counseling through social justice* (pp. 127–146). New York: Springer.

Rogers, C. (1959). A theory of therapy, personality and interpersonal relationships as developed in the client-centered framework. In S. Koch (Ed.), *Psychology: A study of a science. Vol. 3: Formulations of the person and the social context*. New York: McGraw Hill.

Rosenberg, R. S., & Kosslyn, S. M. (2011). *Abnormal psychology* (2nd ed.). New York: Worth.

Rotter, J. B. (1966). Generalized expectancies of internal versus external control of reinforcements. *Psychological Monographs, 80*(1), 1–28 (whole no. 609).

Rotter, J. B. (1975). Some problems and misconceptions related to the construct of internal versus external control of reinforcement. *Journal of Consulting and Clinical Psychology, 43*, 56–67. doi:10.1037/h00776301.

Shin, R. Q. (2015). The application of critical consciousness and intersectionality as tools for decolonizing racial/ethnic identity development models in the fields of counseling and psychology. In R. D. Goodman & P. C. Gorski (Eds.), *Decolonizing "multicultural" counseling through social justice*. New York: Springer Science and Business Media.

Smith, L., & Chamber, C. (2015). Decolonizing psychological practice in the context of poverty. In R. D. Goodman & P. C. Gorski (Eds.), *Decolonizing "multicultural" counseling through social justice* (pp. 73–84). New York: Springer.

Smith, L. C., & Geroski, A. M. (2015). Decolonizing alterity models within school counseling practice. In R. D. Goodman & P. C. Gorski (Eds.), *Decolonizing "multicultural" counseling through social justice* (pp. 99–116). New York: Springer.

Stewart, A. J., & McDermott, C. (2004). Gender in psychology. *Annual Review of Psychology, 55*, 519–544.

Stryker, S. (1968). Identity salience and role performance: The importance of symbolic interaction theory in family research. *Journal of Marriage and the Family, 30*, 558–564.

Stryker, S. (1987). Identity theory: Developments and extensions. In K. Yardley & T. Honess (Eds.), *Self and identity* (pp. 89–104). New York: Wiley.

Sue, D. W. (1978). World views and counseling. *Personnel and Guidance Journal, 56*, 458–462.

Sue, S., & Zane, N. (1987). The role of culture and cultural techniques in psychotherapy: A critique and reformulation. *American Psychologist, 42*, 37–45.

Sundberg, N. D. (1982). Cross-cultural counseling and psychotherapy: A research overview. In A. J. Marsella & P. B. Pedersen (Eds.), *Cross-cultural counseling and psychotherapy* (pp. 28–62). New York: Pergamon Press.

Tate, K. A., Torres Rivera, E., & Edwards, L. M. (2015). Colonialism and multicultural counseling competence research: A liberatory analysis. In R. D. Goodman & P. Gorski (Eds.), *Decolonizing "multicultural" counseling and psychology: Visions for social justice theory and practice*. New York: Springer Science and Business Media.

Torrey, E. F. (1986). *Witchdoctors and psychiatrists: The common roots of psychotherapy and its future* (2nd ed.). New York: Harper-Collins.

US Department of Health and Human Services. (2001). *Mental health: Culture, race, and ethnicity*. Rockville, MD: U.S. Department of Health and Human Services, Public Health Service, Office of the Surgeon General.

Van De Vijver, F. J., & Phalet, K. (2004). Assessment in multicultural groups: The role of acculturation. *Applied Psychology, 53*(2), 215–236.

Weiner, B. (1974). *Achievement motivation and attribution theory*. Morristown, NJ: General Learning Press.

Zane, N., Sue, S., Young, K., Nunez, J., & Hall, G. N. (2004). Research on psychotherapy with culturally diverse populations. In M. J. Lambert (Ed.), *Handbook of psychotherapy and behavior change* (5th ed., pp. 767–804). New York: Wiley.

Chapter 2
Cultural Identity: Components and Assessment

The concept of cultural identity refers to familial and cultural dimensions of a person's identity, and how others perceive him or her, i.e., factors that are salient to a person's identity both as perceived by the individual and how others perceive the person's identity. Interest in understanding cultural identity began with the publication of Cross (1978) theory of nigrescence. This was a novel notion as previously identity was perceived as a unitary variable, and denoted a sense of belonging to a social setting (Stryker, 1987). Cross' (1978) model expanded our thinking to include (a) identity is influenced by positive or negative experiences in a social setting, especially for marginalized individuals, identity can get facilitated, or compromised; (b) it is possible for identity to evolve to higher levels of functioning in spite of challenging life experiences; and (c) the social construction of race, and the history of slavery, segregation, exclusion, and the negative sociopolitical history of a nation can negatively influence identity development with race-related trauma and stress over several generations (Ibrahim & Ohnishi, 2001; Pascoe & Smart Richman, 2009; Shin, 2015). Ibrahim (1993) anchors cultural identity within a person's primary cultural context, it includes ethnicity, gender and gender identity, spiritual assumptions, age and life stage, ability and disability status, family, community, and nation. Culture influences all these dimensions however; the effect varies across various dimensions, including life experiences and time. Hofstede (2001) states "culture is the collective programming of the mind that distinguishes the members of one group or category of people from others" (p. 10). This conception considers culture as a collective phenomenon; he allows that there can be as many different perspectives within each collective as there are individuals.

Hofstede adds that in general the term culture is used for tribes or ethnic groups (in anthropology), or nations (in political science, sociology and management), and for organizations (in sociology and management). The term culture can also be applied to gender, sexual orientation, generations, social classes, etc., although changing the level of aggregation studied can change the nature of the concept of "culture" (Hofstede, 2001; Ibrahim, 1984). Societal, national, and gender cultures

F.A. Ibrahim, J.R. Heuer, *Cultural and Social Justice Counseling*,
International and Cultural Psychology, DOI 10.1007/978-3-319-18057-1_2

are acquired from early childhood, are deeply rooted in the psyche, and are usually acquired and held unconsciously. Given the implicit nature of culture, cultural identity assessment cannot be based on ethnicity alone, or cultural characteristics of a specific group (Ibrahim, 1991; Shin, 2015). Rather, the focus shifts to understanding the intersectionality of a client's various identities, and the meaning of the crisis the client faces in terms of what core values or worldview, and identities are affected (Conwill, 2015; Eklund, 2012; Ibrahim, 2007a, 2007b).

Given the ethical mandates and competency guidelines from mental health professional organizations, it is critical that we honor cultural identity in counseling interventions (American Counseling Association (ACA), 1992, 2014; American Psychiatric Association 2000, 2013a, 2013b, 2013c; American Psychological Association [APA], 2002, 2010; Leong, Leach, & Malikiosi-Loizos, 2012; National Association of Social Workers (NASW), 2008; American Association of Marriage and Family Therapy (AAMFT), 2012). The cultural assessment model presented in this text considers cultural identity multidimensional, and identifies several aspects of a person's identity, that may have different salience and relevance to the person depending on the issues they bring to counseling (Conwill, 2015; Ibrahim, 1991; Shin, 2015). Current thinking on identity has moved from single concept of identity to considering the intersections of identity, which is specifically relevant to counseling and psychotherapy (Ibrahim 1991, 2007a, 2007b; McDowell & Jeris, 2004). Conwill (2015) notes that the intersectionality perspective highlights the way in which there is a simultaneous interaction of discrimination that impinges upon multiple identities of an individual. Given such a conceptualization, it is easy to begin to see the interconnection between culture and power (Reyes Cruz & Sonn, 2015).

The Cultural Identity Check List-Revised© (Ibrahim, 2008) includes the following variables: Age, gender, cultural background, and religion/spirituality as identification variables. The exploration of cultural influences begins with racial/ethnic/national identity, migration or indigenous status, migration pattern of the client's cultural group, dominant or nondominant group status, sociopolitical history, gender, sexual orientation, socioeconomic status of family of origin and the client, religion or spirituality, educational level, birth order in the family of origin, the family the client grew up in (two parents, extended, blended, single parent), ability/disability status, region of the country/world client is from, and where the client resides now. These variables contribute to not only client experiences, but also how the therapist relates to the client. Each of these variables will be discussed in this chapter and why they are presented as relevant to cultural identity. In addition, approaching the client from the multidimensional identity perspective also helps in consideration of those aspects of cultural identity that are relevant to the presenting problem.

Ethnicity

Globally and in US society the concept of ethnicity is gaining attention, as pluralism in societies increases due to economic globalization, and migrations due to wars and conflicts, along with issues of integration of the culturally different in monocultural societies (Leong, Leach, & Malikiosi-Loizos, 2012; Organista, Marin, & Chun, 2009; Verkuyten, 2005). In the USA the growth of ethnic psychology has emerged as a major force, and continues to identify how ethnicity mediates behavior, even after several generations (McGoldrick, Giordano, & Garcia-Preto, 2005; Phinney & Ong, 2007).

Ethnicity is considered a multifaceted variable. An individual's self-identification can change depending on time and space, and the people in the person's environment at any given time (Huot & Rudman, 2010; Spencer, Dupree, & Hartmann, 1997; Thomas, Townsend, & Belgrave, 2003; Umaña-Taylor, 2011). Ethnic identity can be differently defined in various government agencies and states (Jackson, 2006). Many authors argue that it is the reference to descent and common origin that makes a group an ethnic group; it is this idea and belief that a common origin, descent, and history distinguish ethnic identity from other social identities (Verkuyten, 2005). The emphasis on origin and descent in identifying oneself as a member of a specific ethnic group comes from Weber (1968). Another perspective is that it is primarily the political community that dictates a common ethnicity (Verkuyten, 2005). This may be relevant to how different cultures define themselves, politically, instead of ethnically, as the founding fathers of the USA conceived of a new nation with specific ideals and goals, and conceived of a US identity, based on White Anglo Saxon values, distinct from any of the ethnic or national groups that migrated to the USA (Takaki, 1979).

In this context it is important to consider the concept of race, it is a concept that assumes that there are distinct human populations. Helms, Jernigan, and Mascher (2005) note that this is a concept that has no "consensual, theoretical, or scientific meaning in psychology" (p. 27). Racial classifications are rooted in the idea of biological classification of humans according to morphological features such as skin color or facial characteristics. However, biological sciences do not accept the concept of race either; it is considered a social construct that was created by humans and is maintained to create political and social hierarchies (Cavalli-Sforza, Menozzi, & Piazza, 1996; Long & Kittles, 2003). Ethnicity may be related to physical characteristics of people, however the concept does not refer to physical characteristics specifically; it identifies social-cultural traits that are shared by a group. Some traits used for ethnic classification include but are not limited to: nationality, tribe, religious faith, shared language, shared culture, and shared traditions.

According to Hutchinson and Smith (1996) ethnicity is characterized by a common or collective name, a myth of common ancestry or descent, memories of a common past or shared history, elements of common culture, linked with a specific homeland, and a sense of solidarity. Hylland Erickson (2002) considers ethnicity from an anthropological perspective and states "ethnicity is an aspect of social relationships between agents who consider themselves culturally distinctive from members of other groups with whom they have a minimum of regular interaction. It can thus also be defined as a social identity (based on contrast with others) characterized by metaphoric or fictive kinship," (p. 12). Verkuyten (2005) views ethnicity from a social psychological perspective, and states that ethnic identity is not simply the result of social assignments. He believes that ethnic identity is the result of interactions between the individual and society, and has three levels of analysis, based on House's conception (1981), i.e., individual, interactive, and societal. The first level pertains to personal characteristics and refers to the self, sense of identity and cognitive structures. The interactive level is based on understanding emergence and maintenance of identity in situated interactions. The societal level refers to macrosocial variables of history, politics, ideology, culture, and economics. He maintains that it is in the interaction of all these levels that ethnic identity can be understood, and evaluated.

Ultimately, there are many ways to look at the concept of ethnicity. A common thread between all definitions is that it can be seen as a specific and distinct group, which has many common rituals, beliefs, ways of being, etc., and that it is part of a person's social identity. Beyond these three similarities between conceptions of what ethnicity is the opinion on what it means to be a part of an ethnic group or to define one's ethnicity varies widely in the literature. However, sociopolitical history, culture, economics, etc., all influence the development and maintenance of ethnic identity, and the interactions of all three levels result in an individual perception of ethnic identity.

Having a strong ethnic identity indicates that clients are deeply embedded in the rituals, beliefs, and ways of being of their cultural groups. Usually, very strong ethnic identities are found in recent immigrants or sojourners, because they may not have been exposed to other ethnic groups in their culture of origin. Ethnic identity of immigrants is reshaped over several generations, as each generation successively adapts to the host culture. When an ethnic group is excluded from integrating into mainstream society, due to perceived racial or religious differences, ethnic identity can become stronger, in spite of several generations in the USA, e.g., African Americans, Asian Americans, indigenous people of the USA, Mormons, Presbyterians, Muslims, and Jews (Organista et al., 2009).

In cross-cultural counseling encounters it is imperative that the clients are given the opportunity to describe their ethnicity and what they believe about how they are perceived. The US context also has multiracial identities, a term used to describe individuals who have parents from two different racial/ethnic groups (Root, 2000). Given the 400 years of mixing of cultural groups, the idea that only one ethnicity defines a person has been rejected. It is important to accept the client's self-definition and work on a supportive and caring therapeutic relationship. In addition, in counseling and psychotherapy it is necessary to analyze cultural beliefs and values held by clients as a defining variable to understand how their ethnic identity was formed interacting with their primary familial and cultural groups, and the social-cultural context in which they grew up and how their ethnic identity developed (Root, 2000). In addition, given the complexity of the US context, it is necessary to recognize that the worldview held by the client may not be defined by the last name. Taking the stance that the client is the expert on his or her ethnicity conveys respect and acceptance. It also precludes any assumptions the counselor may make about the client, which can lower trust and reduce the possibility of developing a positive and engaged therapeutic relationship.

Age and Developmental Stage

It is important to consider the cognitive, affective, and physical development of the client in the context of developmental theories, and from the perspective of developmental counseling (Ivey, Ivey, Myers, & Sweeney, 2004). Being aware of developmental counseling approaches can be very useful for therapists. Developmental Counseling theory can guide the work we do with clients, as it pertains to their cultural identity. It can help complement cultural information that has been collected, and provide greater specificity in counseling and psychotherapy. Too long the counseling profession has been accused of working with generic counseling models that assume that theoretical frameworks that are available to us would work with every age and developmental stage. Age and development is also mediated by the primary cultural context, not by theoretical formulations offered by theorists who may not be from the client's cultural group. In the last 15 years with the advent of Developmental Counseling theory, and specific efforts by theorists and practitioners to consider age and development stage as critical variables, we have many more resources available to us for working with each generation (Ivey, Ivey, Myers, & Sweeney, 2004; Erikson, 1963, 1968, 1980).

Focusing on culture, age, and developmental stage become significant, because culturally, the expectations for age and developmental stage vary, although, this variable is neglected in training programs, and generic information does exist by ethnicity on expectations and norms for developmental stages, it is not given enough attention by professionals and its use it in counseling interventions (Deal, 2000). Understanding normative expectations for each developmental stage by culture can help make interventions meaningful to clients, and reduce the chances of judgment and negative evaluation of clients by mainstream educated counselors and therapists (Baruth & Manning, 2011).

It is important for mental health professionals recognize that the social structure of the USA segregates people according to age, and this segregation leads to indifferent attitudes toward other generations from one's own (Jun, 2010). The social segregation creates distance between the generations leading to lack of empathy and connection. In recent years, attention has focused on age discrimination both for the older and the younger worker (Hartzler, 2003; Nelson, 2005; Rosigno, Mong, & Tester, 2007). Research shows that mental health, and medical professionals, along with educators hold negative stereotypes about older adults (Ivey, Wieling, & Harris, 2000; Pasupathi & Lockenhoff, 2002; Reyes-Ortiz, 1997; Williams, 2012). Some theorists posit that negative attitudes toward older adults may be due to threatening aspects of confronting one's own old age and possible fear of death (Edwards & Wetzler, 1998; Snyder & Meine, 1994).

Each stage of life presents opportunities and challenges, it is important for mental health professionals to be equipped with appropriate knowledge and skills to provide meaningful services to clients. It is important to understand age and stage of clients and have information about the opportunities and challenges that these phases represent to provide services. The most vulnerable populations tend to be older adults and adolescents. The Centers for Disease Control assesses suicide rates per 100,000 people, and the last reported data were for 2011. The highest suicide rates in the nation tend to be for the 45–64 age range and the 85+ age range (18.6 for every 100,000), adolescents and young adults (ages 15–24) had a suicide rate of 11 for every 100,000 (Hoyert & Xu, 2012). In 2011, the highest suicide rate was among White Americans (11 for every 100,000), followed by Native Americans and Alaskan Natives (10.6), lower rates were reported, but roughly similar were reported for Asian American and Pacific Islanders (5.9), Black (5.3), and Hispanics (5.2). Since the CDC collects data separately on Hispanics as they may also be members of other cultural groups in the USA. Suicide rates for men tend to be four times higher than for women. In 2011, suicide rates were 78 % were men (20.2 per 100,000) and 21.5 % were women (5.4).

Gender

Gender "refers to the attitudes, feelings, and behaviors that a given culture associates with a person's biological sex. Behavior that is compatible with cultural expectations is referred to as gender-normative; behaviors that are viewed as incompatible with societal expectations constitute "gender non-conformity" (APA, 2011)." Gender identity is the internal experience of being either male, female, or transgendered. Usually, it is considered congruent with biological gender; however, as we learn more about transgendered identities, it is clear that in some cases it is not congruent with biological gender (APA, 2011; Gainor, 2000). Stewart and McDermott (2004) note "gender is increasingly recognized as defining a system of power relations embedded in other power relations. Psychological research on gender—which has most often focused on analysis of sex differences, within sex variability, and gender roles—has begun to incorporate this new understanding" (p. 519). They recommend drawing on three resources, to understand the significance of gender for psychological processes: social science theories that link the individual and social levels of analysis; constructs (such as identity) that bridge the social and individual levels; and conceptual tools generated in feminist theory, especially the intersections of aspects of identity.

The sociological perspective on gender refers to social expectations about behavior considered appropriate for members of a gender. It does not refer to the physical attributes on which men and women differ, but to socially formed traits of masculinity and femininity (Giddens, 1997). Gender is considered distinct from biological sex; it refers to the socially constructed categories of masculine and feminine that are differently defined in various cultures. Many contemporary theorists use a broader definition to refer to the set of beliefs and practices about male and female (or other genders), that not only feed into individual identities, and are fundamental to social institutions and symbolic systems (Bilton, Bonnett, Jones, Lawson et al., 2002). Smith and Chambers (2015) present a model for social justice alterity as it pertains to nondominant ethnicity, age/life stage, or gender; this includes (a) identifying colonizing dominant discourses, (b) awareness of tacit collusion in dominant discourses, and (c) advocacy efforts to promote counter-discourses.

Within anthropology, gender is a specialized area of study that emerged in significance during the 1970s and is linked to the advent of the feminist movement. Early research focused on how and why women were subordinated in patriarchal social systems. This was followed by the recognition that men, too, have gender, and it led to a much deeper analysis of the ways in which definitions of gender were constructed (Collier & Rosaldo, 1981; Coltrane, 1994; Connell, 1995). Research focused on different societies produced a variety of religious, kinship, gender, and economic systems (Petchesky, 2000; Sargent & Brettell, 1996). It is generally assumed that sex is the natural given; and gender based on a cultural definition is built upon that base. Additional research raised questions about the relation between sex and sexual orientation, and whether there might be more than two genders, and whether sex itself may to a large extent be a social and cultural construct. Studies of primates, long thought to hold the key to human behavior, have shown results that depend to a significant extent on the theoretical lens through which scientists view their behavior, as well as on which primates are the object of study; these discoveries have destabilized the base on which many assumptions about gender exist. When the critical gender lens has been focused on the archaeological record, old biases and assumptions, such as "man the hunter, woman the gatherer," have been overturned or significantly modified; new approaches to the study of the past and material culture have emerged (Paul, 2014).

Another area relevant to understanding gender in a cultural context comes from linguistic anthropology. This area of research focuses on gendered aspects of linguistic structure, for example, pronouns. It includes a study of the different ways in which women and men use language, to identify the extent to which gender is culturally constituted through linguistic practice over the life cycle. Other researchers have an interest in the way in which language applies connotations of gender to conceptual areas of study such as "soft" versus "hard" sciences, and how these labels may affect the gendered beings working within these fields. Gendered language and its impact on broader systems including worldviews, theology, and cosmology has also emerged, including the consequences for men and women when the deity is symbolically male and the earth is symbolically female (Eckert & McConnell, 2003).

Gender is not adequately addressed in the multicultural counseling literature. Historically in the counseling literature analysis of various cultural groups have focused on generic variables in terms of values, beliefs, assumptions, rituals, life cycle tasks, developmental markers, etc., of different cultures. The focus has been on considering similarity and differences among cultures (Baruth & Manning, 2011; McGoldrick et al., 2005; Sue & Sue, 2013). Gender, however, within each culture has specific meaning that may not emerge as a result of a global analysis of a culture. Although, most cultures of the world appear to be patriarchal, the world of men and women and their socialization tends to be different within social-cultural contexts. Gender roles, and power within a cultural system are influenced by the cultural context including the domains of influence that are allowed for each gender (Carli, 2001; Falbo, 1977). Understanding gender as a social construct helps in not pathologizing the client, or considering the client as resistant to change, it can also prevent misinterpretation of cultural conceptualizations and cultural malpractice (Dana, 1998). Smith and Chambers (2015) present a model for social justice alterity as it pertains to nondominant ethnicity, age/life stage, or gender; this includes (a) identifying colonizing dominant discourses, (b) awareness of tacit collusion in dominant discourses, and (c) advocacy efforts to promote counter-discourses.

Gender Identity

Money (1973) was the first person to define gender identity as composed of three distinct aspects: gender role—the external presentation of gender, gender identity—the internal experience of gender, and core gender identity (the developmental process of the identity that begins around 18 months of age). LaTorre (1976) notes that gender identity can be understood as composed of several parts, and these parts are described differently by theorists; however, there is considerable overlap among the categories subsumed within gender identity. Gender identity is differentiated from biological gender. Gender identity is a sense of awareness, usually beginning in infancy, continuing throughout childhood, and reaching maturity in adolescence, of being male or female. Barker and Kuiper (2003) note that gender identity is "the degree to which an individual takes on the behaviors, personality patterns, and attitudes that are usually associated with male or female *sex roles*" (p. 394). It can be consistent with biological sex, but it does not necessarily have to be, as is the case with people who identify with the other sex. Eagly (2009) emphasizes that gender role beliefs are both descriptive and prescriptive; they identify what men and women usually do, and what they should do. According to her, the descriptive aspects of gender role identify what is expected and are stereotypes about what is typical behavior for a specific gender. The prescriptive aspect of gender roles defines what is worthy of admiration within a culture. This is behavior that is executed to gain social approval and increase self-esteem. In addition, according to Eagly, gender role beliefs are derived from the cultural context and provide a template for culturally normative behavior, and are internalized as gender identities that enact personal dispositions. Studies of gender stereotypes show two main themes ascribed to male and female gender roles and these are communion and agency, with communion being ascribed to women and agency to men, and this appears to be a worldwide phenomenon (Kite, Deaux, & Haines, 2008; Williams & Best, 1990).

In the past psychiatry has considered gender identity when inconsistent from biological gender as pathology. However, it is accepted in psychological circles that gender identity can vary from the defined biological gender, without pathology. Social justice psychological theorists do not accept the pathology assumption, and note that if there is any, it is not the result of a neurological or biological deficit, but the result of societal emotional abuse, and victimization due to not subscribing to descriptive or prescriptive gendered behaviors (Higgins, Barker, & Begley, 2008; Ibrahim & Ohnishi, 2001; Ohnishi, Ibrahim, & Gzregorek, 2006). Stress, trauma, and emotional abuse over the lifespan can lead to severe anxiety, depression, and other psychological problems (Pascoe & Smart Richman, 2009). This analysis points to the need for understanding the issues clients may face in their primary cultural and familial contexts, it clearly shows how oppression and victimization of people can occur in their familial, social, and occupational worlds, creating a need for social justice training on issues of privilege, oppression, and advocacy.

Transgender Identity

A case of gender identity that has not been adequately addressed in the psychological literature pertains to transgendered individuals (Garrett, 2004; Mizock & Lewis, 2008). Transgendered people do not accept their biological gender as their gender identity or outward gender expression (Mizock & Fleming, 2011). Usually, transgendered individuals are misclassified as delusional primarily due to the DSM-IV-TR label of Gender Identity Disorder (American Psychiatric Association, 2000). Although, the DSM-IV-TR clearly differentiates between gender identity and delusional disorders, the label of disorder creates a confusion for the professional. Further, the psychological literature identifies that cultural competence for working with transgendered clients is not the focus in psychology training programs (Israel, Gorcheva, Walther, Sulzner, & Cohen, 2008; Russell & Horne, 2009). Bockting, Benner, and Coleman (2009) appropriately notes in response to the DSM-IV-TR categorization in the editorial to a special issue of *Sexual Relationship Therapy* (2009):

> The disease-based model assumes that normative gender identity development has been compromised and that establishing congruence between biological sex can alleviate the associated distress, gender identity and gender role, if necessary through hormonal and surgical sex reassignment. The identity-based model assumes that gender variance is merely an example of human diversity and that the distress transgender individuals might experience results from social stigma attached to gender variance (p. 103).

In the recent revision of the DSM (5th ed., APA, 2013), this category has been redefined as Gender Dysphoria. The insistence on bringing biological gender into congruence with normative beliefs is an index of societal oppression and emotional abuse that overtime, given the accumulated stress may lead to psychological problems that may have nothing to do with being transgendered; given the heterosexist emphasis in most societies, and especially in the West and the USA. The APA Task Force on Gender Identity and Gender Variance (2008) notes:

> The concerns of transgender and gender variant persons are inextricably tied to issues of social justice, which have historically been important to APA. The stigmatization and discrimination experienced by transgender people affect virtually all aspects of their lives, including physical safety, psychological wellbeing, access to services, and basic human rights. The Task Force report highlights opportunities for APA to advance social justice, as well as to support competent and ethical practice, by promoting research, education, and

> professional development concerning transgender issues among psychologists; by creating a welcoming environment for transgender psychologists and students of psychology; and by supporting the human rights of all transgender citizens (p. 10)

This population is highly vulnerable to social exclusion and isolation, we recommend that initial client assessment needs to take into account relationship history, social support, privilege and oppression of clients and the impact on psychological adjustment prior to establishing therapeutic goals. Ethically, it is important that therapists get supervision and training in working with gender variant individuals, and reflect on their learned biases and feelings toward this vulnerable population (APA, 2009). Recently there has been progress in identifying the exclusion and stressors faced by transgendered individuals as exemplified by the National Center for Transgender Equality (NCTE) and the National Gay and Lesbian Task Force *Survey on Transgender Discrimination* (2011), along with an earlier report on trans health priorities to eliminate health disparities (Xavier et al., 2004). Another positive outcome as a result of the Affordable Health Care Act (US Department of Health & Human Services (HHS.give/HealthCare), 2010) is the ban on sex discrimination in many health care facilities and programs, and has led to the publication of *Health care rights and transgender people* by NCTE in March 2012.

Sexual Orientation

Sexual orientation is important in understanding the impact of the intersection of multiple identities held by individuals, as it creates another category, where privilege and oppression function without recognition by most professionals. We live in a very heterosexist world (APA, 2009) and majority of the world religions with the largest following hold a negative perspective on any sexual behavior that is not in the service of procreation of the species. The norms established for gender roles also overlap with sexual orientation. Behaving in a culturally or socially inconsistent manner with regard to culturally accepted sexual norms leads to victimization and oppressive behavior, exclusion, and emotional abuse. The Institute of Medicine (2011) in their report on Lesbian Gay Bisexual and Transgendered (LGBT) health note that it is important to consider the contextual factors that impact the lives of GLBT groups, including sociopolitical history, societal and religious stigmas, laws and policies, demographic factors, and barriers to care. Gay, Lesbian, and Bisexual individuals are defined by their sexual orientation. Meanwhile transsexual individuals are defined by their gender identity and presentation. The LGBT umbrella is a loose coalition of four distinct and diverse groups. However, they also have commonalities in terms of stigmatization, exclusion, and oppression.

Since the 1970s several models of homosexual identity development have been proposed. These include stage models (Cass, 1979, 1984; Fassinger, 1991; Savin-Williams, 1988, 1990; Troiden, 1979, 1988); theories specific to Bisexual (Fox, 1995; Klein, 1990, 1993), Lesbian (Brown, 1995; Sears, 1989), and nondominant LGBT populations (Boykin, 1996; Crow, Brown, & Wright, 1997; Diaz, 1997;

Espin, 1993; Manalansan, 1993; Wilson, 1996); and lifespan approach to LGBT identity development (D'Augelli, 1994). The stage models did not address the intersectionality of identities, or the multiple influences that impinge upon identity development within a cultural context. However, lifespan development and theories addressing lesbian, bisexual, and nondominant groups identity development theories offer approaches that take into account the multiple factors that impinge upon identity, along with contextual factors (Bilodeau & Renn, 2005; Eklund, 2012). Shin (2015) notes that critical consciousness and intersectionality can be useful tools in decolonizing identity development models. Further, Smith (2015) recommends that it is time to "queer" the multicultural counseling paradigm by "examining taken-for-granted assumptions within the paradigm, challenging the status quo of multicultural competence, deconstructing hegemonic practices, and promoting critical consciousness" (p. 25).

Cultural Background

It is important to understand how the client perceives his or her cultural identity, recognizing the vital aspects of identity and how the client wishes to be perceived (Castillo, 1996). Accepting the client's evaluation of his or her own cultural identity is critical to the process of developing a therapeutic relationship. Hipolito-Delgado (2007) reported on a study of Latino/a college students that several students preferred Hispanic, Latino/a, or Chicano/a as their cultural identity, instead of the politically accepted term Hispanic. Therapists need to respect clients' preferred self-definition and cultural identity, if they hope to develop a working alliance with the client (Dana, 1998).

Castillo (1996) recommends always conducting a cultural identity assessment to understand the meaning of the presenting problem, and the implications of the presenting problem for the client. He also recommends seeking input from the client on what would be the resolution to the dilemma. During the process of counseling or psychotherapy, it may be necessary to correct some of the assumptions by identifying what the clients believe about their cultural background and the influence or lack of it on their cultural identity, especially when negative stereotypes are internalized and accepted (Knapp, Lemoncelli, & VandeCreek, 2010).

Migration Status

The USA, along with a few other countries, such as Australia, Canada, New Zealand, and South Africa, have a sociopolitical history, where indigenous people were outnumbered by immigrants, who were culturally very different from the native people. Although similar attempts were made by other colonial powers, none were as successful as the Western European immigrants in the four nations mentioned above.

The sociopolitical changes that occurred in these cultures made the culture of the colonial rulers the norm, due to the large numbers, and the power they held as invaders of these lands (Diamond, 1999). Understanding migration status, and its impact on identity is much more complex for people who have colonial ancestors, and now constitute the dominant cultural group, due to several hundred years of residence. The Europeans who settled in these lands believe they are indigenous to these societies. If the indigenous populations had not survived, or not retained their culture, languages, rituals, etc., it would have been easier to understand the stance taken by several generations of immigrants, over the last 250–400 years in these societies. There is considerable shame and anxiety when issues of culture, and sociopolitical history are brought up for the dominant groups, due to abuse, extermination, exclusion, forced poverty and lack of opportunities, and several other violations that indigenous populations have undergone. Reyes Cruz and Sonn (2015) note that Western thought has been characterized by dichotomous thinking, and this worldview would have been one of many in general, except for the globalization of the European colonialization that began with the Americas. This movement also led to a "the imposition of a hierarchical articulation of difference (e.g., "civilized/uncivilized," "modern/primitive," "expert knowledge/general knowledge," "development/underdevelopment," "saved/condemn," "European/Other," "White/Other") to the benefit of the ruling classes" (p. 128). Further Reyes Cruz and Sonn identify that coloniality shaped culture and as a result identity, and positioned the West as the only standard of civilization, paving the way for oppression and marginalization. For mental health professionals who are from the dominant cultural in the USA, it is important to approach their sociopolitical history from a reflective dialectical perspective to overcome the anxiety or stress in working with a diverse population (Israel, 2012; Todd & Abrams, 2011).

Recent immigrants face issues of acculturative stress, confusion about adapting to a new culture, and not understanding the rules and norms in the host culture (Sam & Berry, 2010). In addition, when migration is from cultural systems that are collectivistic to Western individualistic cultures, adaptation and adjustment is much more difficult. Historically, people from cultures very different from the host culture retain their culture of origin and either develop a bicultural identity, or choose to stay separate from the dominant culture (Berry, 1980; Rogers-Sirin, Ryce, & Sirin, 2014). Several orthodox religions, such as orthodox Jews and Muslims have had a difficult time developing a bicultural identity postmigration (Sam & Berry, 2010; Rogers-Sirin, Ryce, & Sirin, 2014). Integration into US society has been difficult for immigrants from Africa, Asia, and Latin America because of the anti-miscegenation laws adopted in the USA (and repealed in 1926), people from these cultural groups were forced to form tight social connections in order to survive due to exclusion, and racism (Landrine & Klonoff, 2002, 2004; Portes & Rumbaut, 2006; Rudmin, 2003).

All immigrants whether they are coming from collectivistic or individualistic cultures have significant stress and go through an adjustment process integrating to a new system (Phinney, 1990; Portes & Rumbaut, 2006; Verkuyten, 1998). Immigrants come to their new country with several assumptions and hopes. However, many of these assumptions are based on superficial knowledge or understanding of a culture, and there is always culture shock, despondency, homesickness, or a desire to get back to a familiar world. The immigrant generation generally ends up living in two worlds, culture of origin, and culture of the adopted land, or psychologically staying in the culture of origin and choosing to do a daily "border crossing" when they go to work, or interact with the host culture, e.g., educational, and/or local, state, and national institutions (Portes & Rumbaut). If the cultural system is flexible, and willing to adapt, first generation immigrants tend to adjust better as they are born and educated in a system that they have the ability to comprehend, learn the unwritten norms and rules of society, and have less adjustment issues than their parents. However, in groups that are excluded from mainstream society due to cultural, ethnic, racial, or religious differences, future generations of immigrants have two social-cultural-psychological worlds that they negotiate daily as they interact with mainstream society (Portes & Zhou, 1993; Rudmin, 2003).

Languages

Being bilingual or being able to use several languages with facility is a gift that most cultures value, especially as research in the last 15 years has shown evidence of all the benefits (Grosjean, 2010). In many countries of the world, and within one country there may be more that three or four languages (Allardi, Bak, Duggirala, Surampudi, Shailaja, Shukla et al., 2013; European Commission, 2012). A survey by Eurobarometer estimated that 54 % of Europe was bilingual. Neuroscience, neurolinguistics, and researchers studying the brain have shown that white matter increases in the brain of bilinguals, and that they are able to have better focus during learning, and better recall. Further, bilingual individuals have better decision-making skills; recent research shows that being bilingual delays dementia in older adults by approximately four and a half years, when compared to monolingual individuals (Allardi, Bak, Duggirala, Surampudi, Shailaja, Shukla et al., 2013; Mortimer et al., 2014; Krizman, Marian, Shook, Skoe, & Kraus, 2012; Mechelli et al., 2004; Luk, Bialystok, Craik, & Grady, 2011).

With the monolingual focus adopted by the founding fathers, primarily to create a unified nation in the USA, having more than one language was not seen as an asset (Takaki, 2000). With globalization of economic systems of the world, being bilingual is an asset. Individuals with accents and who had acquired multiple languages were historically not respected for the language skills they possessed. If we approach a client with an accent with a position that obviously they are recent immigrants and English is not their primary language, therefore they are not very "smart." We may be underestimating the knowledge and skills of the client, given that he or she may have additional resources having lived, worked, or functioned in different cultures. Multiple languages are a strength and can be employed as an asset to help the client resolve the issues that brought him or her to counseling. The client may need coaching and assistance coping with US culture, and we as therapists can be very helpful in providing assistance to negotiate cultural impasses as recent immigrants and sojourners acclimate to the culture.

One issue that has been debated significantly in the literature pertains to using a translator when conducting therapy with a non-English speaking client. Current research cautions against using translators as in many cases the translator may not translate culturally sensitive issues that the client is bringing up to "save face," this can actually be harmful to the therapeutic process (DeAngelis, 2010). Further, miscommunications can occur due to cultural misunderstandings, social class differences, and research shows that more severe diagnosis are given to individuals who cannot speak the dominant language (Putsch, 1985; Westermeyer, 1989). In addition, when emotional dialogues are translated, affect can get "flattened" due to the limited words available for emotional expression in the English language and the therapist may not understand the depth of emotion connected to the situation, and what it means to the client (McNamee & Gergen, 1992). Sometimes, highly emotional expression can be intimidating and exhausting for both the therapist and the translator (if they both represent non-emotional cultures), especially in working with traumatized refugees (Lipton, Arends, Bastian, Wright, & O'Hara, 2002).

Tribe and Lane (2009) and DeAngelis (2010) provide excellent recommendations for preparing for a psychological consultation and intervention, when an interpreter is needed. DeAngelis notes that several programs exist for training translators for mental health services, if possible a trained individual should be hired. When working with translators, it is important to set appropriate boundaries, provide information on confidentiality, and protection of clients' rights. Both Tribe and Lane and DeAngelis caution mental health service providers to ensure that the client is comfortable with the arrangement, and understands that the interpreter is part of the treatment team. In taking on clients who are culturally different, therapists must have clarity on their own beliefs, values, and biases, and also consider if a client with minimal English proficiency would be best served by them; in such cases it may be best to refer the client to a therapist who can communicate with a client in his or her native language.

Religion and Spirituality

Religion and spirituality have deep seated emotional meaning for individuals (Cornish, Wade, Tucker, & Post, 2014; Taylor, Chatters, & Jackson, 2007). Hodge and Derezotes (2008) note that religion is a set of shared communal beliefs and practices, which are organized with the goal of spiritual development. Hodge and Derezotes consider spirituality as a subjective, individualistic set of assumptions. They identify two common themes between the two concepts: (a) the existence of a transcendent reality, transpersonal in nature and (b) this reality is personal, existential, and subjective, and involves a connection with the nontemporal, i.e., not related to worldly affairs or time.

Mohr (2006) notes that spirituality and religion are often neglected in mental health assessment, intervention, and care. Further, it is an understudied aspect of client identity, and not addressed in training (Cornish et al., 2014). This gap in focus and especially in training is confounding given that 92 % of people in the USA report a belief in God or a universal entity, and 56 % report that religion is an important part of their lives (Pew Forum on Religion & Public Life, 2008).

When working across religious and spiritual differences, once again, therapists need to be clear on their own worldview and perception of religion and spirituality. Dinham and Jones (2010) note that religious literacy and the ability to communicate one's own religious values, along with critical reflection on religion and recognition of the legitimacy of religious views held by others are very important skills. Counseling at its core is about negotiating deep-seated values, beliefs, and assumptions, acquired very early in life. Usually, our core beliefs and values are derived from religious socialization, which takes place from birth onwards as parents identify right and wrong, and socialize children, within a community and a cultural context. Furseth and Repstad (2006) in their introduction on the concept of religious socialization argue that through this process individuals largely adopt ways of thinking and acting that are transmitted and controlled by the expectations of others, and eventually come to comply with these expectations. Lövheim (2012) notes that empirical studies of socialization place a high value on the role of parents in the process of religious socialization. Most individuals are socialized in their parents' faith or spiritual beliefs (Erikson, 1977). However, commitment to a specific faith or spirituality varies among people, considering the influence of the cyber age and the access to global knowledge bases (Høeg, 2011; Lövheim, 2011; Martin, White, & Perlman, 2003; Pettersson, 2006). Further, the rise of atheism in the USA requires sensitivity and care in therapeutic work, specifically given the lack of attention in the psychological literature to people who do not subscribe to a religion or spirituality (Brewster, Robinson, Sandil, Esposito, & Geiger, 2014).

Religious differences can negatively affect the therapeutic relationship if assumptions are not clarified. Clarity for the client on the therapist's assumptions and beliefs about the client's religion, and how it is perceived are very important. Mental health practitioners are encouraged to have an open dialogue about religion or spiritual beliefs. It is also important to conduct a spiritual assessment to understand the strength of commitment (Hodge & Derezotes, 2008; Ibrahim & Dykeman, 2011; Ibrahim & Heuer, 2013). Clarity on these core assumptions and their importance to the client will facilitate the therapeutic process (Mohr, 2006). Another necessary condition for working in a culturally pluralistic society is to accurately understand the assumptions underlying major religions of the world, and using this as a backdrop to gauge how deeply client may be embedded in a religion (Hodge, Bonifas, & Chou, 2010).

We maintain that religion and spirituality is mediated by the cultural context. Religion and spirituality have core concepts and how these are expressed, accepted, and practiced depends on a culture that has adopted it (Ibrahim & Dykeman, 2011; Ibrahim & Heuer, 2013). Most cultures of the world have had religions imposed upon them by invaders and colonizers of their lands, and assumptions from previous religious or spiritual beliefs are still functioning within the acquired religious context. For example, Latino/a cultures in South America retained several values from their original assumptions and translated Catholic beliefs to fit what they believed, e.g., the concept of Marianismo, is ascribed to Mary, as the ideal Madonna, however, the status of women as mothers is highly revered in Latino culture and that has been translated to fit Catholic assumptions (Garcia-Preto, 2005). Similarly, Jewish religion and culture has been mediated in the US context to create three distinct sets of assumptions that fit the lifestyle of the followers in the USA (Rosen & Weltman, 2005). In addition, Bedouin culture has greatly influenced how Islam is practiced in Saudi Arabia and other nomadic Arab societies. Several assumptions regarding revenge, war, status, and treatment of women are derived from ancient beliefs in Bedouin culture, and do not reflect the values embedded in Islam (Abudabbeh, 2005). We must consider culture of origin, generations in the host culture, depth of commitment to the religion or spirituality, and how the client perceives his/her/zir commitment to the religion or spirituality. It may vary from the traditional assumptions about the religion or the spiritual practice. This process will help facilitate the therapeutic process, because the client knows his or her beliefs best, for us to put our own interpretation on it would be disrespectful, and lead to a break in the therapeutic relationship (Hodge, Bonifas, & Chou, 2010).

Ability/Disability Status

People with disabilities constitute the largest minority group in the USA (Artman & Daniels, 2010). Approximately 54 million Americans (about 1 in 5) have physical, sensory, psychiatric, or cognitive disabilities that interfere with daily living (Bowe, 2000). Olkin (2002) notes that with the increased focus on multicultural counseling, one population has not received adequate attention, i.e., people with disabilities. Although, recently there has been a focus in psychology on disability, Artman and Daniel note that "the disability-related literature in psychology focuses on psychosocial adjustment to disability, rather than strategies for better serving this population" (p. 442). Ability and disability status has an impact on identity. It defines what people can and cannot do, and also addresses the limitations that a lack of ability can have on a person. This plays a meditational role in cultural identity development. Another aspect to consider is the role of intersectionality of identities, and the role of multiple stigmatized aspects of identity, along with disability (Bryan, 2007; Hernandez, Balcazar, Keys, Hidalgo, & Rosen, 2006; Thompson, Noel, & Campbell, 2004). Societal attitudes toward visible disabilities can also pose oppressions for a person with disabilities. Hatzenbuehler, Phelan, and Link (2013) note that stigma influences several physical and mental health outcomes for millions of people in the USA. Sensitivity to issues of ability/disability is critical in creating an accepting therapeutic context (APA, 2014).

Very little research focuses on invisible disabilities, i.e., people may have physical limitations that are not visible, such as deafness, and the problems of aging, difficulty walking, bending, or sitting on the floor (Elliot, Uswatte, Lewis, & Palmatier, 2000; Thompson et al., 2004). These issues create different sociocultural contexts for dealing with limitations, and when these are not acknowledged it affects cultural identity of an individual, and this aspect needs to be explored with clients.

Multicultural movement in applied psychology has given a sense of group identity and pride to disability-rights activists (Artman & Daniels, 2010; Gilson & DePoy, 2000). Gross and Hahn (2004) maintain that disability community identifies as an oppressed group because of the projected embarrassment, hostility, and existential anxiety of the nondisabled in society. As a culture, people with disability share a common history and an outrage at the stigmatization, oppression they experience, placing their plight within the context of civil rights (Gilson & DePoy, 2000; Olkin, 1999; Phemister, 2001). Recent developments in psychology have started to address disability issues (APA, 2014; Cornish et al., 2008; Olkin, 1999, 2002; Olkin & Pledger, 2003).

People born with a disability, generally adjust better to their situation, and achieve a high level of functionality in their lives. However, losing abilities over the lifespan due to accidents, war, aging, or late onset of a debilitating condition makes it much harder for people to accept limitations (Bowe, 2000; Elliot et al., 2000). There is a grieving process that needs to be undertaken, to help the client accept the changes, even when people appear to be doing well despite their ability to cope with the changes that they are encountering (Burke, Hainsworth, Eakes, & Lindgren, 1992; Davis, 1987). Group support with similar people who are also dealing with similar changes is highly recommended as the cultural identity of the individual has changed, and being in a group with people also struggling or coping well with a similar disability reinforces a positive cultural identity for a person with disabilities. For both groups, people born with disabilities or people having to confront loss of abilities, group support helps validate the new cultural identity, which is now mediated by the ability/disability context (Chan, Thomas, & Berven, 2002; Rajeski & Focht, 2002).

Two disability affirmative therapy models exist (Balcazar, Suarez-Balcazar, & Taylor-Ritzler, 2009; Olkin, 2008). These models provide guidance on case formulation and do not over- or under-inflate the role of disability, a common hazard when able-bodied therapists work with individuals with disabilities. Artman and Daniels (2010) provide specific information to achieve cultural competence in working with people with disabilities, along with information for therapists on becoming active advocates for their clients. It is important for therapists to confront their own attitudes toward disability and to review the legal mandates (Americans with Disabilities Act [ADA], 2008), and review the *APA Guidelines for Assessment of and Intervention with people with disabilities* (APA, 2014).

Composition of the Family

The familial context clients come from is an important variable in understanding cultural identity (Fowers & Olson, 1993; Olson & Gorall, 2003). A significant body of research exists on how people negotiate intact, blended, single parent, or two-parent, adoptive, gay or lesbian families; however, it is mostly focused on the majority group culture (Borrine, Handal, Brown, & Searight, 1991; Bray & Berger, 1993; Lansford, Ceballo, Abbey, & Stewart, 2001). How the client perceives the composition of the family and what their primary culture believes is the "ideal" family has an effect on identity development and adjustment in life (Baruth & Manning, 2011; McGoldrick, 2005). Exploration with the clients of the meaning and impact of the type of family they grew up in, is useful in understanding the influence of family dynamics on the client's personality, and outlook (Demo & Acock, 1996; Friedman, Terras, & Kreisher, 1995; Vandewater & Lansford, 1998).

Research indicates considering a person's attachment orientation in infancy predicts the emotional quality of romantic relationships a person will have in early adulthood. A significant association exists between parent–child relationships and adult romantic relationships (Dinero, Conger, Shaver, Widaman, & Larsen-Rife, 2011). All factors that influence developmental processes are useful in understanding strengths and challenges that the client brings to counseling as they work on the presenting problem. It is important for therapists to confront their own experience of growing up in their own family of origin, and how these experiences may influence their work with their clients.

Birth Order

Birth order research addresses how children in specific cultural contexts develop certain behavioral characteristics based on whether they are the first, the middle, or the last child in a family (Booth & Kee, 2009; Iacovou, 2001; Zajonc & Sulloway, 2007). What has not been adequately explored is how gender affects these characteristics, of being a leader, an accommodator, or the baby of the family (Conley, 2000; Stewart, 2012). Rosenblatt and Skoogberg (1974) reported on a study with a worldwide sample of 39 countries that the birth of the first child of either sex resulted in increased status for the parents and marital stability. First-born daughters in adulthood received more respect and had greater influence on siblings than other daughters, or first-born sons. Contrary to this finding, in two specific cultures of the world, if the first child is female, there is open mourning, e.g., in South Asia, because a daughter is seen as a burden, who is a guest in her parents home, until she marries, and her dowry will be a significant cost for the family (Bumiller, 1991). In the Middle East, a mother is not called a mother if she does not have a son, when she has a son, she is referred to as a mother (Brooks, 1995). Obviously, female children who are the oldest child in such cultures would be hampered by these cultural beliefs, and would possibly develop lower self-esteem, because they may view themselves as liabilities, or children who did not bring honor to their mother. The opposite also can occur, where despite their gender, they strive to show their parents that they are capable, dependable, and out-excel their peers and brothers. Educational level of the parents can be a major mediational factor in how the identity of a female child in these cultures develops. It is important for helping professionals to reflect on their own birth order, their role in the family, and cultural beliefs about their own gender.

Geographical Environment

Chandler and Munday (2014) define geographical identity in two ways: (1) an individual or group's sense of attachment to the country, region, city, or village in which they live and (2) the key characteristics with which a particular country, region, city, or village is associated. Individuals have deep attachments to geographical locations, where significant development tasks were completed and/or life cycle events take place, and these locations are romanticized (Brown & Swanson, 2003; Logan, 1996). Socialization in a specific geographical region has an influence on cultural identity; each type of geographical location provides strengths and challenges based on the topography of the region. Moving from one geographical setting to another also provides additional strengths in coping with different geographical environments.

Socialization in urban, suburban, and rural environments has somewhat different dynamics, i.e., rural communities, although fast becoming diverse, tend to not be diverse, professional jobs may be lacking, economy may be dependent on agriculture and retail businesses, income and tax base tends to be lower than in metropolitan centers (Crockett, Shanahan, & Jackson-Newsom, 2000; Yang & Fetsch, 2007). Metropolitan centers provide higher incomes, greater diversity, choice and access to many educational models, and greater options for better health care (Harter, 1999; Yang & Fetsch, 2007). This is an important factor in exploring with a client about the location of their primary identity development and comfort level in current setting. The presenting problem may or may not be occurring due to geographical changes, however coping with urban settings, versus living in a rural setting requires different knowledge and skills (Gimpel & Karnes, 2006). The research available on rural children and youth has often referred to the challenges of rural life (Adams, 2003; Conger & Elder, 1994; MacTavish & Salamon, 2003). However, Yang and Fetsch found children in rural areas in their sample did not have any negative impact, their sense of self-esteem and academic achievements were higher than the norm. The negative findings were similar to children in metropolitan areas (both urban and suburban) these included concerns about physical appearance (Pipher, 1995). Bronfenbrenner (1958) notes that socialization practices flow from urban middle-class families to rural working-class families. This phenomenon of anxiety about appearance and the body may be related to this variable. It could also be due to the increased time youth in the USA are spending online and engaged with the media, as the desire to be out of doors is no longer valued in all geographical areas of the USA reducing physical activity (Strife & Downey, 2009).

Research on psychological implications of growing up in metropolitan areas identifies several negative outcomes, primarily, lack of attachments to grandparents and extended kinship systems, neighborhood connections, along with overcrowding and distance from nature (Kunstler, 1993; Putnam, 2000; Suarez, 1999; Strife & Downey, 2009). However, is no specific evidence has been presented that shows a direct connection with patterns of psychological distress or low levels of happiness in urban, and suburban settings (Argyle, 1999). Research in psychology and sociology has linked the effect of physical environments, such as crowding, noise, pollution, to mood disorders, delinquency and suicide (Freedman 1975; Halpern, 1995) and social isolation (Gable & Nezlek, 1998). Fischer (1984) in a literature review of psychological outcomes of urban and rural areas found no evidence of negative psychological outcomes of living in urban areas. Although, there is evidence of negative psychological consequences due to economic segregation, as noted by Oliver (1999); research shows that affluence reduces community engagement and leads to social isolation and alienation. Understanding client concerns may be limited for a therapist who does not understand what it means to be a person from the suburbs or a densely populated urban area. Once again, we as therapists must explore where we grew up, and our understanding of different geographical environments, and the strengths and challenges of different settings.

Social Class

The concept of social class is an emotionally loaded issue in the USA; the concept that people may be unequal is not readily accepted (Hollingshead & Redlich, 1958; Hooks, 2000; Rothenberg). Baker (1996) has argued that class is difficult to define, because it is a construct used in stratification of societies and is therefore difficult to recognize. Social class, an external variable influences cultural identity based on how one understands one's place in a system, the environment one grows up in, and how others perceive a person. Anderson and Collins (2012) note that social class, similar to race, ethnicity, and sexual orientation, does not reside within the individual, it is the result of a system of power created by institutional structures that create inequities. This coincides with Bourdieu (1989) conception that social structures transform into mental structures, and the mental structures in turn provide social structures, there is a possibility for change with the bidirectional interaction between social and mental structures. How people define or understand their social class is based on economic, cultural, and social capital; these capitals are used to define one's place on a system (Bourdieu, 1989; Whitman-Raymond, 2009). As a subjective variable it is important to understand how an individual perceives his or her social class and despite the objective circumstances (Adler & Snibbe, 2003). This reinforces the client-centered perspective, essential for therapeutic work, especially as therapists work across culture and class boundaries (Castillo, 1997; Dana, 1998; Ibrahim, 1985). The concept of social class has received limited attention in applied psychology research (Ballinger & Wright, 2007; Levy & O'Hara, 2010; Liu, Soleck, Hopps, Dunston, & Pickett, 2004; Smith, 2000, 2005, 2009; Smith & Chambers, 2015). Falconnier (2009) asserts that the practice of counseling and psychotherapy is rooted in middle-class values and may not be relevant for other social classes, especially low income clients.

Neil Altman (1995) introduced the concept of a three-person psychology, instead of the counseling dyad, he asserts the third "person" refers to social context. Liu et al.'s (2004) *Social Class Worldview Model* (SCWM) is a cultural variable that is highly subjective, it not static, and neither is it linked to a place and time. In counseling and psychotherapy it is important for therapists to recognize how they perceive social class and what their assumptions are about the different socioeconomic levels. Therapist assumptions and bias can influence diagnosis, interventions, and the possible outcome of the intervention (Liu, 2002; Liu et al., 2004). The counseling relationship can be compromised when social class issues are ignored and the middle-class model is applied to working, lower social class, or homeless clients (Balmforth, 2009; Rose-Innes, 2006; Liu, 2001; Smith, 2005; Snowden & Yamada, 2005; US Department of Health & Human Services, 2001). When low income clients, who are also from racial-cultural nondominant groups seek mental health assistance they are less likely to receive evidence-based interventions (Le, Zmuda, Perry, & Munoz, 2010; Miranda et al., 2005), and more likely to terminate counseling prematurely (Organista, Munoz, & Gonzalez, 1994; Sue & Zane, 1987). Research suggests that people in lower social classes tend to get more severe diagnosis than people in affluent social classes (Belle, 1990; Hollingshead & Redlich, 1958; Shubert & Miller, 1978; Siegel, Kahn, Pollack, & Fink, 1962). These studies show that there is an implicit assumption that people in upper classes, being affluent, and more educated would be healthier (Baker, 1996; Belle, 1990; Liu, Alt, & Pittinger, 2013).

Kim and Cardemil (2012) note that no one is immune to the influence of class divisions that everyone is institutionalized. Further, interpersonal and internalized classism is displayed in stereotypes, prejudice, and discrimination. Therefore, self-awareness and critical reflection about one's own biases is necessary to address classist behaviors and attitudes. They provide several helpful guidelines for assessment and intervention with lower social class clients. Including guidelines for assessment, explicit and ongoing attention to social class issues (including explicit discussion of social class issues and barriers that clients may face), intersectionality of social class with other dimensions of identity, and attending to needed cultural adaptations to the counseling process (individual, group, family interventions, psychoeducation, and number and frequency of sessions), and a need for increased self-disclosure (Cardemil, 2010; Castro, Barrera, & Holleran Steiker, 2010; Grote, Swartz, & Zuckoff, 2008; Miranda et al., 2005).

Three Key Domains of Identity That Feature in the Presenting Problem

The last question on the Cultural Identity Check List-Revised© requires respondents to identify aspects of cultural identity that are implicated in the presenting problem. This helps in narrowing down the core values involved, and where the distress is located (Castillo, 1997; Dana, 1998; Ibrahim, 1999). Culture usually emerges as a very strong factor in human suffering, because many of life's major dilemmas are focused on an individual's need to do something, and the constraints usually come from learned cultural, gendered, religious, assumptions, or internalized privilege and oppressions (Brody et al., 2006; Caughy, Nettles, O'Campo, & Lohrfink, 2006; Chen & Bargh, 1997). However, we cannot assume that culture is always the issue; exploration of core values, as they affect these domains helps in creating a fuller understanding of the client's cultural identity, and especially on variables that have not been traditionally considered as important (Castillo, 1997; Dana, 1998; Ibrahim, 2003). Frable (1997) notes that the multidimensionality of identity is overlooked in counseling and psychotherapy because the aspects of identity have been studied in a fragmented manner in the psychological literature.

To integrate the social justice perspective in this discussion, it is important to recognize that ethnic, cultural/racial identity, along with the other variables discussed in this chapter, i.e., gender, gender identity, sexual orientation, age and life stage, educational status, religion, ability-disability continuum, and the geographic location one comes from, given the context can be a source of privilege or oppression (Dana, 1998; Frable, 1997; Ibrahim, 2010). Societal values, beliefs, and assumptions can elevate some aspects and down grade other aspects of a person's identity and either provide opportunities or deny access to opportunities for the good life. The constant stress of either high expectations (privilege) or low expectations (oppressions) on a daily basis results in stress-related disorders, which affect the mind and the body (Adams et al., 2013; Ibrahim & Ohnishi, 2001). Epidemiological studies have shown that lifetime exposure to trauma is high, with 50–69 % of people (Hetzel-Riggin & Roby, 2013; Kessler, Sonnega, Bromet, Hughes, & Nelson, 1995; Resnick, Kilpatrick, Dansky, Saunders, & Best, 1993).

When conducting a cultural identity assessment, it is important to also incorporate the *DSM-5* Cultural Formulation Interview (CFI; American Psychiatric Association, 2013a, 2013b, 2013c). This interview will provide the answers to the cultural meaning of the distress for the client, what it represents and how to resolve the problem. It will also highlight what resources the client may have that would support the therapeutic intervention, e.g., support system (familial, kin, or friends, coworkers), occupational status, change in level of functioning at home and on the job (if employed), and current religious or spiritual status (Castillo, 1997; Dadlani, Overtree, & Perry-Jenkins, 2012; Ibrahim, 2010; Ivey, D'Andrea, & Ivey, 2011) This will be useful adjunct to cultural identity assessment in preparation for diagnosis, case formulation, and intervention (APA, 2002).

It is important for mental health professionals to meditate and reflect on each of these categories to identify their own assumptions, and to critically examine the meaning of each of these categories; given individual sociopolitical history, unearned and earned privilege, and oppressions, and actively seek experiential training in working with the dimensions that are unfamiliar and were not addressed in their training program (Collins & Pieterse, 2007; Croteau, Lark, Lidderdale, & Chung, 2005; Hardiman, Jackson, & Griffin, 2007). Critical awareness requires reflection and practice through experiential exercises, meditation and journaling to understand our unconscious and implicit learning (Banaji & Hardin, 1996; DeCoster, Banner, Smith, & Semin, 2006; Jun, 2010). As professionals we are always evolving and growing and incorporating a regular practice on understanding our conscious and unconscious assumptions will prove to be very helpful in enhancing the ability to be culturally responsive.

Conclusion

Each of the cultural identity categories is critical for understanding the client, the presenting problem, and the possible resolutions. It is equally important for therapists to recognize the multidimensionality of their own identity. Both the therapist and the client's identities are interacting within the therapeutic encounter. For therapists, it is very important to be aware of their own identity, their issues, and their privilege and oppressions; if not understood and addressed, these will come up as unguided missiles in the therapeutic encounter (Ibrahim, 2003). Our focus in counseling and psychotherapy has always reduced the client to a single identity, e.g., an American, which usually implies White Anglo Saxon Protestant, as historically, it has been used as a label for European immigrants. However, given that there are 21 distinct White ethnic groups in the USA, from several regions, and geographical settings (McGoldrick et al., 2005), we may be making several erroneous assumptions about the client. This checklist was developed in 1990 to address all possible variables inherent in a cultural identity, and to supplement information gained from the Scale to Assess World View© on core values and assumptions. Without the information from the CICL-R we do not have all the information we need for a personal encounter, which involves helping an individual address serious issues in counseling and psychotherapy.

References

Abudabbeh, N. (2005). Arab families: An overview. In M. McGoldrick, J. Pearce, & N. Garcia-Preto (Eds.), *Ethnicity and family therapy* (3rd ed., pp. 423–436). New York: Guilford Press.

Adams, J. (Ed.). (2003). *Fighting for the farm: Rural America transformed*. Philadelphia, PA: University of Pennsylvania Press.

Adams, M., Blumenfeld, W. J., Castaneda, R., Hackman, H. W., Peters, M. L., & Zuniga, X. (2013). *Readings for diversity and social justice* (3rd ed.). New York: Routledge.

Adler, N. E., & Snibbe, A. C. (2003). The role of psychosocial processes in explaining the gradient between socioeconomic status and health. *Current Directions in Psychological Science, 12*(4), 119–123.

Allardi, S., Bak, T. H., Duggirala, V., Surampudi, B., Shailaja, M., Shukla, et al. (2013). Bilingualism delays age at onset of dementia, independent of education and immigration status. *Neurology, 26*(8), 1938–1944. doi:10.1212/01.wnl.0000436620.33155.a4. Epub 2013 Nov 6.

Altman, N. (1995). *The analyst in the inner city: Race, class, and culture through a psychoanalytic lens*. Hillsdale, NJ: Analytic Press.

American Association of Marriage and Family Therapy (AAMFT). (2012). *Code of ethics*. Alexandria, VA: Author.

American Counseling Association (ACA). (1992). *Multicultural competencies*. Alexandria, VA: Author.

American Counseling Association (ACA). (2014). *Code of ethics*. Alexandria, VA: Author.

American Psychiatric Association. (2000). *Diagnostic and statistical manual of mental disorders-IV-TR*. Washington, DC: Author.

American Psychiatric Association. (2013a). *Diagnostic and statistical manual-5 (DSM-5)*. Washington, DC: American Psychiatric Association.

American Psychiatric Association. (2013b). *Diagnostic and statistical manual of mental disorders* (5th ed.). Washington, DC: Author.
American Psychiatric Association. (2013c). *The principles of medical ethics with annotations especially applicable to psychiatry*. Washington, DC: Author.
American Psychological Association (APA). (2002). *Guidelines on multicultural education, training, research, practice, and organizational change for psychologists*. Washington, DC: Author.
American Psychological Association (APA). (2008). *Report of the task force on gender identity and gender variance*. Washington, DC: Author.
American Psychological Association (APA). (2009). *Report of the task force on appropriate therapeutic responses to sexual orientation*. Washington, DC: Author.
American Psychological Association (APA). (2010). *Ethical principles of psychologists and code of conduct: With 2010 amendments*. Washington, DC: Author (Original work published 2002).
American Psychological Association (APA). (2011). *The guidelines for psychological practice with lesbian, gay, and bisexual clients*. Washington, DC: Author.
American Psychological Association (APA). (2014). *Guidelines for assessment and intervention with persons with disabilities*. Author: Washington, DC. Retrieved from https://www.apa.org/pi/disability/resources/assessment-disabilities.aspx
Americans with Disabilities Act. (2008). *Amendments Act of 2008*, Public Law 110–325, 42 USCA § 12101.
Anderson, M. L., & Collins, P. H. (2007). *Race, class, & gender: An anthology* (8th ed.). Belmont, CA: Cengage Learning.
Argyle, M. (1999). Causes and correlates of happiness. In D. Kahneman, E. Diener, & N. Schwartz (Eds.), *Well being: The foundations of hedonic psychology*. New York: Russell Sage.
Artman, L. K., & Daniels, J. A. (2010). Disability and psychotherapy practice: Cultural competence and practical tips. *Professional Psychology: Research and Practice, 41*(5), 442–448. doi:10.1037/a0020864.
Baker, N. L. (1996). Class as a construct in a "classless" society. *Women and Therapy, 18*(3–4), 13–23.
Balcazar, F. E., Suarez-Balcazar, Y., & Taylor-Ritzler, T. (2009). Cultural competence: Development of a conceptual framework. *Disability and Rehabilitation, 31*, 1153–1160.
Ballinger, L., & Wright, J. (2007). Does class count? Social class and counseling. *Counselling and Psychotherapy Research: Linking Research with Practice, 7*(3), 157–163. doi:10.1080/14733140701571316.
Balmforth, J. (2009). "The weight of class": Clients' experiences of how perceived differences in social class between counsellor and client affect the therapeutic relationship. *British Journal of Guidance & Counselling, 37*, 375–386. doi:10.1080/03069880902956942.
Banaji, M. R., & Hardin, C. D. (1996). Automatic stereotyping. *Psychological Sciences, 7*, 136–141.
Barker, D. K., & Kuiper, E. (2003). *Toward a feminist philosophy of economics*. New York: Routledge.
Baruth, L. G., & Manning, M. L. (2011). *Multicultural counseling and psychotherapy: A lifespan perspective* (5th ed.). Upper Saddle River, NJ: Prentice Hall.
Belle, D. (1990). Poverty and women's mental health. *American Psychologist, 45*, 385–389.
Berry, J. W. (1980). Acculturation as varieties of adaptation. In A. Padilla (Ed.), *Acculturation: Theory, models and some new findings* (pp. 9–25). Boulder, CO: Westview.
Bilodeau, B. L., & Renn, K. A. (2005). Analysis of LGBT identity development models and implications for practice. *New Directions in Student Services, 111*, 25–39.
Bilton, T., Bonnett, K., Jones, P., Lawson, T., Skinner, D., Stanworth, M., et al. (2002). *Introductory sociology* (4th ed.). New York: Palgrave Macmilan.
Bockting, W., Benner, A., & Coleman, E. (2009). Gay and bisexuality identity development among female-male transsexuals in North America: Emergence of a transgender sexuality. *Archives of Sexual Behavior, 38*, 688–701. doi:10.1007/s10508-009-9489-3.
Booth, A., & Kee, H. (2009). Birth order matters: The effect of family size and birth order on educational attainment. *Journal of Population Economics, 22*(2), 367–397.

Borrine, M. L., Handal, P. J., Brown, N. Y., & Searight, H. R. (1991). Family conflict and adolescent adjustment in intact, divorced, and blended families. *Journal of Consulting and Clinical Psychology, 59*, 753–755.

Bourdieu, P. (1989). Social space and symbolic power. *Sociological Theory, 7*, 14–25.

Bowe, F. (2000). *Physical, sensory, and health disabilities: An introduction*. Upper Saddle River, NJ: Merrill.

Boykin, K. (1996). *One more river to cross: Black and gay in America*. New York: Anchor Books.

Bray, J. H., & Berger, S. H. (1993). Developmental issues in stepfamilies research project: Family relationships and parent-child interactions. *Journal of Family Psychology, 7*, 76–90.

Brewster, M. E., Robinson, M. A., Sandil, R., Esposito, J., & Geiger, E. (2014). Arrantly absent: Atheism in psychological science from 2001-2012. *The Counseling Psychologist, 42*(5), 628–663. doi:10.1177/0011000014528051.

Brody, G., Chen, Y., Murray, V. M., Ge, X., Simons, R. L., Gibbon, F. X., et al. (2006). Perceived discrimination and adjustment of African American youths: A five-year longitudinal analysis with contextual moderation effects. *Child Development, 77*, 1170–1189.

Bronfenbrenner, U. (1958). Socialization and social class through time and space. In E. E. Maccoby, T. M. Newcomb, & E. Hartley (Eds.), *Readings in social psychology* (pp. 400–424). New York: Holt.

Brooks, G. (1995). *Nine parts of desire: The hidden world of Islamic women*. New York: Anchor.

Brown, L. S. (1995). Lesbian identities: Concepts and issues. In A. R. D'Augelli & C. J. Patterson (Eds.), *Lesbian, gay and bisexual identities over the lifespan*. New York: Oxford University Press.

Brown, D. L., & Swanson, L. E. (2003). Rural America enters the new millennium. In D. L. Brown & L. E. Swanson (Eds.), *Challenges for rural America in the twenty-first century* (pp. 1–15). University Park, PA: Pennsylvania State University Press.

Bryan, W. V. (2007). *Multicultural aspects of disabilities: A guide to understanding and assisting minorities in the rehabilitation process* (2nd ed.). Springfield, IL: Charles C. Thomas.

Bumiller, E. (1991). *May you be the mother of a 100 sons: A journey among the women of India*. New York: Ballantine Books.

Burke, M. L., Hainsworth, M. A., Eakes, G. G., & Lindgren, C. L. (1992). Current knowledge and research on chronic sorrow: A foundation for inquiry. *Death Studies, 16*, 231–245.

Cardemil, E. V. (2010). Cultural adaptations to empirically supported treatments: A research agenda. *The Scientific Review of Mental Health Practice, 7*, 8–21.

Carli, L. L. (2001). Gender and social influence. *Journal of Social Issues, 57*(4), 725–741.

Cass, V. C. (1979). Homosexual identity formation: A theoretical model. *Journal of Homosexuality, 4*, 219–235.

Cass, V. C. (1984). Homosexual identity formation: Testing a theoretical model. *Journal of Sex Research, 20*, 143–167.

Castillo, R. J. (1996). *Culture and mental illness: A client-centered approach*. Belmont, CA: Cengage.

Castillo, R. J. (1997). *Culture and mental illness*. Belmont, CA: Cengage.

Castro, F. G., Barrera, M. J., & Holleran Steiker, L. K. (2010). Issues and challenges in the design of culturally adapted evidence-based interventions. *Annual Review of Clinical Psychology, 6*, 213–239.

Caughy, M., Nettles, S. M., O'Campo, P. J., & Lohrfink, K. F. (2006). Racial socialization and African American child development. The importance of neighborhood context. *Child Development, 77*, 1220–1236.

Cavalli-Sforza, L., Menozzi, P., & Piazza, A. (1996). *The history and geography of human genes*. Princeton, NJ: Princeton University Press.

Chan, F., Thomas, K. R., & Berven, N. L. (Eds.). (2002). *Counseling theories and techniques for rehabilitation health professionals*. New York: Springer.

Chandler, D., & Munday, R. (2014). Geographical identity. In D. Chandler & R. Munday (Eds.), *Oxford: Dictionary of media and communication*. Oxford, England: Oxford University Press. Retrieved from: http://www.oxfordreference.com/view/10.1093/oi/authority.20110810104955832.

Chen, M., & Bargh, J. A. (1997). Nonconscious behavioral confirmation processes: The self-fulfilling consequences of automatic stereotype activation. *Journal of Experimental Social Psychology, 33*, 541–560.
Collier, J., & Rosaldo, M. (1981). Politics and gender in simple societies. In S. B. Ortner & H. Whitehead (Eds.), *Sexual meanings: The cultural construction of gender and sexuality* (pp. 275–329). Cambridge: Cambridge University Press.
Collins, N. M., & Pieterse, A. L. (2007). Critical incident analysis based learning: An approach to training for active racial and cultural awareness. *Journal of Counseling and Development, 85*, 14–23.
Coltrane, S. (1994). Theorizing masculinities in contemporary social science. In H. Brod & M. Kaufman (Eds.), *Theorizing masculinities*. Thousand Oaks, CA: Sage.
Conger, R. D., & Elder, G. H., Jr. (1994). *Families in troubled times: Adapting to change in rural America*. New York: A. de Gruyter.
Conley, D. (2000). Sibling sex composition: Effects on educational attainment. *Social Science Research, 24*, 441–457.
Connell, R. W. (1995). *Masculinities*. Berkeley, CA: University of California Press.
Conwill, W. L. (2015). De-colonizing multicultural counseling and psychology: Addressing race through intersectionality. In R. D. Goodman & P. C. Gorski (Eds.), *Decolonizing "multicultural" counseling through social justice* (pp. 117–126). New York: Springer.
Cornish, J. A. E., Gorgens, K. A., Monson, S. P., Olkin, R., Palombi, B. J., & Abels, A. V. (2008). Perspectives on ethical practice with people who have disabilities. *Professional Psychology: Research and Practice, 39*, 488–497. doi:10.1037/a0013092.
Cornish, M. A., Wade, N. G., Tucker, J. R., & Post, B. C. (2014). When religion enters the counseling group: Multiculturalism, group processes, and social justice. *The Counseling Psychologist, 42*(5), 578–600. doi:10.1177/001000014527001.
Crockett, L. J., Shanahan, M. J., & Jackson-Newsom, J. (2000). Rural youth: Ecological and life course perspectives. In R. Montemayor, G. R. Adams, & T. P. Gullotta (Eds.), *Adolescent diversity in ethnic, economic, and cultural contexts: advances in adolescent development* (Vol. 10, pp. 43–74). Thousand Oaks, CA: Sage.
Cross, W. E., Jr. (1978). The Thomas and Cross models of psychological nigrescence: A review. *The Journal of Black Psychology, 5*, 13–31.
Croteau, J. M., Lark, J. S., Lidderdale, M. A., & Chung, Y. B. (Eds.). (2005). *Deconstructing heterosexism in the counseling professions: A narrative approach*. Thousand Oaks, CA: Sage.
Crow, L., Brown, L. B., & Wright, J. (1997). Gender selection in two American Indian tribes. In L. B. Brown (Ed.), *Two spirit people: American Indian lesbian women and gay men*. New York: Harrington Park Press.
D'Augelli, A. R. (1994). Identity development and sexual orientation: Toward a model of lesbian, gay, and bisexual development. In E. J. Trickett, R. J. Watts, & D. Birman (Eds.), *Human diversity: Perspectives on people in context*. San Francisco: Jossey-Bass.
Dadlani, M. B., Overtree, C., & Perry-Jenkins, M. (2012). Culture at the center: A reformulation of diagnostic assessment. *Professional Psychology: Research and Practice, 43*(3), 175–182.
Dana, R. H. (1998). *Understanding cultural identity in intervention and assessment*. Thousand Oaks, CA: Sage.
Davis, B. H. (1987). Disability and grief. *Social Casework, 68*, 352–357.
Deal, K. H. (2000). The usefulness of developmental stage models for clinical social work students: An exploratory study. *The Clinical Supervisor, 19*(1), 1–19.
DeAngelis, T. (2010). Found in translation. *Monitor on Psychology, 41*(2), 52.
DeCoster, J., Banner, M. J., Smith, E. R., & Semin, G. R. (2006). On the inexplicability of the implicit: Differences in information provided by the implicit and explicit tests. *Social Cognition, 24*, 5–21.
Demo, D. H., & Acock, A. C. (1996). Family structure, family process, ad adolescent well-being. *Journal of Research on Adolescence, 6*, 457–488.
Diamond, J. (1999). *Guns, steel, and germs: The fates of human societies*. New York: W. W. Norton.

Diaz, R. (1997). Latino gay men and psycho-cultural barriers to AIDS prevention. In M. Levine, J. Gagnon, & P. Nardi (Eds.), *In changing times: Gay men and lesbians encounter HIV/AIDS*. Chicago: University of Chicago Press.

Dinero, R. E., Conger, R. D., Shaver, P. R., Widaman, K. F., & Larsen-Rife, D. (2011). Influence of family of origin and adult romantic partners on romantic attachment security. *Journal of Family Psychology, 22*(3), 622–632.

Dinham, A., & Jones, S. H. (2010). *Religious literacy leadership in higher education: An analysis of challenges of religious faith, and resources for meeting them, for university leaders*. York, England: Religious Literacy Leadership in Higher Education Programme.

Eagly, A. H. (2009). The his and her of prosocial behavior: An examination of the socialpsychology of gender. *American Psychologist, 64*, 644–658.

Eckert, P., & McConnell, S. (2003). *Language and gender*. Cambridge, England: Cambridge University Press.

Edwards, K., & Wetzler, J. (1998). *Too young to be old: The role of self threat and psychological distancing in social categorization of the elderly*. Unpublished manuscript.

Eklund, K. (2012). Intersectionality of identity in children: A case study. *Professional Psychology, 43*(3), 256–264. doi:10.1037/a0028654.

Elliot, T. R., Uswatte, G., Lewis, L., & Palmatier, A. (2000). Goal instability and adjustment to disability. *Journal of Counseling Psychology, 47*, 251–265.

Erikson, E. H. (1963). *Childhood and society* (2nd ed., Rev.). New York: W.W. Norton & Co.

Erikson, E. H. (1968). *Identity: Youth and crisis*. New York: W.W. Norton.

Erikson, E. (1977). *Childhood and society*. St. Albans, England: Triad/Paladin.

Erikson, E. H. (1980). *Identity and the life cycle*. New York: W.W. Norton.

Espin, O. M. (1993). Issues of identity in the psychology of Latina lesbians. In L. S. Garnets & D. C. Kimmel (Eds.), *Psychological perspectives on lesbian and gay male experiences*. New York: Columbia University Press.

European Commission. (2012). *Special Eurobarometer 386: Europeans and their Languages report*. Retrieved from http://ec.europa.eu/public_opinion/index_en.htm

Falbo, T. (1977). Relationships between sex, sex role, and social influence. *Psychology of Women Quarterly, 2*, 62–72.

Falconnier, L. (2009). Socioeconomic status in the treatment of depression. *American Journal of Orthopsychiatry, 79*(2), 148–158.

Fassinger, R. E. (1991). The hidden minority: Issues and challenges in working with Lesbian women and gay men. *The Counseling Psychologist, 19*(2), 157–176.

Fischer, C. (1984). *The urban experience* (2nd ed.). San Diego, CA: Harcourt Brace Jovanovich.

Fowers, B. J., & Olson, D. H. (1993). Five types of marriage: Empirical typology based on ENRICH. *The Family Journal, 1*(3), 196–207.

Fox, R. (1995). Bisexual identities. In A. R. D'Augelli & C. J. Patterson (Eds.), *Lesbian, gay, and bisexual identities over the lifespan: Psychological perspectives* (p. 1995). New York: Oxford University Press.

Frable, D. E. S. (1997). Gender, racial, ethnic, and class identities. *Annual Review of Psychology, 48*, 139–162.

Freedman, J. L. (1975). *Crowding and behavior*. San Francisco: W. H. Freeman.

Friedman, A. A., Terras, A., & Kreisher, C. (1995). Family and client characteristics as predictors of outpatient treatment outcome for adolescent drug abusers. *Journal of Substance Abuse, 7*, 354–356.

Furseth, I., & Repstad, P. (2006). *An introduction to the sociology of religion. Classical and contemporary perspectives*. Farnham, England: Ashgate.

Gable, S. L., & Nezlek, J. B. (1998). Level and instability of day-to-day psychological well being and risk for depression. *Journal of Personality and Social Psychology, 74*, 129–138.

Gainor, K. A. (2000). Including transgender issues in lesbian, gay, and bisexual psychology: Implications for clinical practice and training. In B. Greene & G. L. Croom (Eds.), *Education, practice, and research in lesbian, gay, bisexual, and transgendered psychology: A resource manual* (pp. 111–160). Thousand Oaks, CA: Sage.

Garcia-Preto, N. (2005). Latino families: An overview. In M. McGoldrick, J. Pearce, & N. Garcia-Preto (Eds.), *Ethnicity and family therapy* (3rd ed., pp. 153–165). New York: Guilford Press.
Garrett, N. R. (2004). Treatment of a transgender client with schizophrenia in a public psychiatric milieu: A case study by a student therapist. *Journal of Gay and Lesbian Psychotherapy, 8*, 127–141.
Giddens, A. (1997). *Sociology*. London: Polity Press.
Gilson, S. F., & DePoy, E. (2000). Multiculturalism and disability: A critical perspective. *Disability and Society, 15*, 207–218.
Gimpel, J. G., & Karnes, K. A. (2006). The rural side of the urban-rural gap. *Political Science & Politics, 39*(3), 467–472.
Grosjean, F. (2010). *Bilingual: Life and reality*. Cambridge, MA: Harvard University Press.
Gross, B. H., & Hahn, H. (2004). Developing issues in the classification of physical and mental disability. *Journal of Disability Policy Studies, 15*, 130–134.
Grote, N. K., Swartz, H. A., & Zuckoff, A. (2008). Enhancing interpersonal psychotherapy for mothers and expectant mothers on low incomes: Adaptations and additions. *Journal of Contemporary Psychotherapy, 38*, 23–33.
Halpern, D. (1995). *Mental health and the built environment: More than bricks and mortar?* New York: Taylor & Francis.
Hardiman, R., Jackson, B., & Griffin, P. (2007). Conceptual foundations for social justice education. In M. Adams, L. A. Bell, & P. Griffin (Eds.), *Teaching for diversity and social justice* (2nd ed., pp. 35–66). New York: Routledge/Taylor & Francis.
Harter, S. (1999). *The construction of the self: A developmental perspective*. New York: Guilford.
Hartzler, K. J. (2003). Reverse age discrimination under the age discrimination in employment class. *Valparaiso University Law Review, 38*(1), 217–266.
Hatzenbuehler, M. I., Phelan, J. C., & Link, B. G. (2013). Stigma as a fundamental cause of population health disparities. *American Journal of Public Health, 103*(5), 813–821.
Helms, J. A., Jernigan, M., & Mascher, J. (2005). The meaning of race in psychology and how to change it: A methodological perspective. *The American Psychologist, 60*(1), 27–36. doi:10.1037/0003-066X.60.1.27.
Hernandez, B., Balcazar, F., Keys, C., Hidalgo, M., & Rosen, J. (2006). Taking it to the streets: Ethnic minorities with disabilities seek community inclusion. *Community Development, 37*(3), 13–25.
Hetzel-Riggin, M. D., & Roby, R. P. (2013). Trauma type and gender effects on PTSD, general distress, and peritraumatic dissociation. *Journal of Loss and Trauma, 18*, 41–53.
Higgins, A., Barker, P., & Begley, C. M. (2008). 'Veiling sexualities:' A grounded theory of mental health nurses responses to issues of sexuality. *Journal of Advanced Nursing, 62*(3), 307–317. doi:10.1111/j.1365-2648.2007.04586.x.
Hipolito-Delgado, C. P. (2007). *Internalized racism and ethnic identity in Chicana/o and Latina/o college students* (UNI# 3277390). Doctoral dissertation, University of Maryland, College Park, MD.
Hodge, D. R., Bonifas, R. P., & Chou, R. J.-A. (2010). Spirituality and older adults: Ethical guidelines to enhance service provision. *Advances in Social Work, 11*(1), 1–16.
Hodge, D. R., & Derezotes, D. S. (2008). Postmodernism and spirituality: Some pedagogical implications for teaching content on spirituality. *Journal of Social Work Education, 44*(1), 103–123.
Høeg, I. M. (2011). Religiøs tradering [Religion passed on]. In P. K. Botvar & U. Schmidt (Eds.), *Religion i dagens Norge. Mellom sekularisering og sakralisering* [Religion in Norway today. Between secularization and sacralization] (pp. 181–195). Oslo, Norway: Universitetsforlaget.
Hofstede, G. (2001). *Culture's consequences, comparing values, behaviors, institutions, and organizations across nations*. Thousand Oaks, CA: Sage.
Hollingshead, A., & Redlich, F. (1958). *Social class and mental illness: A community study*. New York: Wiley.
Hooks, B. (2000). *Where we stand: Class matters*. New York: Routledge.

House, J. S. (1981). Social structure and personality. In M. Rosenberg & R. Turner (Eds.), *Sociological perspectives on social psychology*. New York: Basic Books.

Hoyert, D. L., & Xu, J. (2012). Deaths: Preliminary data for 2011. *National Vital Statistics Reports, 61*(6), 1–7.

Huot, S., & Rudman, D. L. (2010). The performances and places of identity: Conceptualizing intersections of occupation, identity and place in the process of migration. *Journal of Occupational Science, 17*(2), 68–77.

Hutchinson, J., & Smith, A. D. (1996). *Ethnicity*. Oxford, England: Oxford University Press.

Hylland Erickson, T. (2002). *Ethnicity and nationalism: Anthropological perspectives*. London: Pluto Press.

Iacovou, M, (2001, June). *Family composition and children's educational outcomes*. Working paper of the Institute for Social and Economic Research, paper 2001–12 (PDF). Colchester, England: University of Essex.

Ibrahim, F. A. (1984). Cross-cultural counseling and psychotherapy: An existential-psychological perspective. *International Journal for the Advancement of Counseling, 7*, 159–169.

Ibrahim, F. A. (1985). Effective cross-cultural counseling and psychotherapy: A framework. *The Counseling Psychologist, 13*, 625–638.

Ibrahim, F. A. (1991). Contribution of cultural worldview to generic counseling and development. *Journal of Counseling and Development, 70*, 13–19.

Ibrahim, F. A. (1993). Existential worldview theory: Transcultural counseling. In J. McFadden (Ed.), *Transcultural counseling: Bilateral and international perspectives* (pp. 23–58). Alexandria, VA: ACA Press.

Ibrahim, F. A. (1999). Transcultural counseling: Existential world view theory and cultural identity: Transcultural applications. In J. McFadden (Ed.), *Transcultural counseling* (2nd ed., pp. 23–57). Alexandria, VA: ACA Press.

Ibrahim, F. A. (2003). Existential worldview theory: From inception to applications. In F. D. Harper & J. McFadden (Eds.), *Culture and counseling: New approaches* (pp. 196–208). Boston: Allyn & Bacon.

Ibrahim, F. A. (2007a, September). *Understanding multiple identities in counseling: Use of the scale to assess worldview© and the cultural identity checklist©*, at the Colorado Psychological Association Society for the Advancement of Multiculturalism and Diversity (SAMD), September 27, 2007, Denver, CO.

Ibrahim, F. A. (2007b). *Cultural identity check list-revised©*, Denver, CO. Unpublished document.

Ibrahim, F. A. (2008). *United States acculturation index©*, Denver, CO. Unpublished document.

Ibrahim, F. A. (2010). Innovative teaching strategies for group work: Addressing cultural responsiveness and social justice. *Journal for Specialists in Group Work, 35*(3), 271–280.

Ibrahim, F. A., & Dykeman, C. (2011). Muslim-Americans: Cultural and spiritual assessment for counseling. *Journal of Counseling and Development, 89*, 387–396.

Ibrahim, F. A., & Heuer, J. R. (2013). The assessment, diagnosis, and treatment of mental disorders among Muslims. In F. A. Paniagua & A. M. Yamada (Eds.), *Handbook of multicultural mental health* (2nd ed., pp. 367–387). New York: Academic Press.

Ibrahim, F. A., & Ohnishi, H. (2001). Posttraumatic stress disorder and the minority experience. In D. R. Pope-Davis & H. L. K. Coleman (Eds.), *The intersection of race, class, and gender in multicultural counseling* (pp. 89–119). Thousand Oaks, CA: Sage.

Institute of Medicine. (2011). *The health of lesbian, gay, bisexual and trangendered people: Building a foundation for better understanding*. Washington, DC: The National Academies Press.

Israel, T. (2012). 2011 society of counseling psychology presidential address: Exploring privilege in counseling psychology: Shifting the lens. *The Counseling Psychologist, 40*(1), 158–180. doi:10.1177/0011000011426297.

Israel, T., Gorcheva, R., Walther, W. A., Sulzner, J. S., & Cohen, J. (2008). Therapists' helpful and unhelpful situations with LGBT clients: An exploratory study. *Professional Psychology: Research and Practice, 39*, 361–368.

Ivey, A. E., D'Andrea, M., & Ivey, M. B. (2011). *Theories of counseling and psychotherapy: A multicultural perspective* (7th ed.). Thousand Oaks, CA: Sage.

Ivey, A. E., Ivey, M. B., Myers, J. E., & Sweeney, T. J. (2004). *Developmental counseling and therapy: Promoting wellness over the lifespan*. New York: Houghton Mifflin.
Ivey, D. C., Wieling, E., & Harris, S. M. (2000). Save the young-the elderly have lived their lives: Ageism in marriage and family therapy. *Family Process, 39*(2), 163–175.
Jackson, S. (2006). Sons of which soil? The language and politics of autochthony in Eastern D.R. Congo. *African Studies Review, 49*, 95–124. doi:10.1353/arw.2006.0107.
Jun, H. (2010). *Social justice, multicultural counseling, and practice: Beyond a conventional approach*. Thousand Oaks, CA: Sage.
Kessler, R. C., Sonnega, A., Bromet, E., Hughes, M., & Nelson, C. B. (1995). Posttraumatic stress disorder in the national comorbidity survey. *Archives of General Psychiatry, 52*, 1048–1060.
Kim, S., & Cardemil, E. (2012). Effective psychotherapy with low-income clients: The importance of attending to social class. *Journal of Contemporary Psychotherapy, 42*, 27–35.
Kite, M. E., Deaux, K., & Haines, E. (2008). Gender stereotypes. In F. Denmark & M. Paludi (Eds.), *Handbook on the psychology of women* (2nd ed., pp. 205–236). Westport, CT: Greenwood Press.
Klein, F. (1990). The need to view sexual orientation as multivariable dynamic process: A theoretical perspective. In D. P. McWhirter, S. A. Sanders, & J. M. Reinisch (Eds.), *Homosexuality/heterosexuality: Concepts of sexual orientation*. New York: Oxford University Press.
Klein, F. (1993). *The bisexual option* (2nd ed.). New York: Haworth Press.
Knapp, S., Lemoncelli, J., & VandeCreek, L. (2010). Ethical responses when patient's religious beliefs appear to harm their wellbeing. *Professional Psychology: Research and Practice, 41*(5), 405–412.
Krizman, J., Marian, V., Shook, A., Skoe, E., & Kraus, N. (2012). Subcortical encoding of sound is enhanced in bilinguals and relates to executive function advantages. *Proceedings of the National Academy of Sciences of the United States of America, 109*(20), 7877–7881.
Kunstler, J. H. (1993). *The geography of nowhere: The rise and decline of America's man-made landscape*. New York: Simon & Schuster.
Landrine, H., & Klonoff, E. A. (2002). *African American acculturation: Deconstructing race and reviving culture*. Thousand Oaks, CA: Sage.
Landrine, H., & Klonoff, E. A. (2004). Culture change and ethnic-minority health behavior: An operant theory of acculturation. *Journal of Behavioral Medicine, 27*(6), 527–555.
Lansford, J. E., Ceballo, R., Abbey, A., & Stewart, A. J. (2001). Does family structure matter? A comparison of adoptive, two-parent biological, single-mother, stepfather, and stepmother households. *Journal of Marriage and Family, 63*, 840–851.
LaTorre, R. A. (1976). The psychological assessment of gender identity and gender role in Schizophrenia. *Schizophrenia Bulletin, 2*(2), 266–285.
Le, H.-N., Zmuda, J., Perry, D. F., & Munoz, R. F. (2010). Transforming an evidence-based intervention to prevent perinatal depression for low-income Latina immigrants. *American Journal of Orthopsychiatry, 80*(1), 35–45. doi:10.1111/j.1939-0025.2010.01005.x.
Leong, F. T. L., Leach, M. M., & Malikiosi-Loizos, M. (2012). Internationalizing the field of counseling psychology. In F. T. L. Leong, W. E. Pickren, M. M. Leach, & J. Marsella (Eds.), *Internationalizing the psychology curriculum in the United States*. New York: Springer.
Levy, L. B., & O'Hara, M. W. (2010). Psychotherapeutic interventions for depressed, low-income women: A review of the literature. *Clinical Psychology Review, 30*, 934.
Lipton, G., Arends, M., Bastian, K., Wright, B., & O'Hara, P. (2002). The psychosocial consequences experienced by interpreters in relation to working with torture and trauma clients: A West Australian pilot study. *Synergy, 3–7*, 14–17.
Liu, W. M. (2001). Expanding our understanding of multiculturalism: Developing a social class worldview model. In D. B. Pope-Davis & H. L. K. Coleman (Eds.), *The intersection of race, class, and gender in counseling psychology* (pp. 127–170). Thousand Oaks, CA: Sage.
Liu, W. M. (2002). The social class-related experiences of men: Integrating theory with practice. *Professional Psychology: Research and Practice, 33*, 355–360.

Liu, W. M., Alt, M. C., & Pittinger, R. F. (2013). The role of social class worldview model in assessment, diagnosis, and treatment of mental and physical health. In F. A. Paniagua & A.-M. Yamada (Eds.), *Handbook of multicultural mental health* (2nd ed., pp. 111–125). Amsterdam: Academic.

Liu, W. M., Soleck, G., Hopps, J., Dunston, K., & Pickett, T., Jr. (2004). A new framework to understand social class in counseling: The social class worldview model and modern classism theory. *Journal of Multicultural Counseling and Development, 32*(2), 95–122. doi:10.1002/j.2161-1912.2004.tb00364.x.

Logan, J. R. (1996). Rural America as a symbol of American values. *Rural Development Perspectives, 12*, 19–21.

Long, J. C., & Kittles, R. A. (2003). Human genetic diversity and the nonexistence of biological races. *Human Biology, 75*, 449–471.

Lövheim, M. (2011). Mediatisation of religion: A critical appraisal. *Culture and Religion, 12*(2), 153–166.

Lövheim, M. (2012). Religious socialization in a media age. *Nordic Journal of Religion and Society, 25*(2), 151–168.

Luk, G., Bialystok, E., Craik, F. I., & Grady, C. L. (2011). Lifelong bilingualism maintains white matter integrity in older adults. *Journal of Neuroscience, 31*(46), 16808–16813.

MacTavish, K., & Salamon, S. (2003). What do rural families look like today? In D. L. Brown & L. E. Swanson (Eds.), *Challenges for rural America in the twenty-first century* (pp. 73–85). University Park, PA: Pennsylvania State University Press.

Manalansan, M. (1993). (Re)locating the gay Filipino: Resistance, postcolonialism, and identity. *Journal of Homosexuality, 26*(2/3), 53–73.

Martin, T. F., White, J. M., & Perlman, D. (2003). Religious socialization: A test of the channeling hypothesis of parental influence on adolescent faith maturity. *Journal of Adolescent Research, 18*(2), 169–187. doi:10.1177/0743558402250349.

McDowell, T., & Jeris, L. (2004). Talking about race using critical race theory: Recent trends in the journal of marital and family therapy. *Journal of Marital and Family Therapy, 30*, 81–94. doi:10.1111/j.1752-0606.2004.tb01224.x.

McGoldrick, M. (2005). Overview: Ethnicity and family therapy. In M. McGoldrick, J. Giordano, & N. Garcia-Preto (Eds.), *Ethnicity and family therapy* (3rd ed., pp. 1–43). New York: Guilford Press.

McGoldrick, M., Giordano, J., & Garcia-Preto, N. (2005). *Ethnicity and family therapy* (3rd ed.). New York: Guilford Press.

McNamee, S., & Gergen, K. (Eds.). (1992). *Therapy as social construction*. London: Sage.

Mechelli, A., Crinion, J. T., Noppeney, U., O'Doherty, J., Ashburner, J., Frackowiak, R. S., et al. (2004). Neurolinguistics: Structural plasticity in the bilingual brain. *Nature, 431*(7010), 757.

Miranda, J., Bernal, B., Lau, A., Kohn, L., Hwang, W., & LaFromboise, T. (2005). State of the science on psychosocial interventions for ethnic minorities. *Annual Review of Clinical Psychology, 1*, 113–142.

Mizock, L., & Fleming, M. Z. (2011). Transgender and gender variant populations with mental illness: Implications for clinical care. *Professional Psychology: Research and Practice, 42*(2), 208–213. doi:10.1037/a0022522.

Mizock, L., & Lewis, T. K. (2008). Trauma in transgender populations: Risk, resilience, and clinical care. *Journal of Emotional Abuse, 8*, 335–354.

Mohr, W. K. (2006). Spiritual issues in psychiatric care. *Perspectives in Psychiatric Care, 42*(3), 174–183.

Money, J. (1973). Gender role, gender identity, core gender identity: Usage and definition of terms. *Journal of the American Academy of Psychoanalysis, 1*, 397–403.

Mortimer, J. A., Alladi, S., Bak, T. H., Russ, T. C., Shailaja, M., & Duggirala, V. (2014). Bilingualism delays age of onset of dementia, independent of education and immigration status. *Neurology, 82*(21), 1936. doi:10.1212/WNL.0000000000000400.

National Association of Social Workers (NASW). (2008). *Code of ethics*. Washington, DC: National Association of Social Workers.

National Center for Transgender Equality (NCTE). (2012). *Health care rights and transgendered people*. Washington, DC: NCTE.
National Center for Transgender Equality (NCTE) and National Gay and Lesbian Task Force. (2011). *Injustice at every turn: A report of the national transgender discrimination survey, executive summary*. Washington, DC: NCTE.
Nelson, T. D. (2005). Ageism: Prejudice against our feared future self. *Journal of Social Issues, 61*(2), 207–221.
Ohnishi, H., Ibrahim, F. A., & Gzregorek, J. L. (2006). Intersection of identities: Counseling LGBT Asian Americans. *Journal of LGBT Counseling, I*(3), 77–94.
Oliver, J. E. (1999). The effects of metropolitan economic segregation on local civic participation. *American Journal of Political Science, 43*, 186–212.
Olkin, R. (1999). *What psychotherapists should know about disability*. New York: Guilford Press.
Olkin, R. (2002). Could you hold the door for me? Including disability in diversity. *Cultural Diversity and Ethnic Minority Psychology, 8*, 130–137. doi:10.1037/1099-9809.8.2.130.
Olkin, R. (2008). Disability-affirmative therapy and case formulation: A template for understanding disability in a clinical context. *Counseling & Human Development, 39*, 1–20.
Olkin, R., & Pledger, C. (2003). Can disability studies and psychology join hands? *American Psychologist, 58*, 296–304. doi:10.1037/0003-066X.58.4.296.
Olson, D. H., & Gorall, D. M. (2003). Circumplex model of marital and family systems. In F. Walsh (Ed.), *Normal family processes* (3rd ed., pp. 514–547). New York: Guilford Press.
Organista, P. B., Marin, G., & Chun, K. M. (2009). *The psychology of ethnic groups in the United States*. Thousand Oaks, CA: Sage.
Organista, K. C., Munoz, R. F., & Gonzalez, G. (1994). Cognitive behavioral therapy for depression in low-income and minority medical outpatients: Description of a program and exploratory analyses. *Cognitive Therapy and Research, 18*, 241–259.
Pascoe, E. A., & Smart Richman, L. (2009). Perceived discrimination and health: A meta-analytic review. *Psychological Bulletin, 135*(4), 531–554. doi:10.1037/a0016059.
Pasupathi, M., & Lockenhoff, C. (2002). Ageist behavior. In T. D. Nelson (Ed.), *Ageism: Stereotyping and prejudice against older persons* (pp. 201–246). Cambridge, MA: MIT Press.
Paul, R. A. (2014). The study of gender. *Encyclopedia Britannica*. http://www.britannica.com/EBchecked/topic/27505/anthropology/23685
Petchesky, R. P. (2000). Sexual rights: Inventing a concept, mapping an international practice. In R. Parker, R. M. Barbosa, & P. Aggleton (Eds.), *Framing the sexual subject: The politics of gender, sexuality, and power* (pp. 81–103). Berkeley, CA: University of California Press.
Pettersson, P. (2006). Religious belonging and life rites without confession and regular practice. In H.-G. Zeibert & W. K. Kay (Eds.), *Youth in Europe II: An international empirical study about religiosity* (pp. 139–158). Münster, Germany: LIT.
Pew Forum on Religion and Public Life. (2008, February). *U.S. Religious landscape survey*. Retrieved from http://religionspewforum.org/pdf/report-religious-landscape-study-full.pdf
Phemister, A. A. (2001). Revisiting the principles of free will and determinism: Exploring conceptions of disability and counseling theory. *Journal of Rehabilitation, 67*, 5–12.
Phinney, J. S. (1990). Ethnic identity in adolescents and adults: Review of research. *Psychological Bulletin, 10*(3), 499–514.
Phinney, J. S., & Ong, A. D. (2007). Conceptualization and measurement of ethnic identity: Current status and future directions. *Journal of Counseling Psychology, 54*(3), 271–281. doi:10.1037/0022-0167.54.3.271.
Pipher, M. B. (1995). *Reviving Ophelia: Saving the selves of adolescent girls*. New York: Ballantine.
Portes, A., & Rumbaut, R. G. (2006). *Immigrant America: A portrait*. Berkeley, CA: University of California Press.
Portes, A., & Zhou, M. (1993). The new second generation: Segmented assimilation and its variants. *The Annals of the American Academy of Political and Social Science, 530*, 74–96.
Putnam, R. (2000). *Bowling alone: The collapse and revival of American community*. New York: Simon & Schuster.

Putsch, R. (1985). Cross-cultural communication. The special case of interpreters in health care. *Journal of the American Medical Association, 254*(23), 3344–3348.
Rajeski, W. J., & Focht, B. C. (2002). Aging and physical disability: On integrating group and individual counseling with promotion of physical activity. *Exercise and Sport Sciences Reviews, 30*(4), 166–170.
Resnick, H. S., Kilpatrick, D. G., Dansky, B. S., Saunders, B. E., & Best, C. L. (1993). Prevalence of civilian trauma and posttraumatic stress disorder in a representative national sample of women. *Journal of Consulting and Clinical Psychology, 61*, 984–991.
Reyes Cruz, M., & Sonn, C. C. (2015). (De)colonizing culture in community psychology: Reflections from critical social science. In R. D. Goodman & P. C. Gorski (Eds.), *Decolonizing "multicultural" counseling through social justice* (pp. 127–146). New York: Springer.
Reyes-Ortiz, C. (1997). Physicians must confront ageism. *Academic Medicine, 72*(10), 831.
Rogers-Sirin, L., Ryce, P., & Sirin, S. R. (2014). Acculturation, acculturative stress, ad cultural mismatch and their influences on immigrant children and adolescents' wellbeing. In R. Dimitrova, M. Bender, & F. Van de Vijver (Eds.), *Global perspectives on wellbeing in immigrant families* (pp. 11–30). New York: Springer Science+Business Media.
Root, M. P. P. (2000). Rethinking racial identity development. In P. Spickard & W. J. Burroughs (Eds.), *We are a people: Narrative and multiplicity in constructing ethnic identity* (pp. 206–220). Philadelphia, PA: Temple University Press.
Rose-Innes, O. (2006, October). Sociocultural aspects of AIDS. Health24. Retrieved from http://www.health24.com/Medical/HIV-AIDS/The-South-African-culture/Sociocultural-aspects-of-HIVAIDS-20120721.
Rosen, E. J., & Weltman, S. F. (2005). Jewish families: An overview. In M. McGoldrick, J. Pearce, & N. Garcia-Preto (Eds.), *Ethnicity and family therapy* (3rd ed., pp. 667–679). New York: Guilford Press.
Rosenblatt, P. C., & Skoogberg, E. L. (1974). Birth order in cross-cultural perspective. *Developmental Psychology, 10*(1), 48–54.
Rosigno, V. J., Mong, S., & Tester, G. (2007). Age discrimination, social closure and employment. *Social Forces, 86*(1), 313–334. doi:10.1353/sof.2007.0109.
Rudmin, F. W. (2003). Critical history of the acculturation psychology of assimilation, separation, integration, and marginalization. *Review of General Psychology, 7*, 3–37.
Russell, G. M., & Horne, S. G. (2009). Finding equilibrium: Mentoring, sexual orientation, and gender identity. *Professional Psychology: Research and Practice, 40*, 194–200.
Sam, D. L., & Berry, J. W. (2010). Acculturation: When individuals and groups of different cultural backgrounds meet. *Perspectives on Psychological Science, 5*(4), 472–481.
Sargent, C. F., & Brettell, C. (Eds.). (1996). *Gender and health: An international perspective.* Upper Saddle River, NJ: Prentice Hall.
Savin-Williams, R. C. (1988). Theoretical perspectives accounting for adolescent homosexuality. *Journal of Adolescent Health, 9*(6), 95–104.
Savin-Williams, R. C. (1990). Gay and lesbian adolescents. *Marriage and Family Review, 14*, 197–216.
Sears, J. (1989). The impact of gender and race on growing up lesbian and gay in the South. *National Women's Studies Association Journal, 1*, 422–457.
Shin, R. Q. (2015). The application of critical consciousness and intersectionality as tools for decolonizing racial/ethnic identity development models in the fields of counseling psychology. In R. D. Goodman & P. C. Gorski (Eds.), *Decolonizing "multicultural" counseling through social justice* (pp. 11–22). New York: Springer.
Shubert, D., & Miller, S. I. (1978). Social class and psychiatric diagnosis: Differential findings in lower-class sample. *International Journal of Social Psychiatry, 24*, 117–124.
Siegel, N. H., Kahn, R. L., Pollack, M., & Fink, M. (1962). Social class, diagnosis, and treatment in three psychiatric hospitals. *Social Problems, 10*, 191–196.
Smith, J. M. (2000). Psychotherapy with people stressed by poverty. In A. N. Sabo & L. Havens (Eds.), *The real world guide to psychotherapy practice* (pp. 71–92). Cambridge: Harvard University Press.

Smith, L. (2005). Psychotherapy, classism and the poor: Conspicuous by their absence. *American Psychologist, 60*, 687–696.
Smith, L. (2009). Enhancing training and practice in the context of poverty. *Training and Education in Professional Psychology, 3*, 84–93.
Smith, L. C. (2015). Queering multicultural competence in counseling. In R. D. Goodman & P. C. Gorski (Eds.), *Decolonizing "multicultural" counseling through social justice* (pp. 23–40). New York: Springer.
Smith, L., & Chambers, C. (2015). Decolonizing psychological practice in the context of poverty. In R. D. Goodman & P. C. Gorski (Eds.), *Decolonizing "multicultural" counseling through social justice* (pp. 73–84). New York: Springer.
Snowden, L., & Yamada, A. M. (2005). Cultural differences in access to care. *Annual Review of Clinical Psychology, 1*, 143–166.
Snyder, M., & Miene, P. K. (1994). Stereotyping of the elderly: A functional approach. *British Journal of Social Psychology, 33*, 63–82. doi:10.1111/j2044-8309.1994.tbo01011.x.
Spencer, M. B., Dupree, D., & Hartmann, T. (1997). A phenomenological variant of ecological systems theory (PVEST): A self-organization perspective in context. *Development and Psychopathology, 9*, 817–833. doi:10.1017/S0954579497001454.
Stewart, A. E. (2012). Issues in birth order research methodology: Perspectives from individual psychology. *The Journal of Individual Psychology, 68*(1), 75–106.
Stewart, A. J., & McDermott, C. (2004). Gender in psychology. *Annual Review of Psychology, 55*, 519–544.
Strife, S., & Downey, L. (2009). Childhood development and access to nature: A new direction for environmental inequality. *Organization & Environment, 22*(1), 99–122. doi:10.1177/1086026609333340.
Stryker, S. (1987). Identity theory: Developments and extensions. In K. Yardley & T. Honess (Eds.), *Self and identity* (pp. 89–104). New York: Wiley.
Suarez, R. (1999). *The old neighborhood: What we lost in the great suburban migration, 1966-1999.* New York: Free Press.
Sue, D. W., & Sue, D. (2013). *Counseling the culturally diverse: Theory and practice* (6th ed.). New York: Wiley.
Sue, S., & Zane, N. (1987). The role of culture and cultural techniques in psychotherapy: A critique and reformulation. *American Psychologist, 42*, 37–45.
Takaki, R. (1979). *Iron cages*. New York: Oxford University Press.
Takaki, R. T. (2000). *Iron cages: Race and culture in 19th-century America.* Oxford, England: Oxford University Press.
Taylor, R. J., Chatters, L. M., & Jackson, J. S. (2007). Religious and spiritual involvement among older African Americans, Caribbean Blacks, and non-Hispanic Whites: Findings from the National Survey of American Life. *Journal of Gerontology, 62B*(4), S238–S250.
Thomas, D. E., Townsend, T. G., & Belgrave, F. Z. (2003). The influence of cultural and racial identification on the psychosocial adjustment of inner-city African American children in school. *American Journal of Community Psychology, 32*, 217–228. doi:10.1023/B:AJCP.0000004743.37592.26.
Thompson, V. L. S., Noel, J. G., & Campbell, J. (2004). Stigma, discrimination, and mental health. *American Journal of Orthopsychiatry, 74*(4), 529–544.
Todd, N. R., & Abrams, E. A. (2011). White dialectics: A new framework for theory, research, and practice with White students. *The Counseling Psychologist, 39*(3), 353–395. doi:10.1177/0011000010377665.
Tribe, R., & Lane, P. (2009). Working with interpreters across language and culture in mental health. *Journal of Mental Health, 18*(3), 233–241.
Troiden, R. R. (1979). Becoming homosexual: A model of gay identity acquisition. *Psychiatry, 42*, 362–373.
Troiden, R. R. (1988). Homosexual identity development. *Journal of Adolescent Health Care, 9*, 105–113.

Umaña-Taylor, A. J. (2011). Ethnic identity. In S. J. Schwartz, K. Luyckx, & V. L. Vignoles (Eds.), *Handbook of identity theory and research* (pp. 791–801). New York: Springer. doi:10.1007/978-1-4419-7988- 9-33.

US Department of Health and Human Services. (2001). *Mental health: Culture, race, and ethnicity—A supplement to mental health: A report of the surgeon general*. Rockville, MD: Author. Retrieved September 26, 2004, from http://media.shs.net/ken/pdf/SMA-01-3613/sma-01-3613.

US Department of Health and Human Services (HHS.give/HealthCare). (2010). *Affordable care act*. Washington, DC: HHS.gove/HealthCare. Retrieved from http://www.hhs.gov/healthcare/rights/index.html.

Vandewater, E. A., & Lansford, J. E. (1998). Influences of family structure and parental conflict on children's well-being. *Family Relations, 47*, 323–330.

Verkuyten, M. (1998). Perceived discrimination and self-esteem among ethnic minority adolescents. *Journal of Social Psychology, 138*, 479–493.

Verkuyten, M. (2005). *The social psychology of ethnic identity*. New York: Routledge.

Weber, M. (1968). Basic sociological terms. In G. Roth & C. Wittich (Eds.), *Economy and society* (pp. 3–62). Berkeley, CA: University of California Press.

Westermeyer, J. (1989). *Psychiatric care of migrants: A clinical guide*. Washington, DC: American Psychiatric Press.

Whitman-Raymond, L. M. (2009). The influence of class in the therapeutic dyad. *Contemporary Psychoanalysis, 45*(4), 429–433.

Williams, P. W. (2012). Age discrimination in the delivery of health care services to our elders. *Marquette Elder's Advisor, 11*(1), 1–46. Article 3.

Williams, J. E., & Best, D. L. (1990). *Sex and psyche: Gender and self-concepts viewed cross-culturally*. Newbury Park, CA: Sage.

Wilson, A. (1996). How we find ourselves: Identity development in two-spirit people. *Harvard Educational Review, 66*(2), 303–317.

Xavier, J. M., Hitchcock, D., Hollinshead, S., Keisling, M., Lewis, Y., & Lombardi, E., et al. (2004). *An overview of U.S. trans health priorities: A report by the Eliminating Disparities Working Group*. Retrieved May 10, 2010, from http://www.lgbthealth.net, (http://en.wikibooks.org).

Yang, R. K., & Fetsch, R. J. (2007). The self-esteem of rural children. *Journal of Research in Rural Education, 22*(5). Retrieved July 3, 2014, from http://jrre.psu.edu/articles/22-5.pdf.

Zajonc, R. B., & Sulloway, F. J. (2007). The confluence model: Birth order as a within-family or between-family dynamic. *Personality and Social Psychology Bulletin, 33*(9), 1187–1194.

Chapter 3
Worldview: Implications for Culturally Responsive and Ethical Practice

This chapter focuses on the concept of worldview, the current research and available information on worldview. Originally, my research on cultural competence in counseling and psychotherapy focused on the concept of worldview. This was considered a key variable in working across cultures, and understanding the client's world and experiences (Ibrahim, 1984). After developing the Scale to Assess World View© (SAWV; Ibrahim & Kahn, 1984, 1987), and using the SAWV in training, the feedback I received convinced me that core values and assumptions are one element that helps us understand our clients, but we had to go beyond worldview to comprehend the client's identity and world. This section will focus on understanding the concept of worldview, and how to use it in counseling and psychotherapy.

Worldview Defined

Worldview pertains to the lenses we wear to see the world (Ivey, Ivey, & Simek-Morgan, 1997). The concept of worldview is explained as "mental lenses that are entrenched ways of perceiving the world" (Olsen, Lodwick, & Dunlap, 1992, p. 4). The term worldview is derived from the German word "Weltanschauung," and indicates a view of the world, or a person's total outlook on life, social world, and institutions (Wolman, 1973). It represents beliefs, values, and assumptions about people, relationships, nature, time, and activity (Ibrahim & Kahn, 1987; Ibrahim & Owen, 1994). Worldview refers to core values, beliefs, and assumptions that govern decision-making and problem solving in everyday life; it is derived from one's primary culture, and the socialization process that a person undergoes from childhood to adulthood (Hart, 2010; Ibrahim, 2003). It is mediated by the experiences that people have and it is modified as one confronts issues and challenges over the life-span. Worldview tends to be fairly constant over the life-span and the core values are sustained, unless there is dramatic life changing events, such as a near death

F.A. Ibrahim, J.R. Heuer, *Cultural and Social Justice Counseling*,
International and Cultural Psychology, DOI 10.1007/978-3-319-18057-1_3

experiences (Furn, 1987). Every individual has an ethnic-cultural background, and this plays a significant role in shaping a person's worldview, especially a strong influence on core values from the socialization process (McGoldrick, 2005). Along with variability of worldviews within a society or culture, societies also have dominant and alternative worldviews (Cieciuch & Ibrahim, 2011; Ibrahim, Siquera de Frietas, & Owen, 1993; Kluckhohn, 1951; Olsen et al., 1992). Individuals with an alternative worldview from the mainstream, within a dominant society will have some dominant assumptions, exemplified by national, secular, or religious values, and values derived from their primary ethnic-cultural socialization, along with assumptions held in communities they grow up in.

Hart (2010) notes that worldview is a cognitive, perceptual, and affective map that is used to understand and make sense of the social world, he agrees that it develops over the life-span, tends to be unconscious, and uncritically taken for granted to assume that this is the way things are, and rarely alters in any significant way. Although, he allows that change can happen. There can be incongruences in beliefs and values within a worldview. Koltko-Rivera (2004) defines worldview as a set of beliefs and assumptions that describe reality and encompasses a heterogeneous set of assumptions pertaining to human nature, nature of life, and the composition of the universe, to list a few. Koltko-Rivera (2004) notes that the concept of worldview has been described in several different ways, e.g., Jung refers to it as one's philosophy of life (1942/1954); Maslow (1987) speaks of a world outlook; and Kottler and Hazler (2001) refer to self-and world-construct systems. The term worldview has been used over time to describe how people perceive their world, culture, religion or spirituality, etc. It can be used to describe the behavior and attitudes of other cultures. It has also been conceptualized in many different ways given the perspective of the theorist or the researcher (Ibrahim, Roysircar-Sodowsky, & Ohnishi, 2001; Koltko-Rivera, 2004).

Several researchers have focused on core values to understand how people understand their world, behave, make decisions, and resolve conflicts in interpersonal relationships, in organizational settings, and in conflict between countries. The struggle to identify core values among cultures has historical significance, given the work of Kluckhohn (1951) in anthropology, Williams (1968) in sociology, and Rokeach (1973) in psychology. Originally, Kelly (1963) addressed the concept of worldview in psychology, specific to personality; he noted that people use certain constructs, which were personal to them, to understand and make meaning of their world. Cross-cultural and cross-national research was initiated by Hofstede (1980), followed by Schwartz and Bilsky (1987, 1990); they sought to identify a universal structure for understanding compatibility or conflict among values held by the cultures of the world, which would allow for comparison across cultures. Now we have access to universal aspects of value content and structure, and this has laid the foundations for investigating culture-specific aspects in research, and to conduct comparisons across cultures. Schwartz's empirically derived structure and content of values, and the common meaning within and among cultures correlate well with Kluckhohn's universal value orientations, the comparison is presented in Table 3.1

Table 3.1 Comparison of Kluckhohn's existential value orientations and Schwartz's empirically derived universal values

Kluckhohn	Schwartz
Human nature: Good	Equality; politeness; self-respect; reciprocation of favors; self-discipline; mature love; family security; true friendship; broadminded; humble; honest; obedient; responsible; forgiving; curious; self-discipline; helpful; healthy
Human nature: Bad	Social power; pleasure; an exciting life; wealth; detachment; social recognition; ambitious; authority; daring; choosing own goals; preserving public image
Human nature: Combination of good and bad	Equality; politeness; self-respect; reciprocation of favors; self-discipline; mature love; family security; true friendship; broadminded; humble; honest; obedient; responsible; forgiving; curious; social power; pleasure; an exciting life; wealth; detachment; social recognition; ambitious; authority; daring; choosing own goals; preserving public image
Social relationships: Lineal-hierarchical	Social power; social order; respect for tradition; self-discipline; family security; authority; loyal; honoring of parents and elders; preserving public image; responsible; helpful
Social relationships: Collateral-mutual	Equality; a sense of belonging; self-respect; reciprocation of favors; true friendship; moderation; broadminded; humble; helpful
Social relationships: Individualistic	Independent; enjoying life; seeking an exciting life; preserving public image; daring; ambitious; a varied life; social recognition; detachment; self-discipline
Nature: Harmony	Unity with nature; a world of beauty; protecting the environment; curious
Nature: Control of nature	Social power; pleasure
Nature: Accept the power of nature	Humble; accepting life and the natural order; inner harmony
Time: Past	Honoring parents and elders; wisdom; respect for tradition
Time: Present	Enjoying life; seeking adventure and risk; family security; a world at peace; reciprocation of favors; pleasure; freedom; meaning in life; creativity
Time: Future	Devout; protecting the environment; a varied life; family security; social recognition; a mature love; national security; a spiritual life; social order; a world at peace
Activity: Being	Pleasure; an exciting life; creativity; daring; choosing own goals; accepting my portion in life; enjoying life; curious; forgiving; helpful; detached
Activity: Being in becoming	Inner harmony; a spiritual life; meaning in life; mature love; self-discipline; family security; a varied life; wisdom; true friendship; social justice; moderation; influential; loyal; broadminded; humble; choosing own goals; capable; devout; curious; responsible; helpful; creativity
Activity: Doing	Wealth; self-discipline; social recognition; independent; ambitious; daring; influential; capable; preserving public image; responsible; successful

Worldview and Counseling

Grieger and Ponterotto (1995) note that worldview is one of the most popular constructs in the multicultural counseling literature. Understanding core values and beliefs in the counseling process reduces the chance of oppressing the client by imposing therapist values and assumptions, which is considered cultural malpractice (Dana, 1998). Ibrahim and Arredondo (1986) note clarifying client and counselor core assumptions is critical to meaningful and positive outcomes in counseling and psychotherapy. Considering the hierarchies and the diversity that exists in the US population, and internationally, there are very few cultures that have completely monolithic cultural assumptions. Worldview as a concept has existed in several disciplines as a construct to understand how people understand their world, people, individuals, or cultures.

Although in conducting psychotherapy, guidelines for developing a therapeutic relationship are primarily effective for mainstream US (White Anglo Saxon middle class) populations. These guidelines have encountered difficulties in helping the culturally different (Seligman, 1995; Smith, Glass, & Miller, 1980; Wampold, 2001). To engage in a therapeutic relationship with culturally different clients, Sue (1978) proposed that understanding client worldview is most helpful. Sue used two psychological theoretical frames to understand the client's worldview, i.e., Locus of Control (Rotter, 1966) and Locus of Responsibility (Kanouse, Kelley, Nisbett, Valins, & Weiner, 1972). Locus of control and responsibility help identify whether a person has an individualistic or a collectivistic perspective, and can help identify a person's cultural orientation. Although an assessment measure exists for Locus of Control (Rotter), there is no measure for locus of responsibility. This conceptualization is left much to the counselor's discretion in terms of identifying cultural perspectives of clients. Sue also recommended that understanding the client's sociopolitical history and how it has affected the client was important. We recommend a comprehensive cultural assessment, which includes an assessment of worldview to prevent the possibility of bias that can function unconsciously in cross-cultural, or multicultural encounters. Further, to reduce the possibility of cultural bias, it is critical to involve the client in the process, and explain how the assessments will help provide information for counseling and psychotherapy, i.e., information that would make the counseling process client-specific.

Worldview needs be understood within the cultural identity of the client, to understand the mediating variables that have created the perspectives that a person holds, which may become facilitating or negating factors in the therapeutic process. Understanding cultural identity means acknowledging all the multifaceted dimensions of identity (all the variables identified in the Cultural Identity Check List-Revised© (CICL-R; Ibrahim, 2008)), and including areas of privilege, oppression, and acculturation level. Core beliefs and values have a significant place in the counseling and psychotherapy process; these are linked to the central components of one's identity, and the decisions that are being made in counseling must be consistent with the values and assumptions of the client to be meaningful (Ibrahim, 2010, 2011).

The concept of worldview as it is used in this text was conceptualized from the perspective of beliefs, values, and assumptions that are derived from a cultural context and was based within an existential values model (Kluckhohn, 1951, 1956; Kluckhohn & Strodtbeck, 1961). Kluckhohn proposed a model of universal existential values that are relevant to all cultural contexts; however, the emphasis within each culture varies (Table 3.1). Ibrahim, in collaboration with Kahn, developed the Scale to Assess Worldview© (SAWV; Appendix B; Ibrahim & Kahn, 1984, 1987) to provide a measure to assess worldview, i.e., beliefs, values, and assumptions, in an effort to operationally assess worldview in cross-cultural, and multicultural counseling and psychotherapy. This effort resulted in creating increased specificity in counseling and psychotherapy (Cunningham-Warburton, 1988; Sadlak, 1986). Cultural responsiveness and sensitivity to client assumptions requires cultural assessments, instead of relying only on information about the client's cultural group's assumptions, which is general information about a cultural group, and may not accurately describe a specific client's worldview.

In using the SAWV, core beliefs, values and assumptions can be assessed for an individual, a family, a social group, a nation, or society. Dana (1998) notes that the concept of worldview includes group identity, individual identity or self-concept, values, beliefs, and language. Knowledge of client worldview can facilitate both the therapeutic relationship and the delivery of counseling services. We believe mental health professionals convey respect and acceptance for the client's perspectives by accepting their cultural identity and worldview. Both Dana (1998) and Ibrahim (1999) note that cultural identity, and worldview provide a blueprint for understanding the client's core assumptions in cross-cultural therapeutic encounters. However, these two variables provide a partial window into the client's world given that cultural identity until recently was considered a univariate construct. Cultural identity is multidimensional; it includes the intersection of ethnicity, culture, gender, sexual orientation, client's experiences, and other socializing agents that mediate worldview.

Multicultural competencies (American Counseling Association (ACA), 1992; Association for Multicultural Counseling and Development (AMCD), 1992; Ibrahim & Arredondo, 1986) emphasize that helping professionals must clarify their own cultural identity, and worldview to avoid imposing their own values, beliefs, and assumptions on clients. Effective multicultural training incorporates assessment and understanding of both client and counselor worldviews. Although many theorists and researchers use the term worldview to understand between-group and within-group worldview differences, they may or may not agree on what it means to them (Claiborn, 1986; Fisher, Jome, & Atkinson, 1998; Ibrahim, 1985; Ibrahim et al., 2001).

The concept of worldview focusing on values, beliefs, and assumptions is important in understanding the client's cultural perspectives (Ibrahim, 1985). Although this was a significant movement forward toward specificity in therapeutic encounters, it was not enough. Over the last 30 years it has become apparent that core values do not provide all the information that is needed to understand a client, because cultural identities are mediated by several variables, these include ethnicity, gender, sexual orientation, socialization process, religion/spirituality, privilege, oppression, and acculturation (Ibrahim, 2007, 2008, 2011). These variables help us clarify the client's identity development over the life-span, and assumptions critically important to the client that need to be considered when setting goals and seeking outcomes that are consistent with the client's socialization.

Conducting Worldview Assessment

Worldview assessment using the SAWV can be conducted face-to-face, in groups, online, or using an interview format for individuals who are not comfortable with paper-pencil instruments. The scale originally had 45 items, after empirical testing, the items that had adequate reliability and validity were retained based on a factor analysis (Ibrahim & Owen, 1994). The current scale has 30 items, and provides four distinct worldviews. These were named *Optimistic*, *Traditional*, *Here-and-Now*, and *Pessimistic*. The hypothesis that all people have a primary and a secondary worldview was retained from Kluckhohn's (1951) theoretical proposition. The two highest scores obtained reflect the worldview held by an individual. The worldview with the highest score is the primary worldview, and the worldview with second highest score represents the secondary worldview. According to Kluckhohn's theory, individuals use the primary worldview to understand their world, make decisions, and solve problems. However, when they cannot explain a phenomenon, or are struggling with a decision, they tend to fall back on their secondary worldview.

Research on the SAWV shows that most cultures have a dominant value system and a secondary value system (Ibrahim, Roysircar-Sodowsky, & Ohnishi, 2001). With the US sample, the primary worldview is *Optimistic*, and considering the values inherent in this worldview, it is consistent with cultural assumptions that are institutionalized through the educational system, and these assumptions are an important part of the socialization process, and homogenization of cultural assumptions in the USA (Takaki, 1979). Table 3.2 identifies the values inherent in each worldview.

Table 3.2 Four worldviews derived for the US sample (Ibrahim & Owen, 1994)

Optimistic	Traditional	Here-and-now	Pessimistic
Human nature: Good	Time: Future orientation	Activity: Being	Human nature: Combination of good and bad
Activity: Being-in-becoming	Social relationships: Lineal-hierarchical	Time: Present orientation	Human nature: Bad
Activity: Being	Time: Past orientation	Time: Past orientation	Nature: Power of nature
Nature: Harmony with nature	Social relationships: Collateral-mutual		
Nature: Accept the power of nature	Human nature: Bad		
Activity: Doing	Nature: Control of nature		

Using Worldview Information in Counseling

The information gathered from understanding worldview can be very helpful in (a) establishing a positive therapeutic relationship and (b) in helping clients recognize and understand their values and assumptions, and keeping this information in the forefront as issues, concerns, and decisions are addressed in counseling, will help make counseling interventions client and context specific for an individual client. In addition, understanding the client's worldview and cultural identity will help in establishing a positive therapeutic relationship, and facilitate counseling interventions.

Establishing a Positive Therapeutic Relationship

Mental health professionals, who have objectively assessed their own worldview, will be able to recognize the similarities and differences between clients and themselves. Knowing the similarities helps in building a connection with clients; this helps in creating a *shared worldview* and increases trust for clients leading to a positive therapeutic relationship (Fisher et al., 1998; Ibrahim, 1985, 1993, 1999). Shared worldview in Ibrahim's conceptualization is derived from finding commonalities in values, sociopolitical history, acculturation level, privilege, and oppression (Ibrahim, 2011; Ibrahim & Heuer, 2013). A shared worldview helps in establishing similar understanding of the issues, and conditions that led to the presenting problem, further, it enhances trust, and hope, that a resolution is possible (Frank & Frank, 1991; Torrey, 1986). Recognizing value differences also facilitates the helping professional's ability to be careful, as these areas may lead to a lowering trust, and create stress for clients if the helping professional imposes her/his/zir assumptions on the client (Ibrahim, 1985, 1999). The goal of counseling and psychotherapy is to help the client find resolution within her/his/zir own value system and cultural identity, and for helpers to assist in the process without imposing their own cultural assumptions (Dana, 1998; Ibrahim & Arredondo, 1986).

Dana (1998) considers it cultural malpractice when therapists are unable to recognize that they are imposing their own assumptions and values on the client. We believe that such a scenario creates stress for the client, and it is the reason why clients who are culturally different from the therapists terminate by the third session (Sue & Zane, 1987; Sue, Zane, Nagayama Hall, & Berger, 2009). It is also important to attend to nonverbal behavior of the client, to recognize signs of discomfort, and to address the nonverbal communication by following up with an empathic query, e.g., "I sense something I said has made you uncomfortable, and I would like to know what you heard me say, in an effort to clarify my statement." Taking the lead to address client discomfort results in renewed trust by the client, and helps the therapist get a better perspective on what may be creating discomfort, or conflict for a client. Further, it reduces the chances of creating a rupture in the therapeutic relationship, which is highly likely in working across cultures and contexts (Gaztambide,

2012; Owen, Imel, Tao, Wampold, Smith, & Rodolfa, 2011). Understanding values and cultural identity is not enough, because the therapeutic environment also needs to be supportive and caring. If a client is distressed by a statement or believes that the therapist was not being supportive, or has misunderstood a comment, it is important to seek clarification, and follow-up with an apology, or a restatement that is more affirming to the client, and exploring the misunderstanding (Ivey, Pedersen, & Ivey, 2009). Professionals need to have courage and own their behavior to create a meaningful and supportive therapeutic relationship (Corey, Corey, Corey, & Callanan, 2014).

Knowledge of worldviews can assist in matching professionals with clients who may have similar worldviews. When client-counselor values are congruent, trust develops quickly and the therapeutic relationship is facilitated (Ibrahim, 1999; Tyler, Sussewell, & Williams-McCoy, 1985). The more the professional and client have in common the easier it is to work together. Beutler and Bergan (1991) note that research on value similarity, and counseling efficacy suggests two conclusions: (a) Value convergence between counselor-client beliefs, and attitudes is directly related to positive outcome in counseling and psychotherapy and (b) a "complex pattern of similarity and dissimilarity between client and counselor values is conducive to enhancing the strength of this convergence" (p. 18). This implies that, for a positive outcome in therapy, counselor and client cognitive and cultural schemas must have certain points of convergence. S. Sue (1988) supports cultural matching; which he believes is more relevant than ethnic matching. He notes that ethnic matching does not necessarily imply cultural similarity, because there are multiple factors mediating client worldviews. Previously, it was assumed that only helping professionals with similar cultural backgrounds could have a positive therapeutic relationship with clients. However, assuming that cultural similarity alone (such as culture, gender, and sexual orientation) will help in creating a strong therapeutic relationship has not proven to be an effective strategy, and research has not supported this assumption (Pedersen, Fukuyama, & Heath, 1989; Tyler et al., 1985).

Recommendations encouraging therapists to be culturally sensitive and to know the culture of the client have also not proven effective (Boysen & Vogel, 2008; Sue & Zane, 1987). In addition, when culture-specific techniques are applied across cultures, without attention to appropriateness of the techniques for a specific client, this poses a threat of cultural oppression (Dana, 1998; Ibrahim, 1993, 1999, 2003; Sadlak & Ibrahim, 1986). Educating counselors to assess and understand cultural assumptions of clients has shown promise in building the therapeutic relationship (Cunningham-Warburton, 1988; Sadlak & Ibrahim, 1986).

Stanley Sue (1988) notes that cultural factors in the treatment of nondominant ethnic clients have received the greatest attention among therapists, yet services for culturally different clients remain inadequate. The training protocols employed today were originally developed to provide services to the dominant cultural group (Beutler & Bergan, 1991; Nagayama Hall, Lopez, & Bansal, 2001; Sue, Zane, Nagayama Hall, & Berger, 2009). Although there are several recommendations to diversify training models, the problem of academic acculturation and its effect on what therapists actually believe or say when working with clients seems to differ

(Beck, Rush, Shaw, & Emery, 1979; Nagayama Hall et al., 2001). It is also important to recognize that although counselor and client worldviews appear similar, without consideration of oppression and exclusion, the implications for the client can be very different from the counselor. Characteristics, such as culture, gender, sexual orientation, religion, age, and disability, mediate worldviews, and result in integration or alienation from the cultural context. Within this context, it is important to recognize issues of privilege and oppression helps the professional in identifying challenges that the client faces, and design interventions to not only address the presenting problem, but also focus on empowerment on issues that pertain to racial, cultural, gender, age, sexual orientation, and disability status (Ibrahim, 2010; Ibrahim, Julie, Estrada, & Michael D'Andrea, 2011).

Using Worldview Information to Facilitate Counseling Interventions

The worldview profiles derived from the SAWV can be helpful in responding to client-specific values and in understanding the cultural values that are most meaningful to a client. This information helps the counseling process in both diagnosis and treatment planning. In arriving at a diagnosis, it is important to first conduct a cultural evaluation to identify the client's cultural context, assumptions, beliefs about the presenting problem and the possible resolutions (American Psychiatric Association, 2013; Castillo, 1977; Lonner & Ibrahim, 2008). Understanding core values and assumptions helps clarify the client's cultural identity. The USA is a highly diverse country with several ethnic and cultural groups, to complicate matters further, within and between the 21 White ethnic groups and the four identified nondominant cultural groups there is variability in values, beliefs, and assumption, mediated by social class, gender, age, sexual orientation, geographic location, religion/spirituality, educational level, and ability/disability status. When values information is viewed within the multidimensional intersections of an individual's identity, it creates specificity, and movement away from imposing cultural assumptions of the client's primary cultural group. The information about a cultural group is a general framework that identifies core cultural assumptions of a cultural group; however, without taking the client's specific cultural socialization, and the influence of various identity variables (such as gender and sexual orientation) it becomes cultural malpractice.

Values are at the core of cultural identity and how life experiences are understood and integrated into a person's ongoing reality, and the meditational forces of privilege and oppression result in creating either a commonality or distance from the primary cultural group, and clarifies the uniqueness of each individual cultural identity (Ibrahim, 2010). Clarification of worldview can make the counseling process meaningful to a client and ethical. Knowledge of worldview can assist in all phases of counseling and psychotherapy, from diagnosis to treatment planning and execution to evaluation of the intervention by keeping the whole process within the client's belief and value perspectives (Ibrahim, 1999, 2003). Understanding client worldview can facilitate counselor understanding of the presenting problem, and the reason why the presenting problem is causing distress (Diener, Shigehiro, & Lucas, 2003). All presenting problems may not have equal significance for helping professionals, as their perceptions of these issues are guided by their own cultural identity, worldview, acculturation, privilege, oppression, and life experiences. Having client cultural information eases the process of understanding client concerns and reduces the possibility of misunderstanding, ruptures in the therapeutic process, or misdiagnosing a client. Our proposition is that worldview interacts with all client variables and, consequently, must be central in understanding the presenting problem, and treatment interventions in multicultural and cross-cultural counseling.

Knowledge of worldview can be a critical facilitator of the common factors that are attributed to therapeutic success, primarily, therapist and relationship factors (Grencavage & Norcross, 1990; Imel & Wampold, 2008; Lambert & Barley, 2002). Garfield (1995) identified change factors that are common to all therapeutic approaches in producing positive change, which include (a) the therapeutic alliance, (b) interpretation, insight, and understanding, (c) cognitive modifications, (d) catharsis, emotional expression, and release, (e) reinforcement, (f) desensitization, (g) relaxation, (h) information, (i) reassurance and support, (j) expectancies, (k) exposure to and confronting of a problem situation, (l) time, and (m) the placebo response. We contend that without a therapeutic alliance and a perceived bond with the therapist, based on convergence of assumptions, and genuine acceptance using the skills of empathy, and cultural intentionality, other change factors would not follow (Ibrahim, 2003, 2010; Ibrahim & Heuer, 2013; Ivey, Normington, Miller, Morrill, & Haase, 1968). Having an understanding of the client's worldview, and conveying genuine acceptance would lead to a strong therapeutic alliance, create hope that resolution is possible, and lead to a positive outcome (Vajari & Ghaedi, 2011). Two research studies used the SAWV to educate the counselors about their own worldview and assessment of client worldviews, and using the information facilitated a therapeutic alliance with positive outcomes (Cunningham-Warburton, 1988; Sadlak, 1986).

The discussion on using the information gained from the SAWV in counseling interventions will be limited to the data derived from the US sample in this chapter. The SAWV identified four worldview profiles for the sample, and these were named: Optimistic, Traditional, Here-and-Now or Spontaneous, and Pessimistic (Ibrahim & Owen, 1994). These examples will help exemplify how worldview information in any context can be applied appropriately. The information gained can help in deciding on the process to use and the goals that would be most meaningful for the client in resolving the presenting problem (Fisher et al., 1998; Ibrahim, 1993, 1999, 2003). The process and goals need to be consistent with the client's cultural identity (as assessed by the CICL-R©), acculturation level, privilege, and oppression issues, along with other important dimensions, such as racial identity development level, for example. Values, although very important, alone cannot provide all the information needed to develop client-specific interventions (Ibrahim & Heuer, 2013). A discussion follows regarding each worldview, and implications for counseling and psychotherapy.

Optimistic Worldview

The items in this worldview are: Human nature is essentially good, activities that people engage in should empower them to grow spiritually, and should also provide for material needs. There is a desire to live in harmony with nature, and an acceptance of the power of nature. This is a balanced perspective on life, work, people, and nature. Values show how a person apprehends the world, and other people, and these values influence how the individual relates to people, life and work, and nature (Binswanger, 1962, 1963; Ibrahim, 2003).

The *Human Nature* value orientation ranges from people are basically good, to people are a combination of good and bad qualities, to people are basically bad. Each of these variations indicates how an individual would relate to other people in her or his world. In the Optimistic Worldview (OWV), the perception that people as essentially good indicates that the person enters counseling with a positive expectation, trusting that the therapist would know what needs to be done, and would be able to develop trust, because the person is entering counseling with positive assumptions about people.

The *Activity* value orientation varies from Being (a preference for spontaneous expression of the self) to Being-in-Becoming (an emphasis on development of all aspects of the self, as an integrated being, including the spiritual domain), to Doing (a preference for activities that result in measurable accomplishments by external standards). The two activity domains in the Optimistic Worldview emphasize the need for humans to seek meaning in their lives (Frankl, 1978; Hillman, 1997). Frankl identifies the midlife crisis as a crisis of meaning, coming to counseling indicates a similar crisis of meaning, where an individual who was managing her or his life, is overwhelmed by a dilemma, that has become unresolvable. Yalom (1980) supports this perspective, and notes that most clients are suffering from a lack of meaning in their lives; the therapist must function as a catalyst to help clients find meaning in their lives. Existential philosophy has traditionally addressed the issue of meaning of life, within the context of the finiteness of life, and the desire to answer the ultimate question, i.e., what is the meaning of life (Hillman, 1997; Ibrahim, 1984; Sartre, 1953).

The *Nature* dimension ranges from accepting the power of nature, living in harmony with nature, to controlling nature, these vary based on the cultural context (Kluckhohn, 1951). Binswanger (1962, 1963) notes that the way people perceive their physical world affects how they relate to it, and further, it helps explain how they choose to live their lives in relation to the physical world. To ignore this aspect results in oversimplification of the issues clients bring to counseling, simply knowing where people were socialized, and where they live now is not enough. The challenge for helpers is to understand the "meaning" of the environment for clients (Kemp, 1971). For example, considering indigenous cultures and nature, Maweu (2011) asserts that divergent perceptions, interactions, and knowledge are determined by different worldviews and the underlying environmental ethics; for many traditional societies, indigenous knowledge forms a holistic worldview. Indigenous worldviews have many commonalities, and these have emerged from the close relationships between people and their environment (Fitznor, 1998; McKenzie &

Morrissette, 2003). Clients with the *Optimistic* worldview prefer to live in harmony with the cycles of nature, and also recognize the power of nature, they tend to prefer to work with nature, rather than go against it, or disregard the cycles of nature. This perspective may also indicate a concern for the environment (Wesley Schultz & Zelezny, 1999).

OWV: Implications for Process and Goals

Considering this worldview, the communication process that would be most useful and productive would be relationship oriented (Garfield, 1995; Ivey, Ivey, & Zalaquett, 2013). Primarily, because clients with OWV see human nature as basically good, they will not have difficulty establishing a trusting relationship with the counselor, who is genuine, warm, caring, and interpersonally responsive. Initially, the focus needs to be on establishing a positive relationship, identifying strengths, while gathering information, would also help both relationship building and trust (Ivey, Ivey, & Zalaquett, 2013). Once trust is established, the focus can shift to developing goals. Goals for this client must reflect both inner development (moral/ethical concerns) and success as measured by external standards (community, society, work site, etc.). The client will also value therapeutic interventions that help clarify the role of the self, family, cultural group, and her/him/zir sociopolitical history. Getting a sociohistorical perspective, and how the events may have influenced the client's life, and specifically the presenting problem, would be very important. Clients with this profile will be fairly easy to work with for a counselor or therapist trained in a traditional program that emphasizes mainstream US culture, and assumptions. However, clients with OWV may have a tendency to respond in a culturally appropriate manner, or social desirability, their responses may not be truly reflective of their perspectives. With OWV clients it would be important to listen carefully to client narratives, to ascertain if their stated position matches the cognitive, affective, and behavioral aspects displayed. Clients with this profile match the assumptions of modern first world counseling and psychotherapy expectations.

Traditional Worldview

This worldview is composed of items from *Social Relations*, *Time*, and *Nature*. Social Relations vary from Lineal-Hierarchical (power rests with authority figures, and everyone must comply with authority) to Collateral-Mutual (if you treat me well, I will treat you well), to Individualistic (the individual is responsible for all decisions, what others require is of no importance) modes of relating to people. The Traditional Worldview (TWV) is primarily focused on two domains of social relations, i.e., Lineal-Hierarchical and Collateral-Mutual schemas. Time orientation varies from Past Time orientation (a focus on the past), Present Time orientation (being in the here-and-now), to Future Time orientation (emphasis on future goals and plans). The TWV perspective on Time shows a very strong focus on the Future dimension and some attention to the Past (history, events). TWV perceives nature as something humans can control. The primary characteristics of this perspective are that relationships are primarily lineal-hierarchical, implying that lines of authority are clearly defined, power comes from the top, and traditional gender roles are accepted. Lineal-hierarchical implies ordered positional succession within the group, continuity through time, and primacy given to group goals. Collateral-mutual implies that primacy is given to the goals and welfare of lateral extended groups, and the self is enhanced through mutual relationships. There is a strong future orientation, which implies a focus on long-range planning, and an emphasis on delayed gratification. There is a belief that humans can control and overpower the elements of nature (Ibrahim, 1993, 1999).

Existential philosophers such as Binswanger, Buber, Fromm, and Yalom have addressed the importance of relationships to humans. Existentialists view social relationships as the interpersonal world (Binswanger, 1962, 1963). Buber (1970) considers relationships one of the most important aspects of human existence and defined people as creatures of the in-between, who need relationships. Fromm (1963) and Yalom (1980) agree that the greatest fear for people is existential isolation. This according to Yalom (1980) is an "unbridgeable gap between oneself and other beings" (p. 355). The isolation is the source of all anxiety and a major psychological task that counselors face is to help clients to work through this anxiety within counseling and psychotherapy (Fromm, 1963). Time is a critical variable in existential philosophy as it focuses on the finiteness of human life and the anxiety associated with issues of death and the denial of death (Becker, 1973; Frankl, 1978; Yalom, 1980). Existentialists believe that the profound human experiences of life (joy, tragedy, etc.) occur in the dimension of time rather than space (Kemp, 1971). Yalom (1980) notes that recognition of the finiteness of life generally results in a major shift of perspective and can be a catalyst for positive human growth.

The TWV indicates a traditional perspective on life, and the welfare of the group may be more important than the needs of an individual. The emphasis is on respecting tradition and authority, to create order in society, which will eventually lead to well-being for the individual (Ibrahim, 1993, 1999). TWV reflects a cultural orientation found in more traditional societies except for the control of nature perspective. Kluckhohn and Strodtbeck (1961) in their research show that US cultural values differed from Mexican value orientations on issues of authority, and social positioning, and welfare of the group over welfare of an individual, as these were found in traditional societies, such as Mexico. In their research they found that control of nature was attributed to US culture, which at the time was thriving during the industrial revolution, and it was a prevalent belief among US citizens in the 1960s. Recent research has linked the control of nature as a self-enhancement perspective (Wesley Schultz & Zelezny, 1999). Control of nature within the constellation of assumptions in TWV could indicate considering nature useful for the benefits it could provide for society (Gagnon Thompson & Barton, 1994).

TWV: Implications for Process and Goals

Clients with TWV require both relationship and task-oriented approaches. This assumption is based on the values underlying ordered social relationships, and importance of the future (Ivey et al., 2013; Lambert & Barley, 2002). Role boundaries will be important for a client with this worldview, especially, in using respectful, culturally appropriate mode of address and formal communication with clients, and recognition of their cultural contexts (Corey et al., 2014; Ibrahim, 1999). Developing a genuine, empathic, and warm relationship with a client with TWV is important. Given that source credibility is important for clients with this worldview, helpers need to recognize that clients come to them because they are seen as experts (LaCrosse, 1980). In selecting an expert, clients with TWV, value the opinions of the counselor as an expert. The most beneficial process would involve mutual respect, and the client's involvement in generating goals and making decisions. Clients with this worldview value long-term goals, and accept working with short-term interim goals; the usefulness of this approach needs to be explained to get buy-in. In addition, since TWV client have a lineal-hierarchical assumptions, clients will be influenced by traditional, historical assumptions, and will value the therapist's attention to traditional values, and goals.

The communication process for TWV clients also needs to be both relationship and task oriented. With TWV clients it is important to give them respect for what they have achieved personally and professionally in their lives. In resolving the presenting problem they would prefer a task-oriented approach, and would have greater respect for the therapist if the focus were on the problem and the solutions rather than on the personality of the client. The best process to use in counseling would be action oriented, such as in Solution-Focused therapy (Murphy, 2008). TWV clients will value confrontation when there are discrepancies in beliefs, goals, and progress toward resolution, otherwise they will lose respect for the counselor. Long-term goals would be beneficial, along with interim short-term goals (Ibrahim, 1993, 1999).

The decision-making model again must be action oriented and directive, to be consistent with the role of the expert. We consider directive to imply staying on task, moving the process along, and not telling the client what would be the most useful way to approach resolution. Furthermore, TWV clients prefer task-focused therapeutic approach. The final decisions must rest with the client. The outcomes that a TWV client would prefer are ones that will emphasize needs of their larger system, family, or group. Too much focus on the client will create discomfort, as TWV place the needs of the group above individual needs. For a helper to be successful in working with TWV clients, it would be necessary to work from a perspective that respects authority, and accepts client assumptions, and works from the TWV perspective.

Here-and-Now/Spontaneous Worldview

Originally this worldview was named the Here-and-Now perspective, it is more relevant to call it Spontaneous Worldview; the emphases in this worldview is on two elements, Time and Activity. In the time dimension, all three items from the present orientation, and one item from the past orientation are emphasized. The main characteristic of this worldview is that client with Here-and-Now/Spontaneous Worldview (SWV) would require a focus on the presenting problem, which may shift from session to session. There may be no possibility of long-term goals. In each session, the concerns presented would require immediate attention. The therapist needs to respect the client's urgency, as it is critical to maintaining the therapeutic relationship. The Being orientation in this worldview demands that the client's needs are met, and the spontaneity is respected. This could be a challenge for a counselor trained, and educated in traditional counseling or psychotherapy as the mainstream values that guided counseling and psychotherapy programs assumed that people would be focused on the future instead of the present (Nagayama Hall et al., 2001). From an existential perspective, the client with SWV is influenced by past events, including historical issues (i.e., the client's family, group, and national sociopolitical history, this is also not consistent with mainstream US culture it is more consistent with perspectives found in collectivistic cultures (Castillo, 1977)). Furthermore, the being dimension requires exploration of the client's present concerns, including the finiteness of life and the meaning a client's ascribes to his or her life (Abdoli & Safavi, 2010; Ibrahim, 1993, 1999; Sartre, 1953). The focus on the here-and-now to the exclusion of other issues may create some dissonance for a helper, because it may seem like the client is escaping from the responsibility of confronting the original presenting problem, and basic psychological tasks that are relevant to create equilibrium. This may be another area of exploration for the therapist, to understand the immediate goals for the session (Ibrahim, 1999).

SWV: Implications for Process and Goals

The communication process needs to focus on the client, with an emphasis on relationship building in the present. The process needs to be nondirective, with the therapist following the client's lead. The decision-making model should be mutual. The outcomes that the client will possibly seek will be on the presenting problem of the day. A problem-focused approach or a crisis intervention model, or a solution-focused approach would be the most appropriate (Burwell & Chen, 2006; LeCroy, 2008; Murphy, 2008).

A client with this worldview could pose the greatest challenge to a mainstream counselor with traditional counseling training (future planning and goals). From a process perspective, counseling this client would be a relatively positive experience for the counselor, because the here-and-now focus would allow both the counselor and the client to stay with the issue at hand, and closure in each session, with no unfinished business. It is recommended that goal setting for each session needs to be addressed formally at the beginning of the session, with a summary at the end of what was accomplished and any unfinished business (Ibrahim, 1999).

Pessimistic Worldview

The Pessimistic Worldview (PWV) perspective perceives human nature as basically bad. Alienation (from self and others) can be a factor in creating a negative self-evaluation and perception of others. An understanding of how individuals see themselves and others can be of tremendous value in understanding the quality of their lives and the meaningfulness of their relationships (Ibrahim, 1993, 1999). The second main characteristic is that PWV acknowledges the Power of Nature, and accepts the vulnerability of humans to the forces of nature. This finding among US majority population is contrary to C. Kluckhohn's (1956) assumptions about mainstream culture. This finding highlights a change in values, beliefs, and assumptions, among the US population, specific to the nature dimension (Ibrahim & Owen, 1994). In previous research, mainstream culture viewed nature as something that could be controlled and managed (Kluckhohn & Strodtbeck, 1961). The Social Relations orientation in PWV is collateral mutual (one item): that is, "do unto others as they do to you." This assumption implies a degree of mutuality in relationships. People with PWV consider how others treat them, and formulate their response to people accordingly. Given the perception of human nature, one must view this orientation with caution (1999). The research on the SAWV consistently shows that people who are vulnerable or second class citizens based on their lack of privilege, generally opt for the PWV as their secondary worldview, although their primary worldview is usually OWV, which is consistent with the overarching assumptions in US culture (Ibrahim et al., 2001).

PWV: Implications for Process and Goals

Clients with PWV will pose a challenge to a counselor primarily in the process domain. Trust development will be difficult with this population, due to their perception of human nature. It is important to focus on relationship building in each session with empathic responding and working to always be there for the client (Ivey et al., 2013). Considering the client's low evaluation of human nature, it is critical to focus on the task, i.e., the presenting problem. This will facilitate trust development, as it will help a client with PWV to accept that the therapist is following through on the contract. This perspective could be common among clients in the immersion-emersion stage of racial identity development (Cross, 1995; Helms, 1990). It may be important to have a secondary goal of racial/cultural/gender/sexual orientation/gender identity development for clients with PWV.

Clients with PWV have a slight propensity toward the collateral-mutual orientation, they will need to be respected for their beliefs and will reciprocate with respect for the counselor (LeCroy, 2008). The client's feelings of vulnerability also mediate their perception of nature, and their low trust of human nature. The therapist needs to be able to work with both these dimensions, respecting the client's core assumptions, without negative evaluation of the person with a PWV perspective. Acceptance and understanding of the PWV is important and must be communicated appropriately. Goal development needs to be a mutual process. This will demand a great deal of flexibility on the part of the counselor who has been educated in traditional counseling and psychotherapy approaches.

Research Overview: The Scale to Assess Worldview

The therapeutic community strongly recommends "understanding" client worldviews (American Counseling Association (ACA), 1992; Association for Multicultural Counseling and Development (AMCD), 1992; American Psychological Association, 2002; Beutler & Bergan, 1991; Fisher et al., 1998; Ibrahim & Arredondo, 1986). This indicates that helping professionals need to understand client assumptions, and this recommendation could lead to erroneous conclusions, unless formal assessment is conducted (Ibrahim, 1999). Formal assessments have not been used to understand client worldview, formal assessment measures designed to assess core values measures do not exist, except for The Scale to Assess World View, specific to assessing basic values, beliefs, and assumptions (Ibrahim & Kahn, 1984, 1987), and Carter and Helms (1990) Intercultural Values Inventory. Both these instruments are based on the original research on core values was conducted by Kluckhohn and Strodtbeck (1961), who developed an open-ended questionnaire developed on Kluckhohn's (1951) model of existential value orientations, and collected data in the USA and Mexico. Koltko-Rivera (2004) provides an extensive review of the literature on the construct of worldview, and finds several conceptions of worldview in the literature however, specific assessment measures that focused on values and an attempt to assess them empirically in therapeutic encounters were not identified, except for two mentioned above that specifically addressed the core values. There are also assessment measures available in the intercultural communication domain, and the most prominent is *The Intercultural Development Inventory* (Hammer, Bennett, & Wiseman, 2003).

Research on Worldview

Over the last 30 years several research studies have employed the construct of worldview using the SAWV. These studies show that cultural differences in values can be identified using the SAWV (Ibrahim et al., 2001). This research also shows that comparison of core values and assumptions can be conducted and used to develop appropriate programs and interventions for organizations, families, and individuals. Studies reviewed were on the Kluckhohn and Strodtbeck model of existential values orientation. Instruments for assessing beliefs, values, and assumptions varied in these studies, primarily they included the *Intercultural Values Inventory* (Carter & Helms, 1990; Carter & Parks, 1992; Kohls, 1996) and the *Scale to Assess Worldview©* (SAWV; Ibrahim & Kahn, 1984, 1987; Ibrahim & Owen, 1994). The SAWV was used in 29 studies (Berkow, Richmond, & Page, 1994; Cheng, O'Leary, & Page, 1995; Chu-Richardson, 1988; Cieciuch & Ibrahim, 2011; Cunningham-Warburton, 1988; D'Rozario, 1996; Furn, 1986; Gerber, 1998; Gordon, 1997; Hansman, Grant, Jackson, & Spencer, 1999; Hickson, Christie, & Shmuklcr, 1990; Ibrahim et al., 1993; Ibrahim & Kahn, 1987; Ibrahim & Owen, 1994; Lin, 2008; Lo, 1996, 1996; Lockney, 1999; Lopez, Salas, Arroya-Jurado, & Chinn, 2004; Ngumba, 1996; Ohnishi, 1998; Russell, 2005; Sadlak & Ibrahim, 1986; Sodowsky, Maguire, Johnson, Kohles, & Ngumba, 1994; Tarricone, 1999; Thompson, 1997; Toczyska, 1996; Tonnessen, 2001). Two additional studies used the SAWV Short-Form (1994); SAWV items were reduced to the two dominant factors (Ihle, Sodowsky, & Kwan, 1996; Kwan, Sodowsky, & Ihle, 1994).

In a previous publication Ibrahim et al. (2001) had discussed the issue of American (US) cultural identity, given that several cultures are represented in both the dominant and nondominant cultural groups in the USA. Carter and Parks (1992) had also noted the issue of an American (US) identity, as several of the participants in their study identified as "American" when the responded to the demographic questionnaire regarding ethnicity. In the studies conducted on the SAWV in the USA, regardless of ethnicity, dominant or nondominant group membership, the primary worldview is Optimistic, it is the secondary worldview that discriminates members of vulnerable cultural groups as they always identify the secondary worldview as "Pessimistic." Ibrahim (2003) notes that this worldview needs to be renamed as "Realistic" given that it shows that all US participants aspire to the same cultural assumptions as exemplified by the Optimistic worldview, however, members of vulnerable groups, which included women, LGBTQ, nondominant cultural ethnic groups both indigenous to the USA and immigrants, and people with disabilities, and nondominant religions or spirituality, recognize that they may not be able to achieve their goals in a dominant society that does not value their identities, or undervalued nondominant cultures, genders, sexual orientations, etc.

The findings across studies indicate that there are cultural differences among and between societies, specifically on the cultural orientations of individualism and collectivism, and the dimensional variations on the East–west continuum (Green, Deschamps, & Paez, 2005; Hofstede, 1980; Van de Vijver & Leung, 1997). Studies comparing US cultural assumptions with other countries and cultures showed cultural differences consistent with the assumptions of each given society (Berkow et al., 1994; Cheng et al., 1995; Cieciuch & Ibrahim, 2011; Ibrahim et al., 1993; Schwartz, 1994). Research comparing US and Brazilian assumptions highlights cultural differences in values that are consistent with cultural assumptions in both countries (Ibrahim et al., 1993). Research with the SAWV discriminates on cultural assumptions within cultures and between cultures (Cieciuch & Ibrahim, 2011; Furn, 1986; Ibrahim et al., 1993; Ibrahim & Kahn, 1987; Ibrahim & Owen, 1994).

The SAWV has been used in several research studies research within group cultural values, and variations (Cieciuch & Ibrahim, 2011; Gerber, 1998; Hickson et al., 1990; Ibrahim & Kahn, 1987; Ibrahim & Owen, 1994; Lo, 1996; Lockney, 1999; Thompson, 1997), for cross-cultural comparisons of cultural assumptions (Boatswain, 1997; D'Rozario, 1996; Ibrahim et al., 1993), disability worldview (Gordon, 1997); therapeutic interventions and counselor efficacy as perceived by clients (Cunningham-Warburton, 1988; Sadlak & Ibrahim, 1986), gender differences (D'Rozario, 1996; Furn, 1986), comparison of international and US students worldview (Berkow et al., 1994; Cheng et al., 1995; Ihle et al., 1996; Kwan et al., 1994; Sodowsky et al., 1994; Thompson, 1997), variations in worldview by social class (Gerber, 1998); and academic and organizational culture (Chu-Richardson, 1988; Hansman et al., 1999; Toczyska, 1996). In most cases the findings have been consistent with the cultural values and assumptions of the cultural groups within societies, and their contexts. The SAWV provides the information on the client's and the professional's subjective reality (Ibrahim, 1985; Lin, 2008; Saenz-Adames, 2014). This information is critical in expanding the professional's knowledge base and in developing meaningful interventions that are culturally sensitive and humanistic (Hickson et al., 1990).

The SAWV can be useful in developing a shared frame of reference and when a shared frame of reference was established between the counselor and the client, counselor effectiveness and perceived efficacy leads to successful engagement in counseling (Cunningham-Warburton, 1988; Sadlak & Ibrahim, 1986). The SAWV can be successfully used as a training tool to enhance cross-cultural counselor effectiveness in addressing existential dilemmas that people face, and can help them cope with life's challenges. The scale can also be used in different cultures to compare groups as well as to compare differences within each cultural group and to gain important information on cross-cultural differences and similarities. The SAWV addresses some universal concerns pertaining to core values and thus compensates for the deficits of limited, Western-based assessment research (Sue, Ito, & Bradshaw, 1982; Triandis & Brislin, 1984; Triandis, Malpass, & Davison, 1973). The scale also attempts to address the lack of attention to individual differences within cultural groups, a major drawback in cross-cultural research of the 1970s and 1980s (Atkinson, 1985; Hilliard, 1985).

Conclusion

This chapter reviewed the concept of worldview in general and specifically the conceptualization the authors use to understand core values, and assumptions of clients. It includes information on understanding client worldviews as assessed by the Scale to Assess World View© and using the information gained in counseling and psychotherapy. The chapter concludes with a review of research conducted using the Scale to Assess World View.

References

Abdoli, S., & Safavi, S. S. (2010). Nursing students' immediate responses to distressed clients based on Orlando's theory. *Iranian Journal of Nursing and Midwifery Research, 15*(4), 178.

American Counseling Association (ACA). (1992). *Multicultural counseling competencies.* Alexandria, VA: Author.

American Psychiatric Association. (2013). *Diagnostic and statistical manual of mental disorders-5: DSM-5* (5th ed.). Arlington, VA: Author.

American Psychological Association (APA). (2002). *Guidelines on multicultural education, training, research, practice, and organizational change for psychologists.* Washington, DC: Author.

Association for Multicultural Counseling and Development (AMCD). (1992). *Multicultural counseling competencies.* Alexandria, VA: American Counseling Association.

Atkinson, D. R. (1985). A meta-review of research on cross-cultural counseling and psychotherapy. *Journal of Multicultural Counseling and Development, 13*, 138–153.

Beck, A. T., Rush, A. J., Shaw, B. F., & Emery, G. (1979). *Cognitive therapy of depression.* New York: Guilford Press.

Becker, E. (1973). *The denial of death.* New York: Simon & Schuster.

Berkow, D. N., Richmond, B., & Page, R. C. (1994). A cross-cultural comparison of worldviews: American and Fijian counseling students. *Counseling and Values, 38*, 121–135.

Beutler, L. E., & Bergan, J. (1991). Value change in counseling and psychotherapy: A search for scientific credibility. *Journal of Counseling Psychology, 38*(1), 16–24.

Binswanger, I. (1962). *Existential analysis and psychotherapy.* New York: Dutton.

Binswanger, I. (1963). *Being-in-the-world: Selected papers.* New York: Basic Books.

Boatswain, B. (1997). The relationship between cultural values and job satisfaction among African-American managers and higher level professionals. *Dissertation Abstracts International, 58-11B*, 62–64.

Boysen, G. A., & Vogel, D. L. (2008). The relationship between level of training, implicit bias, and multicultural competency among counselor trainees. *Training and Education in Professional Psychology, 2*(2), 103–110.

Buber, M. (1970). *I and thou.* New York: Scribner.

Burwell, R., & Chen, C. P. (2006). Applying the principles and techniques of solution-focused therapy to career counseling. *Counselling Psychology Quarterly, 19*(2), 189–203.

Carter, R. T., & Helms, J. E. (1990). *The intercultural values inventory (ICV). Tests in microfiche test collection.* Princeton, NJ: Educational Testing Service.

Carter, R. T., & Parks, E. E. (1992). White ethnic group membership and cultural values preferences. *Journal of College Student Development, 33*, 499–506.

Castillo, R. J. (1977). *Culture and mental illness: A client-centered approach.* Pacific Grove, CA: Brooks/Cole.

Cheng, H., O'Leary, E., & Page, R. C. (1995). A cross-cultural comparison of the world-views of American, Chinese (from Taiwan), and Irish graduate counseling students and implications for counseling. *Counseling and Values, 40*, 45–54.

Chu-Richardson, P. B. (1988). *World view, learning style, and locus of control as factors of institutional culture differentiating academically unsuccessful students, academically successful students, and faculty.* Unpublished doctoral dissertation, University of Connecticut, Storrs.

Cieciuch, J., & Ibrahim, F. A. (2011, August). *Polish worldviews: Using the scale to assess worldview.* Presentation at the American Psychological Association annual conference, Washington, DC.

Claiborn, C. D. (1986). Social influence: Toward a general theory of change. In F. J. Dora (Ed.), *Social influence processes in counseling and psychotherapy* (pp. 65–74). Springfield, IL: Charles C Thomas.

Corey, G., Corey, M., Corey, C., & Callanan, P. (2014). *Issues and ethics in the helping professions.* Belmont, CA: Cengage Learning.

Cross, W. M. (1995). The psychology of Nigrescence: Revising the Cross model. In J. G. Ponterrotto, J. G. Ponterotto, J. M. Casas, L. A. Suzuki, & C. M. Alexander (Eds.), *Handbook of multicultural counseling* (pp. 93–122). Thousand Oaks, CA: Sage.

Cunningham-Warburton, P. A. (1988). *A study of the relationship between cross-cultural training, the scale to assess world views, and the quality of care given by nurses in a psychiatric setting.* Unpublished doctoral dissertation, University of Connecticut, Storrs.

D'Rozario, V. A. (1996). Singaporean and United States college students' worldviews, expectations of counseling, and perceptions of counselor effectiveness based on directive and nondirective counseling style. *Dissertation Abstracts International, 56*, 2564.

Dana, R. H. (1998). *Understanding cultural identity in intervention and assessment.* Thousand Oaks, CA: Sage.

Diener, E., Shigehiro, O., & Lucas, R. E. (2003). Personality, culture, and subjective well-being: Emotional and cognitive evaluation of life. *Annual Review of Psychology, 54*, 403–425.

Fisher, A. R., Jome, L. M., & Atkinson, D. R. (1998). Reconceptualizing multicultural counseling: Universal healing conditions in a culturally specific context. *The Counseling Psychologist, 26*, 525–588.

Fitznor, L. (1998). The circle of life: Affirming aboriginal philosophies in everyday living. In D. C. McCance (Ed.), *Life ethics in world religions.* Atlanta, GA: Scholars Press.

Frank, J. D., & Frank, J. B. (1991). *Persuasion and healing: A comparative study of psychotherapy.* Baltimore: Johns Hopkins University Press.

Frankl, V. (1978). *The unheard cry for meaning: Psychotherapy and humanism.* New York: Simon & Schuster.

Fromm, E. (1963). *The art of loving.* New York: Bantam Books.

Furn, B. G. (1986). The psychology of women as a cross-cultural issue: Perceived dimensions of worldviews. *Dissertation Abstracts International, 48-OlA*, 234.

Furn, B. G. (1987). Adjustment and the near death experience: A conceptual and a therapeutic model. *Journal of Near-Death Studies, 6*, 4–19.

Gagnon Thompson, S. C., & Barton, M. A. (1994). Ecocentric and anthropocentric attitudes toward the environment. *Journal of Environmental Psychology, 14*(2), 149–157.

Garfield, S. L. (1995). *Psychotherapy: An eclectic-integrative approach.* New York: Wiley.

Gaztambide, D. J. (2012). Addressing cultural impasses in rupture resolution strategies: A proposal and recommendation. *Professional Psychology: Research and Practice, 43*(3), 183–189. doi:10.1037/a0026911.

Gerber, M. H. (1998). Worldview, social class, and psychosocial development. *Dissertation Abstracts International, 60*, 2983.

Gordon, R. D. (1997). Worldview, self-concept, and cultural identity patterns of deaf adolescents: Implications for counseling. *Dissertation Abstracts International, 58*, 4448.

Green, E. G. T., Deschamps, J. C., & Paez, D. (2005). Variation of individualism and collectivism within and between 20 countries a typological analysis. *Journal of Cross-Cultural Psychology, 36*(3), 321–339.

Grencavage, L. M., & Norcross, J. C. (1990). Where are the commonalities among the therapeutic common factors. *Professional Psychology: Research and Practice, 21*(5), 372.

Grieger, I., & Ponterotto, J. C. (1995). A framework for assessment in multicultural counseling. In J. G. Ponterotto, J. M. Casas, L. A. Suzuki, & C. M. Alexander (Eds.), *Handbook of multicultural counseling* (pp. 357–3741). Thousand Oaks, CA: Sage.

Hammer, M. R., Bennett, M. J., & Wiseman, R. (2003). Measuring intercultural sensitivity: The intercultural development inventory. *International Journal of Intercultural Relations, 27*, 421–443.

Hansman, C. A., Grant, D. F., Jackson, M. H., & Spencer, L. (1999). Implications of students' worldviews in graduate professional preparation programs. *Education, 119*(3), 551–559.

Hart, P. (2010). No longer a 'little added frill': The transformative power of environmental education for educational change. *Teacher Education Quarterly, 37*(4), 155–178.

Helms, J. (1990). *Black and white racial identity: Theory, research, and practice.* Westport, CT: Greenwood.

Hickson, J., Christie, C., & Shmuklcr, D. (1990). A pilot study of Black and White South African adolescent pupils: Implications for cross-cultural counseling. *South African Journal of Psychology, 20*, 170–177.

Hilliard, A. B. (1985). Multicultural dimensions of counseling and human development in an age of technology. *Journal of Non-White Concerns in Personnel and Guidance, 13*, 17–27.

Hillman, J. (1997). *The soul's code: IN search of character and calling*. New York: Random House.

Hofstede, G. H. (1980). *Culture's consequences: International differences in work related values*. Thousand Oaks, CA: Sage.

Ibrahim, F. A. (1984). Cross-cultural counseling and psychotherapy: An existential-Psychological perspective. *International Journal for the Advancement of Counselling, 7*, 159–169.

Ibrahim, F. A. (1985). Effective cross-cultural counseling and psychotherapy: A frame-work. *The Counseling Psychologist, 13*, 625–638.

Ibrahim, F. A. (1993). Existential worldview theory: Transcultural counseling. In J. McFadden (Ed.), *Transcultural counseling: Bilateral and international perspectives* (pp. 25–58). Alexandria, VA: American Counseling Association.

Ibrahim, F. A. (1999). Transcultural counseling: Existential worldview theory and cultural identity. In J. McFadden (Ed.), *Transcultural counseling* (2nd ed., pp. 23–58). Alexandria, VA: American Counseling Association.

Ibrahim, F. A. (2003). Existential worldview theory: From inception to applications. In F. D. Harper & J. McFadden (Eds.), *Culture and counseling: New approaches* (pp. 196–208). Boston: Allyn & Bacon.

Ibrahim, F. A. (2007). *Cultural identity check list-revised©*, Denver, CO. Unpublished Document.

Ibrahim, F. A. (2008). *United States acculturation index©*, Denver, CO. Unpublished Document.

Ibrahim, F. A. (2010). Innovative teaching strategies for group work: Addressing cultural responsiveness and social justice. *Journal for Specialists in Group Work, 35*(3), 271–280.

Ibrahim, F. A. (2011). Teaching strategies for group work: Addressing cultural responsiveness and social justice. In A. Singh & C. Salazar (Eds.), *Social justice in group work* (pp. 188–215). London: Routledge/Taylor & Francis Group.

Ibrahim, F. A., & Arredondo, P. M. (1986). Ethical standards for cross-cultural counseling: Preparation, practice, assessment, and research. *Journal of Counseling and Development, 64*, 349–351.

Ibrahim, F. A., & Heuer, J. R. (2013). The assessment, diagnosis, and treatment of mental disorders among Muslims. In F. A. Paniagua & A.-M. Yamada (Eds.), *Handbook of multicultural mental health* (2nd ed., pp. 367–388). New York: Academic.

Ibrahim, F. A., Julie, D., Estrada, D., & Michael D'Andrea, M. (2011). Counselors for social justice: Ethical standards. *Journal for Social Action in Counseling and Psychology, 3*(2), 29–43. http://jsacp.tumblr.com.

Ibrahim, F. A., & Kahn, H. (1984). *Scale to assess world view©*. Storrs: University of Connecticut.

Ibrahim, F. A., & Kahn, H. (1987). Assessment of worldviews. *Psychological Reports, 60*, 163–176.

Ibrahim, F. A., & Owen, S. V. (1994). Factor-analytic structure of the scale to assess World view. *Current Psychology, 13*, 201–209.

Ibrahim, F. A., Roysircar-Sodowsky, G., & Ohnishi, H. (2001). Worldview: Recent developments and needed directions. In J. G. Ponterotto, J. M. Casas, L. A. Suzuki, & C. M. Alexander (Eds.), *Handbook of multicultural counseling* (pp. 425–456). Thousand Oaks, CA: Sage.

Ibrahim, F. A., Sequiera de Frietas, K., & Owen, S. V. (1993, August). *Comparison of Brazilian and American worldviews*. Paper presented at the annual meeting of the American Psychological Association, New York.

Ihle, G. M., Sodowsky, G. R., & Kwan, K. (1996). Worldviews of women: Comparisons between White American clients, White American counselors, and Chinese international students. *Journal of Counseling and Development, 74*, 300–306.

Imel, Z., & Wampold, B. (2008). The importance of treatment and the science of common factors in psychotherapy. In S. D. Brown & R. W. Lent (Eds.), *Handbook of counseling psychology* (pp. 249–262). New York: Wiley.

Ivey, A. E., Ivey, M. B., & Simek-Morgan, L. (1997). *Counseling and psychotherapy: A multicultural perspective*. Boston: Allyn & Bacon.

Ivey, A. E., Ivey, M. B., & Zalaquett, C. P. (2013). *Intentional interviewing and counseling: Facilitating client development in a multicultural society* (8th ed.). Belmont, CA: Brooks/Cole.

Ivey, A. E., Normington, C. J., Miller, C. D., Morrill, W. H., & Haase, R. F. (1968). Microcounseling and attending behavior: An approach to pre-practicum counselor training. *Journal of Counseling Psychology, 15*, 1–12 (Monograph).

Ivey, A. E., Pedersen, P. B., & Ivey, M. B. (2009). *Intentional group counseling: A Microscounseling approach*. Belmont, CA: Cengage.

Jung, C. G. (1942). A psychological approach to the dogma of the trinity. *Collected Works, 11*, 175.

Jung, C. G. (1954). *The development of personality* (Vol. 17). Princeton, NJ: Princeton University Press. The collected works.

Kanouse, D. E., Kelley, H. H., Nisbett, R. E., Valins, S., & Weiner, B. (1972). *Attribution: Perceiving the causes of behavior* (pp. 79–94). Morristown, NJ: General Learning Press.

Kelly, G. (1963). *A theory of personality: The psychology of personal constructs*. New York: W. W. Norton.

Kemp, C. G. (1971). Existential counseling. *The Counseling Psychologist, 2*, 171–186.

Kluckhohn, C. (1951). Values and value orientations in the theory of action. In T. Parsons & E. A. Shields (Eds.), *Toward a general theory of action* (pp. 388–433). Cambridge, MA: Harvard University Press.

Kluckhohn, C. (1956). Towards a comparison of value-emphasis in different cultures. In L. D. White (Ed.), *The state of social sciences* (pp. 116–132). Chicago: University of Chicago Press.

Kluckhohn, F. R., & Strodtbeck, F. L. (1961). *Variations in value orientations*. Evanston, IL: Row, Petersen.

Kohls, L. R. (1996). *Survival kit for overseas living*. Yarmouth, ME: Intercultural Press.

Koltko-Rivera, M. E. (2004). The psychology of worldviews. *Review of General Psychology, 8*(1), 3–58. doi:10.1037/1089-2680.8.1.3.

Kottler, J. A., & Hazler, R. J. (2001). The therapist as a model of humane values and humanistic behavior. In K. J. Schnieder, J. F. T. Bugental, & J. F. Pierson (Eds.), *The handbook of humanistic psychology: Leading edges in theory, research, and practice* (pp. 355–370). Thousand Oaks, CA: Sage.

Kwan, K. L. K., Sodowsky, G. R., & Ihle, G. M. (1994). Worldviews of Chinese international students: An extension and new findings. *Journal of College Student Development, 35*, 190–197.

LaCrosse, M. B. (1980). Perceived counselor social influence and counseling outcomes: Validity of the counselor rating form. *Journal of Counseling Psychology, 27*(4), 320–327.

Lambert, M. J., & Barley, D. E. (2002). Psychotherapy relationships that work: Therapist contributions and responsiveness to patients. In J. C. Norcross (Ed.), *Research summary on the therapeutic relationship and psychotherapy outcome* (2nd ed., pp. 17–32). New York: Oxford University Press.

LeCroy, C. W. (2008). *Handbook of evidence-based treatment manuals for children and adolescents*. New York: Oxford University Press.

Lin, S. A. (2008). The imposter phenomenon among high-achieving women of color: Are worldview, collective self-esteem and multigroup ethnic identity protective? Fordham University Dissertation. Retrieved from http://www.proquest.com/products-services/pqdt.html.

Lo, Y. H. (1996). The role of culture and subculture in worldviews: The impact of Western influence and profession in Taiwan. *Dissertation Abstracts International, 57*, 2948.

Lockney, J. P. (1999). Worldview: Accuracy of interpersonal perceptions on diversity. *Dissertation Abstracts International, 6006B*, 3018.

Lonner, J., & Ibrahim, F. A. (2008). Assessment in cross-cultural counseling. In P. B. Pedersen, J. Draguns, W. J. Lonner, & J. Trimble (Eds.), *Counseling across cultures* (6th ed., pp. 37–57). Thousand Oaks, CA: Sage.

Lopez, E. J., Salas, L., Arroya-Jurado, E., & Chinn, K. (2004). Current practices in multicultural assessment by school psychologists. *Forum: Qualitative Social Research, 5*(3), 1. Article 23, Retrieved from http://nbn-resolving.de/urn:nbn:de:0114-fqs0403231.

Maslow, A. H. (1987). *Motivation and personality* (3rd ed.). New York: Harper & Row.

Maweu, J. M. (2011). Indigenous ecological knowledge and modern Western ecological knowledge: Complementary, not contradictory. *Thought and Practice: A Journal of the Philosophical Association of Kenya, 3*(2), 35–47.

McGoldrick, M. (2005). Preface. In M. McGoldrick, J. M. Giordano, & N. Preto-Garcia (Eds.), *Ethnicity and family therapy* (3rd ed.). New York: Guilford Press.

McKenzie, B., & Morrissette, V. (2003). Social work practice with Canadians of aboriginal background: Guidelines for respectful social work. *Envision: The Manitoba Journal of Child Welfare, 2*(1), 13–39.

Murphy, J. J. (2008). *Solution-focused counseling in schools*. Alexandria, VA: American Counseling Association.

Nagayama Hall, G. C., Lopez, I., & Bansal, A. (2001). Academic acculturation. In D. Pope-Davis & H. Coleman (Eds.), *The intersection of race, class, and gender in multicultural counseling* (pp. 171–188). Thousand Oaks, CA: Sage.

Ngumba, E. W. (1996). The relationship between worldview, African self-consciousness, and adjustment of African and African-American students: A comparative study. *Dissertation Abstracts International, 57*, 2877.

Ohnishi, H. (1998). *A comparison of Japanese and United States women on identity status and level of depression*. Doctoral dissertation, University of Connecticut, Storrs.

Olsen, M. E., Lodwick, D. G., & Dunlap, R. E. (1992). *Viewing the world ecologically* (p. 4). Boulder, CO: Westview Press.

Owen, J., Imel, Z., Tao, K. W., Wampold, B., Smith, A., & Rodolfa, E. (2011). Cultural ruptures in short-term therapy: Working alliance as a mediator between clients' perceptions of microaggressions and therapy outcomes. *Counseling and Psychotherapy Research, 11*(3), 204–2011.

Pedersen, P. B., Fukuyama, M., & Heath, A. (1989). Client, counselor, and contextual variables in multicultural counseling. In P. B. Pedersen, W. J. Lonner, J. G. Draguns, & J. Trimble (Eds.), *Counseling across cultures* (3rd ed.). Honolulu, HI: University of Hawaii Press.

Rokeach, M. (1973). *The nature of human values* (Vol. 438). New York: Free Press.

Rotter, J. C. (1966). *Locus of control: Current trends in theory and research*. New York: Wiley.

Russell, E. (2005). *The relationship of worldview to career intervention strategies among African Americans*. Doctoral dissertation, Howard University, Washington, DC.

Sadlak, M. J. (1986). *A study of the impact of training in cross-cultural counseling on counselor effectiveness and sensitivity*. Doctoral dissertation, University of Connecticut, Storrs.

Sadlak, M. J., & Ibrahim, F. A. (1986). *Cross-cultural counselor training: Impact on counselor effectiveness and sensitivity*. Presentation at the annual meeting of the American Psychological Association, Washington, DC.

Saenz-Adames, M. (2014). A phenomenological study examining worldview, acculturation and perceptions of pre-service and in-service educators related to at-risk minority youth who are identified with a disability. New Mexico State University. Retrieved from http://www.proquest.com/products-services/pqdt.html.

Sartre, J. P. (1953). *Existential psychoanalysis*. Chicago: Henry Regnery.

Schwartz, S. H. (1994). Are there universal aspects in the structure and contents of human values? *Journal of Social Issues, 50*(4), 19–45.

Schwartz, S. H., & Bilsky, W. (1987). Toward a universal psychological structure of human values. *Journal of Personality and Social Psychology, 53*, 550–562.

Schwartz, S. H., & Bilsky, W. (1990). Toward a theory of the universal content and structure of values: Extensions and cross-cultural replications. *Journal of Personality and Social Psychology, 58*, 878–891.

Seligman, M. E. P. (1995). The effectiveness of psychotherapy: The consumer reports study. *American Psychologist, 50*(12), 965–974. doi:10.1037/0003-066X.50.12.965.

Smith, M. L., Glass, G. V., & Miller, T. I. (1980). *The benefits of psychotherapy*. Baltimore: Johns Hopkins University Press.

Sodowsky, G. R., Maguire, K., Johnson, P., Kohles, R., & Ngumba, W. (1994). Worldviews of White American, Mainland Chinese, Taiwanese, and African students in a Midwestern university: An investigation into between-group differences. *Journal of Cross-Cultural Psychology, 25*, 309–324.

Sue, D. W. (1978). Worldviews and counseling. *The Personnel and Guidance Journal, 56*, 458–462.

Sue, S. (1988). Psychotherapeutic services for ethnic minorities: Two decades of research findings. *American Psychologist, 43*(4), 301.

Sue, S., & Zane, N. (1987). The role of culture and cultural techniques in psychotherapy: A critique and reformulation. *American Psychologist, 42*(1), 37–45.

Sue, S., Ito, J., & Bradshaw, C. (1982). Ethnic minority research: Trends and directions. In C. E. Jones & S. J. Korchin (Eds.), *Minority mental health* (pp. 47–61). New York: Praeger.

Sue, S., Zane, N., Hall, G. C. N., & Berger, L. K. (2009). The case for cultural competency in psychotherapeutic interventions. *Annual Review of Psychology, 60*, 525–548.

Takaki, R. T. (1979). *Iron cages, race and culture in the 19th century*. Oxford, England: Oxford University Press.

Tarricone, D., (1999) Relationship between homophobia and worldview with respect to attitudes and perceptions of women in sports. *Doctoral Dissertations,* Paper AAI9926298. http://digitalcommons.uconn.edu/dissertations/AAI9926298

Thompson, M. L. (1997). Traditional worldview, interpersonal flexibility, and marital satisfaction among interethnic couples. *Dissertation Abstracts International, 58,07A*, 2864.

Toczyska, M. A. (1996). Worldview and perception of organizational culture: Factors distinguishing dominant cultures from subcultures and managers from non-managers in Northeastern United States workplaces. *Dissertation Abstracts International, 57*, 1737.

Tonnessen, L. (2001). *Cultural identity, worldview and communication style among Norwegian-Americans: Implications for counseling and psychotherapy*. Doctoral Dissertation, Storrs, University of Connecticut.

Torrey, E. F. (1986). *Witchdoctors and psychiatrists: The common roots of psychotherapy and its future*. New York: Harper & Row.

Triandis, H. C., & Brislin, R. W. (1984). Cross-cultural psychology. *American Psychologist, 39*, 1006–1016.

Triandis, H. C., Malpass, R. S., & Davison, A. R. (1973). Psychology and culture. *Annual Review of Psychology, 60*, 355–378.

Tyler, F. B., Sussewell, D. R., & Williams-McCoy, J. (1985). Ethnic validity in psychotherapy. *Psychotherapy: Theory, Research, Practice, Training, 22*(2), 311.

Vajari, M. D., & Ghaedi, Y. (2011). The cultural influences and client expectations in counseling process. *International Journal on Social Science, Economics and Art, 1*(4), 268–271.

Van de Vijver, F., & Leung, K. (1997). *Methods and data analysis of comparative research*. Boston: Allyn & Bacon.

Wampold, B. E. (2001). *The great psychotherapy debate: Model, methods, and findings*. Mahwah, NJ: Lawrence Erlbaum.

Wesley Schultz, P., & Zelezny, L. (1999). Values as predictors of environmental attitudes: Evidence for consistency across 14 countries. *Journal of Environmental Psychology, 19*(3), 255–265.

Williams, R. M. (1968). Values. In D. I. Sills (Ed.), *International encyclopedia of social sciences*. New York: Macmillan.

Wolman, B. B. (1973). *Concerning psychology and the philosophy of science*. Englewood Cliffs, NJ: Prentice Hall.

Yalom, I. D. (1980). *Existential psychotherapy*. New York: Basic Books.

Chapter 4
Understanding Acculturation and Its Use in Counseling and Psychotherapy

A review of acculturation theory and practice issues will be provided in this chapter. In working with clients in a diverse society such as the USA, and internationally, it is emphasized that the cultural assumptions underlying US institutions, legal system, government, and other public entities is not the same as the 22 White ethnic groups in the country subscribe to, or the four main nondominant cultural groups. Given the diversity and cultural pluralism, we cannot assume that everyone is acculturated to the core assumptions of the founding fathers that represent how the nation is set up. The US Acculturation Index (USAI; Ibrahim, 2008) will be introduced as a tool that can be used to assess the individual client's assumptions on White Anglo-Saxon Protestant values that undergird the official culture of the USA. The USAI is included in the text (Appendix C).

Introduction

This chapter discusses the concept of acculturation and its relevance in counseling and psychotherapy in a diverse world. Acculturation refers to understanding the process of adaptation to a new culture for immigrants, refugees, and sojourners. In counseling and psychotherapy acculturation and its relationship to cultural/ethnic identity has not been addressed; however, in social psychological research it has repeatedly emerged as a significant issue (Persky & Birman, 2005; Phinney, 2003; Suzuki, Ponterotto, & Meller, 2001). There is human diversity in plural societies, such as the USA, and in many cultures today, very few societies are completely monolithic. Therefore, it is important to understand how people within a social system relate to the overarching assumptions of that cultural-social system. This information has significance for adaptation and psychological health (Berry & Sabatier, 2010; Persky & Birman, 2005; Phinney & Flores, 2002). Given the cultural differences that exist in all societies, but not to the extent found in the USA, it is important

F.A. Ibrahim, J.R. Heuer, *Cultural and Social Justice Counseling*, International and Cultural Psychology, DOI 10.1007/978-3-319-18057-1_4 to acknowledge that people may have different acculturation levels to the dominant perspectives found in a society and these differences may result in conflicts, confusion, and stress that is not evident to the individual (Trinh, Rho, Lu, & Sanders, 2009). In counseling and psychotherapy it is important to assess the acculturation level of clients, and how they relate to the dominant cultural system(s). This chapter will provide an overview of acculturation in general, its relationship to cultural/ethnic identity, and how to use the concept in counseling and psychotherapy.

Rationale for Incorporating Assessment of Acculturation

Over 175 million people live outside their country of origin (Poston, 2001). According to the National Center for Education Statistics (2013) statistics for the USA are quite impressive: 12 % of residents were born in another nation, as was 14 % of the labor force. One-fifth of US newborns have at least one immigrant parent; about half of the students in New York, Los Angeles, Dallas, and other major cities speak a language other than English at home, as did 19 % (9.9 million) of all US school children in 2003, up from 9 % (3.8 million) in 1979. The numbers surpass all previous total figures, although the proportion of immigrants in the population peaked in 1910, when 15 % of US residents were born elsewhere. Marsella and Ring (2003) note that the global changes account for the unprecedented movements of individuals across the world in search of a better life The assumption is that the people who move and adapt to new settings, change (Suarez-Orozco & Suarez-Orozco, 2001). However, these are not the only people who change; change also occurs for the dominant culture, and for people who are colonized. Indigenous people are affected by contact with outsiders, and outsiders are affected by contact with local culture (Richman, Gaviria, Flaherty, Birz, & Wintrob, 1987).

Cultural competency (i.e., awareness, knowledge, and skills) in working with diverse clients is a requirement for all mental health professions (American Counseling Association (ACA), 1992; American Psychological Association (APA), 2002; American Association of Marriage and Family Therapy (AAMFT), 2012; National Association of Social Workers (NASW), 2008) and mandated by local, state, and federal agencies (Sue, Zane, Hall, & Berger, 2009). To meet the challenge of working ethically with culturally diverse clients, it is important to understand all factors that influence the lives of clients. Locke (1992) and Ramos (2005) note one such variable is acculturation level, and understanding to what extent a person has acquired and adapted to new cultural information as a result of contact with the values, behaviors, and institutions of the host culture is important in helping clients resolve the issues they bring to counseling (Locke, 1992). Furthermore, identity as originally conceptualized in the psychological literature was unidimensional; we need to go beyond hyphenated labels to understand the multidimensionalality of identity (Ibrahim, 2008).

Van de Vijver and Phalet (2004) note that most of the Western European countries that have had waves of migration from the Africa, Asia, Eastern Europe, and the Middle East are no longer monolithic cultures, and are now multicultural societies. They note that several researchers are studying the issue of intercultural contact; however, this would imply that both parties in the encounter are equal, and this is not the case, because the dominant population is much more powerful than the immigrants, and therefore they are not interacting as equals, in a true multicultural society, there would be no social and cultural hierarchies. Previously, assimilation was the model that was considered healthy and immigrants were asked to modify their behavior, attitude, and assumptions to fit in with the host culture. However, this trend has been reversed given the negative outcome for immigrants who were asked to give up their identities to take on the assumptions of the host culture to negotiate their daily life; giving up one's primary socialized identity is not possible and leading a double life or living in two world and crossing borders between home and majority culture, leads to severe psychological distress, leading to drug and alcohol abuse, and mental illness. Van de Vijver and Phalet note that immigrants are choosing other options; they are choosing to retain critical components of their own culture, e.g., in the US Latino/a population has gained a place for themselves in the dominant US society due to their sheer numbers, and have established culturally vital institutions to sustain their culture and identity.

Acculturation

The earliest definition of acculturation was offered by Redfield, Linton, and Herskovits (1936) "Acculturation comprehends those phenomena, which result when groups of individuals having different cultures come into continuous first-hand contact, with subsequent changes in the original cultural patterns of either or both groups" (p. 149). Graves (1967) coined the term *psychological acculturation* to describe the process an individual goes through as a result of acculturation or adaptation to a new cultural setting. Szapocznik, Scopetta, Kurtines, and Aranalde (1978) elaborated on the concept of psychological acculturation by identifying that change occurs along two dimensions: behavioral (language, ad participation in cultural activities) and values (relational style, beliefs about human nature, nature, and time orientation). Padilla (1980) added cultural awareness of host culture, and ethnic loyalty to the concept of acculturation. Berry (1980) identified six dimensions of psychological functioning directly affected by acculturation; these include (a) language, (b) cognitive styles, (c) personality, (d) identity, (e) attitudes, and (f) acculturative stress. These functions are affected at different rates and times, all changes do not occur simultaneously (Birman & Trickett, 2001; Birman, Trickett, & Vinokurov, 2002). Cuéllar, Arnold, and Maldonado (1995) defined acculturation in terms of change at three levels: behavior, affect, and cognitions. Change can be positive or negative, and there are marked differences in acculturation based on mobility, permanence, context, and voluntariness. Involuntary acculturation occurs with refugees and asylum seekers, and indigenous populations who are forced to have contact with others. A key component of efforts to negotiate various cultural contexts is *acculturative stress* (Berry, Kim, Minde, & Mok, 1987). Whether migration is voluntary or involuntary, there is stress related to change, adaptation, and adjustment. In addition, acculturative stress is higher when the two cultural contexts are incompatible, or very different.

Although ethnic identity is an important part of the acculturation process, Liebkind (2001) notes that the distinctions between the constructs of acculturation and ethnic identity are not clear, and sometimes they are used interchangeably. Acculturation, however, is a broader construct, given that it encompasses a much wider range of behaviors that change with intercultural contact (Phinney, 1998). Ethnic identity is a person's sense of self, as a member of an ethnic group (Liebkind, 1992). Similar to culture, ethnic identity is dynamic and mediated by developmental phases, and contextual variables (Marcia, Waterman, Matteson, Archer, & Orlofsky, 1993). The concept of acculturation has been applied to both immigrant and nonimmigrant cultural groups (Pope-Davis, Liu, Ledesma-Jones, & Nevitt, 2000; Saxton, 2001; Suleiman, 2002). Ethnic nondominant groups deal with acculturation challenges in negotiating everyday life, and adhering to the cultural assumptions of the dominant group. According to Schwartz, Montgomery, and Briones (2006) the process of acculturation is different for nonimmigrants from what immigrants and refugees experience.

Several research studies show marked acculturation changes occur over generations in a host culture, both at the individual and group levels (Phinney, 1990; Segall, Dasen, Berry, & Poortinga, 1999). Padilla (1980) believes adherence to culture of origin cultural values is the key to understanding acculturation status. Original research on acculturation focused on understanding the experiences and changes in immigrants. It was assumed that in an effort to reduce acculturative stress, people who migrated adapted to new cultural contexts (Trimble, 2001). However this adaptation varies based on age, allegiance to culture of origin, identity formulation, and desire or need to adapt to a new setting, along with how people are received in the host culture (Dahlberg, 1998; Verkuyten, 2003).

The key to understanding multiple identities in a culturally diverse society is to understand acculturation level of clients to mainstream culture, along with cultural identity, ethnic identity, and worldview (Ibrahim & Heuer, 2013; Phinney, 1992; Van de Vijver & Phalet, 2004). Researchers have noted psychosocial changes in ethnic identity as individuals negotiate the psychosocial developmental tasks in a new setting, as identified by Erikson's developmental theory of psychosocial stages (Erikson, 1993; Hertz, 1988). In addition, the acculturation process also relates to the concept of "achieved identity status a similar process to coming into one's ethnic/racial identity" (Cross, 1995; Helms, 1990). Phinney (1990) notes that nondominant ethnic identity is retained much longer over time and generations due to external forces that continue to label the individual as a "hyphenated American." This leads to feelings of marginalization, exclusion, and stigma, which interferes with acculturation to host or dominant culture.

Similar marginalization also influences the acculturation of African Americans, along with a social stratification and poverty (Landrine & Klonoff, 1996). Discrimination and prejudice are additional factors that influence socialization of most hyphenated Americans. Parents from nondominant cultural groups work on empowering their children to negate the effect of racism, prejudice, and exclusion, by teaching them about the politics of race and giving them knowledge and skills to contradict racist assumptions, to prevent internalization of negative societal assumptions (Chun & Akutsu 2003).

Given the diversity among Latino/as and Asian cultures, it is difficult to arrive at definitive conclusions; however, core cultural values tend to be preserved across Asian and Latino cultures (Edgerton & Karno, 1971; Negy & Woods, 1992). Greater acculturation in both groups leads to increased conflict in families, especially among couples, and parent–child dyads (Szapocznik & Kurtines, 1980; Tang & Dion, 1999). Acculturation among women in both these groups leads to moving beyond traditional gender roles to more egalitarian roles (Leaper & Valin, 1996; Rosenthal, Rainieri, & Klimdis, 1996; Tang & Dion, 1999). For Native American families, LaFromboise, Trimble, and Mohatt (1990) proposed four types of acculturation categories: Traditional, transitional (have characteristics of both systems, but do not identify with either), bicultural, and assimilated (this type is most rewarded in US society, however, it creates the greatest amount of alienation from self and society). Asian Americans are a very diverse cultural groups and it is difficult to categorize acculturation levels due to vast variations among the groups (Lee & Zane, 1998). Although certain core cultural values tend to be retained and perpetuated through generations, with the impact lessening over several generations.

Acculturation: Conceptual Approaches

Berry (2001) notes that although the study of acculturation is a key domain of cross-cultural psychology, there are several perspectives on how it should be conceptualized and measured. Several researchers agree on the difficulties with assessing acculturation because of a lack of consistency in indicators and across the scales, and sometimes within a scale (Chun & Akutsu, 2003; Kim & Abreu, 2001). In measuring acculturation there is the issue of cognitive or behavioral acculturation, along with the dynamic nature of acculturation, and the question arises, do static tools have the capacity to evaluate ongoing change (Zane & Mak, 2003). There are two critical perspectives that appear to be at the core of the confusion and these relate to: (a) if acculturation affects all groups that come in contact and (b) is acculturation unidimensional/unidirectional or multidimensional. Berry offers to establish some common ground among the various perspectives on acculturation to help researchers advance the research on acculturation.

Berry (2001) notes that acculturation has been studied from both cultural and a psychological perspectives. Further, he discriminates between attitudinal and behavioral adherence to culture of origin values and assumptions. He proceeds to link both these two perspectives to create a framework for future research. The model reviews culture and how change occurs when two cultures come in contact. Berry asserts that one must know the cultures involved very well to be able to calibrate and assess change. At the psychological level, he considers how individuals change, adapt, and experience acculturative stress. In conceptualizing acculturation, Berry identifies dimensionality as a key factor and notes that the debate about directionality and dimensionality needs to identify how assessment of acculturation can be done.

Berry (1997) contends that competing cultural frameworks need not result in an identity crisis or conflict. He states that there are four outcomes to acculturative stress, these are: (a) integration, resulting in both change and maintenance; (b) assimilation, implies adoption of a new identity; (c) separation, is opting for maintenance of the original cultural identity, exclusively; and (d) marginalization, where there is neither cultural identity maintenance nor adaptation to new culture. Berry maintains that the best outcome for people who move across cultures or live in a society with a dominant cultural system is integration or a bicultural identity. Research on Berry's model and the importance of integration has been challenged by Rudmin (2006); he notes that it is a shared belief by researchers that this is the best mode of acculturation; however, analysis of the research conducted by the same researchers who present this hypothesis does not support this perspective.

Sociologists have expressed similar concerns and questions, such as, when is each trajectory followed, by whom, and why? All agree that the process is "multidimensional and multidirectional" and the melting pot metaphor no longer applies (Rumbaut, 2005). Berry proposes using attitudinal dimensions that have a yes/no response format will help identify the four acculturative strategies, i.e., assimilation, separation, integration, and marginalization. He further notes that integration and separation are collectivistic, and assimilation is individualistic. Additionally, he notes that separation when required by the dominant culture is segregation; when marginalization is imposed, it is exclusion.

Poston (2001) provides three conceptual models to understand acculturation; these include (a) Psychological models of stress and coping, (b) culture-learning models derived from the social psychology of intercultural encounters, and (c) social identification theories from research on intergroup relations. Psychological models of stress and coping view cross-cultural adaptation resulting from the stress encountered due to transitions and the coping responses that people use to adapt to a new environment. The main explanatory model is called culture shock and the U-curve, which explains adaptation occurring over an 18-month period after relocation. At the point of entry at the top of the U-curve, there is excitement, and positive expectations about the new culture; however, it soon turns to stress, due to the adaptation and learning in a new setting, and at the 9-month point turns to despair, homesickness, and loneliness. However as culture shock sets in, they lose their initial excitement and begin to recognize that the change is stressful, as people are confronted with new rules, and new expectations that they were not aware of, and as the stress builds, optimism fades, the lowest point is at the base of the U, and then as they adapt and learn new rules, and adjust, they start to move up to moderate to low stress, and eventually achieve equilibrium.

According to this model, people who come from highly stressful or trauma situations such as wars and refugee camps are the most disadvantaged as they have few resources to deal with culture shock and stress of adaptation. This model can also explain the chronic stressors experienced by indigenous people, such as deprivation, and changes due to the arrival of others in their world who set the rules, such as colonizers. Developmentally, adolescents and older adults experience the highest stress levels. The most important resource is social support for people going through adaptation to a new culture, or a new system. Not all social support is considered beneficial, it depends on the client's culture and specific situation, which determines who can provide the most beneficial support. Research on this model has reviewed mental and physical health separately; however, the results show that the results are similar on both indices.

Acculturative stress and mental health data for the nondominant cultural group of the USA and acculturation data tends to be inconsistent across cultural groups. Primary stressors appear to be colonization (Native Americans, Latino/a, and Puerto Ricans), due to systematic oppression by the government involving exclusion and racism. African Americans have the highest rate of depression and mental illness compared to Whites and Mexican Americans; this is consistent with the sociopolitical history of their experience in the USA (Landrine & Klonoff, 2002). For US born Latino/as, acculturation was associated with higher rate of mental health issues (Portes & Zhou, 1993).

The Culture Learning model emphasizes learning new skills to adapt rapidly to a new situation. Ward and Rana-Deuba (1999) note that sociocultural adaptation is the key to adjustment to a new situation, and refer to it as the ability to fit into, or negotiate aspects of the new environment by interacting with it. For most clients coming to counseling with social-emotional problems, it is important to query about time in the new environment, because more than likely they are dealing with acculturation issues, and they need to reduce the stress by learning culturally appropriate skills to manage interactions with the new sociocultural environment. There are several techniques and strategies available to build intercultural skills from intercultural training resources (Byram, Barrett, Ipgrave, Jackson, & Mendez Garcia, 2009; Deardorff, 2006; Spitzberg & Changnon, 2009).

Social identity theory does not rely on one theory to understand acculturation. It combines several theories and models to address both individual level analysis of cultural or ethnic identity and group level analysis of intergroup perceptions and relations. Theories focusing on ethnic identity include Phinney's (1990) ethnic identity theory, Tafel's (1981) social identity theory, Stephan and Stephan's (2000) integrated threat theory, and Esses, Jackson, and Armstrong's (1998) instrumental model of group conflict.

Baumeister (1986) believes that identity conflict is the result of an inner struggle. It requires individuals to choose between two or more different identities that may prescribe incompatible behaviors and commitments. Phinney (1990) notes that ethnic identity is a dynamic multidimensional construct that refers to a sense of self in the context of a larger social system. She conceives of identity as dynamic, it is modified over time, and through generations. Modification also occurs as individuals become aware of differences among ethnic groups around them. Change is the critical factor in understanding both ethnic identity and acculturation. For people who relocate to new cultures and specifically for ethnocultural nondominant group members, the conflict between their heritage culture, and the normative culture of the larger social system is the challenge, as they present contradictory cultural assumptions (Thompson, Lightfoot, Castillo, & Hurst, 2010).

Schwartz, Montgomery, and Briones (2006) addressed the theoretical relationship between acculturation and identity, they note that acculturation results in changes in cultural identity, however, personal identity serves as an anchor for immigrants, as they adapt to a new cultural context. They note that nonimmigrant cultural groups also face acculturation challenges; because the majority group subjects them to pressures to adapt to dominant cultural assumptions, within their own country (Pope-Davis et al., 2000; Saxton, 2001; Suleiman, 2002). Schwartz (2001) considers identity a synthesis of personal, social, and cultural self-conceptions. Personal identity refers to goals, values, and beliefs (Schwartz (2001)); social identity is composed of the group one identifies with, and self-identified ideals, mores, conventions, and labels; and the extent to which this leads to identification with a specific group and perceives other groups as outgroups (Erikson, 1968; Tajfel & Turner, 1986). Schwartz considers cultural identity as a special case of social identity (Padilla & Perez, 2003), which refers to the interface between the person and the cultural context (Bhatia & Ram, 2001). The purpose of identity is to work as a self-regulatory, social-psychological mechanism (Adams & Marshall, 1996). Identity evolves as a result of one of two processes: (a) imitation and identification prevalent in collectivistic cultures or (b) exploration, construction, and experience in individualistic cultures (Serafini & Adams, 2002). Schwartz et al. note that acculturation leads to changes in cultural identity; cultural identity may be similar to ethnic identity, but conceptually it is much broader (Jensen, 2003).

Changing Assumptions

Considering Berry's acculturation model, in essence there are two choices for an immigrant, one, to adapt to host culture and two, to maintain their culture of origin (Berry & Sam, 1997). Van de Vijver and Phalet (2004) note that research conducted in Belgium and the Netherlands shows that immigrants want to combine their primary culture with the dominant mainstream culture (Phalet & Hagendoorn, 1996; Phalet, Van Lotringen, & Entzinger, 2000; Van de Vijver, Helms-Lorenz, & Feltzer, 1999). Acculturation also occurs both with respect to the new culture and culture of origin (Trickett, Ryerson Espino, & Persky, 2006). Persky and Birman (2005) note that there are a multitude of possibilities and multiple cultural identities are possible instead of assuming that there are only a couple of possibilities. If immigrants choose to retain their own culture exclusively, this is identified as separation, or segregation, it implies that they are not willing to relate to host culture and that the host culture is not important to them. The opposite strategy is to assimilate to the host culture and lose the original culture; this mode eventually leads to psychological damage and distress (LaFromboise et al., 1990; Phinney, 1990). The original unilinear model of acculturation offered by Gordon (1964) maintains that assimilation is the only option for immigrants. The last acculturation category is marginalization, which Van de Vijver and Phalet (2004) maintain is rare, results in not feeling connected to culture of origin, or the host culture. Rudmin (2006) presents data that the measurement strategies used in several of the studies on Berry's model of acculturation were faulty; therefore, Berry's theory needs to be researched with better instruments.

Van de Vijver and Phalet (2004) agree that there is a need to identify appropriate assessment strategies for pluralistic societies that have had a huge influx of immigrants or have a dominant cultural group and several nondominant cultural groups. They question that any available test would be appropriate, and this is a challenge for mental health service delivery. They also note that it is unfortunate that assessment of acculturation is not a component of assessment strategy used for all cultural (dominant and nondominant) groups in pluralistic society. We believe assessment of acculturation is critical to service delivery as it helps in understanding the person-environment fit, and allows for empowerment, advocacy, and skill building in counseling and psychotherapy leading to adjustment and a sense of well-being.

Psychological Well-Being and Acculturation

Some researchers have posited that psychological well-being and acculturation are associated (Phinney, 1990; Rogler, Cortes, & Malgady, 1991; Suinn, Richard-Figueora, Lew, & Vigil, 1987). Coping with acculturative stress and subsequent adaptation is influenced by a number of factors, at both personal and social levels (Berry, 1997; Ward & Kennedy, 1994). These factors include personal (personality, self-esteem, cognitive style) and environmental variables (social, cultural, and political). According to researchers, bicultural or integration acculturation style is the most positive mode for immigrants and for ethnic nondominant group members (Birman, 1998; de Domanico, Crawford, & De Wolfe, 1994; Donà & Berry, 1994; Ward & Rana-Deuba, 1999). Except with Native Americans and Latino/as this caused the greatest level of stress (Berry, 1997; Eyou, Adair, & Dixon, 2000; LaFromboise et al., 1990; Murray & Lopez, 1996; Ramos, 2005; Verkuyten & Kwa, 1994; Ward & Rana-Deuba, 1999). Marginalization and separation are associated with high levels of acculturative stress, assimilation is considered to have an intermediate level of stress. Psychological adjustment and well-being has been assessed from the perspective of stability of self-concept and happiness (Verkuyten & Kwa, 1994; Yasuda & Duan, 2002; Zheng, Sang, & Wang, 2004), and psychosocial functioning (de Domanico et al., 1994; Eyou et al., 2000; Haritatos & Benet-Martinez, 2002; Lang, Muñoz, Bernal, & Sorensen, 1982; Verkuyten & Kwa, 1994).

Ward and Rana-Deuba (1999) recommend a distinction between psychological and sociological adjustment; according to them, psychological adjustment is associated with emotional well-being, focusing on stress and coping, and sociocultural adjustment pertaining to negotiating and interacting with the host or mainstream culture, essentially, social learning. Ward (1996) indicates that although, these two processes are interrelated, they are conceptually distinct. Research shows that the two processes can be predicted from different variables, psychological adjustment is considered in terms of depression, or mood disorders, which are related to personality and developmental changes over the life-span; whereas sociocultural adjustment is evaluated from the perspective of length of residence, cultural distance, language ability, and degree of contact with host or mainstream culture (Searle & Ward, 1990; Stone Feinstein & Ward, 1990; Ward & Kennedy, 1992; Ward & Searle, 1991). Another reason for differentiating these two processes is the fact that sociocultural issues and concerns level off over time; however, psychological problems are more variable over time (Ward, Okura, Kennedy, & Kojima, 1998). Considering Schwartz et al.'s (2006) notion of personal, social, and cultural identities, it is possible that a coherent personal identity would have favorable psychological outcomes than a less coherent personal identity. Schwartz (2001) notes that Erikson (1950) maintains that a certain level of identity confusion is adaptive, because a person with too much certainty about his or her personal identity may be closed-off and rigid. According to Stephen, Fraser, and Marcia (1992) an adaptive identity evolves over the life-span and cannot be complete at adolescence. Therefore acculturation outcomes vary based on who is migrating to what context, and how valued the individual's cultural group is in the new context. The evolution of identity depends on negotiation with the context, and how people are received or perceived.

Psychological Assessment: Conceptual and Methodological Issues

Lonner and Ibrahim (2008) have addressed the difficulties in using psychological assessments that may not be relevant to the client's cultural context. They note that before assessments are conducted, it is important to understand the client's cultural context and socialization. Although, this is difficult given dominant and nondominant populations. People within a culture may share several cultural assumptions, but this does not imply that the instruments are valid for everyone in a specific context. The problems inherent in assessment in culturally pluralistic are the effects of social hierarchies, along with discrimination and exclusion, which cannot be calibrated using the current assessment tools for acculturation.

Lonner and Ibrahim (2008) and Van de Vijver and Phalet (2004) have identified several methodological issues in assessing acculturation with nondominant populations, given that there may not be adequate commonality between mainstream soci ety and its assumptions, and subcultures in a given society. They list the following: conceptual or construct bias (a construct that may not apply across cultures); method bias (sample not comparable); and item bias (anomalies at the item level), this can be particular problem when people are at varying levels of dominant culture language proficiency (Van der Maesen de Sombreff & Abell, 2001).

In psychological assessment, another confounding factor is social desirability, which also results in method bias, either in the direction of "ethnic affirmation" (direction of the primary group) or "social correction" towards the norms of the dominant group (Triandis, Kashima, Shimada, & Villareal, 1986). The degree of social desirability depends on both the acculturation level of the respondent and also the social cues that a situation may evoke (Georgas & Kalantzi-Azizi, 1992). There are additional concerns about equivalence of unit of measurement and scalar equivalence or full score comparability. Van de Vijver and Leung (1997) have proposed ways to handle these issues; however, arriving at reliable and valid results is difficult. Doucerain, Dere, and Ryder (2013) maintain current research on acculturation provides incomplete information on the psychological changes that take place in multicultural societies, both at individual and group levels.

Given the issues inherent in using standardized psychological assessments across cultures, it may be useful to use qualitative assessments to understand client acculturation level for the purpose of counseling. If culturally sensitive instruments were available, these would be preferred; however, with the level of variation within and between cultures, it is important to have some methods to understand acculturation. An additional concern is the rate at which change occurs during acculturation, as evidenced by research on immigrants resulting in method bias (Marin, Gamba, & Marin, 1992). To understand the meaningfulness of client-specific cultural constructs and how clients construe the world, especially with varying acculturative status, variables such as acculturation are important for the purpose of providing culture-specific counseling interventions. Carr, Marsella, and Purcell (2002) note interest in qualitative methods has increased in recent years, because the goal is to study life in its true context. This is obviously very important in counseling because the goal is to understand the client and provide the most culturally responsive services. Several cultural psychologists have supported the use of qualitative approaches to understand client-specific information (Neimeyer, 1993; Raskin, 2002; Shweder et al., 2007; Wertsch, 1991).

Assessment of Acculturation

Currently several instruments are available to assess acculturation; however, some have been developed for specific populations. Few can address the changing dynamic of acculturation among immigrants, sojourners, and nondominant populations within a multicultural society (Van de Vijver & Phalet, 2004). Kang (1996) reviewed acculturation scale formats and language competence, and noted that features found in bidimensional acculturation instruments create strong inverse relationships between the two cultural orientations (host and original cultures). Trickett, Persky, and Ryerson Espino (2002) share this concern and note "proxy variables" used to assess acculturation, i.e., group data to understand the multidimensional nature of individual identity does not provide meaningful data. In addition, there is evidence that the concept of acculturation is a "black box" that it does not take into account unequal access for individuals in hierarchical societies, and in essence tends to blames the victim (Escobar & Vega, 2000; Hunt, Schneider, & Comer, 2004).

Berry and Sabatier (2010) summarized the three approaches available for assessing acculturation attitudes; these are: (a) development of four individual scales for the four acculturation outcomes (Berry et al., 1987; Bourhis, Moise, Perreault, & Senecal, 1997). This approach provides four independent scores, although the four attitudes are not independent (Rudmin & Ahmadzadeh, 2001; Unger et al., 2002); (b) creating vignettes to assess the four acculturation outcomes, and to have participants respond to the vignettes to help identify the acculturation attitude (Van Oudenhoven, 2006); and (c) assessment of acculturation on the two underlying dimensions, ethnic or national culture orientation (Donà & Berry, 1994; Sabatier & Berry, 1994; Ward & Kennedy, 1994). In the third approach, scores on the two dimensions are split, into high or low on the two dimensions, and classified into the four acculturation modes based on the scores. Berry and Sabatier note there is a risk of losing information in this approach; however, cross-validation can be done using other measures. Several reviews of measures for acculturation are available in the research literature, outlining the domains assessed, outcomes to expect, and reliability and validity. These include Arends-Tóth and Van de Vijver (2008), Celenk and Van de Vijver (2011), Kang (1996), Taras (2013), and Zane and Mak (2003). Although several studies have been conducted to identify the best approach to (a) understand what acculturation means and (b) what is the best mode of acculturation, it appears the field is rife with confounding items, statistical errors, and a shared belief that bicultural or integration is the best model (Rudmin, 2006). In spite of data challenging the assumption that integration is the best mode, especially for US nondominant cultural groups (LaFromboise, Trimble, & Mohatt, 1990; Murray & Lopez, 1996; Ramos, 2005). Rudmin (2003) notes that in the case of cultural similarity, a bicultural approach may not be overly difficult, but in situations where acculturation to a culture that's quite different (e.g., when the heritage culture is primarily collectivist and the receiving culture is primarily individualist), a bicultural attitude may be not only difficult but also distressing.

Our approach is to use an individualism/collectivism continuum to assess acculturation level, by comparing client acculturation attitude to the overarching cultural paradigm prevalent in the USA, as identified by Takaki (1989). Green, Deschamps, and Paez (2005) state that individualism and collectivism are the most popular, theoretically, and empirically sound concepts in cross-cultural psychology. Individualism and collectivism are complex constructs and have both been defined in several ways (Bellah, Madsen, Sullivan, Swidler, & Tipton, 1985; Hofstede, 2001; Kagitçibasi, 1997; Markus & Kitayama, 1991; Triandis, 1995, 1996). Typically, individualism is attributed to the following characteristics: independence, self-reliance, autonomy, achievement, and competition. Individual socialization emphasizes control over and taking responsibility for one's actions. Collectivism is associated with a sense of duty toward the primary group, interdependence and harmony in relationships, close and extended family, and conformity with group norms. Green, Dechamps, and Paez note that people can have both individual and collectivistic characteristics; these two attitudes are not mutually exclusive.

With the prevalent diversity in the USA, a significant stressor for cultural nondominant and vulnerable cultural groups is because of the hidden dimensions of the culture as they negotiate their life, work, and relationships (Landrine & Klonoff,

1996; Thompson et al., 2010). There is an assumption that everyone is aware of the overarching national and mainstream culture, their origins, and structures. However, this is not the case for everyone. As Takaki (1979) explains, the culture established in the USA by the founding fathers, reflects White Anglo Saxon male perspectives designed to create an ideal nation, and an example for the world. This is the superordinate culture that is institutionalized through the public schools, and the values and beliefs that are inculcated are highly individualistic. The unacknowledged indigenous cultures of the USA, Native and Chicano/a or Latino/a were not part of this formulation. The indigenous people of the Americas are collectivistic. The first two waves of migration were from Europe, and although, many came from collectivistic cultural systems (Eastern, Central, and Southern Europe and several groups were Catholics, i.e., collectivistic), the assimilation model of acculturation was imposed and the immigrants were asked to abandon their culture of origin, and give up their language, and embrace US cultural assumptions, i.e., White Anglo-Saxon Protestant and male (Davidson, Pyle, & Reyes, 1995; Weaver, 1999).

Several cultural oppressions have resulted from requiring assimilation, primarily loss of identity, or going underground and posing as someone else, is a good example of the "Imposter phenomenon" (Clance, 1985; Matthews & Clance, 1985). As noted in the research literature, assimilation, or trying to "pass," results in several negative mental health problems, e.g., perfectionism and several stress-related, and anxiety disorders (Cokley, McClain, Enciso, & Martinez, 2013; Henning, Ey, & Shaw, 1998; Thompson et al., 2010). Current research links acculturation and maladjustment, to psychopathology, and substance use (Al-Issa & Tousignant, 1997; Delgado Bernal, 1998; Gil, Wagner, & Vega, 2000; Ramos, 2005; Robinson & Goodpaster, 1991; Rogler et al., 1991; Smokowski, Rose, & Bacallao, 2008; Szapocznik & Kurtines, 1980; Vega & Gil, 1998). When highly acculturated Latino/a are compared to their less acculturated peers they display higher levels of alcohol use, less consumption of balanced, healthy meals, and more consumption of marijuana, cocaine, or both (Goel, McCarthy, Phillips, & Wee, 2004; Marks, Garcia, & Solts, 1990; Vega, Kolody, Valle, & Weir, 1991).

We believe, aligning the information gained from Ibrahim's (2008; Appendix C) US Acculturation Index© with cultural identity, worldview, and privilege and oppression information, we can begin to understand both endogenous and exogenous factors, that are important to understand client assumptions, stressors, and their relationship to the presenting problem. We believe it is important to listen to the client's narrative to corroborate the information gathered from the cultural assessments. There is limited recognition of the importance of acculturation in counseling and psychotherapy. Although several studies exist on acculturation and its outcomes, both positive and negative, there is limited discourse regarding counseling interventions, and the complex dynamics of the presenting problem, social justice, and cultural responsiveness in the therapeutic process. The focus on social justice and cultural responsiveness expands theoretical statements on cultural competence. We believe, abstract statements about competence do not provide the specific tools to implement strategies to empower clients, addressing the client's complex multidimensional identity, separating out intrapsychic, and extrapsychic factors that are embedded in the presenting problem is the key to effective practice.

Counseling Implications

Acculturation information can help in designing interventions by incorporating information about what the client needs beyond solving the presenting problem. A multisystemic approach is needed to address the concerns presented. Once the distance between the client's acculturation level and mainstream or dominant societal culture is identified, incorporation of bicultural skills and strategies, along with self-advocacy skills would be useful. Psychological well-being is greatly enhanced if a sense of self-efficacy is inculcated, along with a strong support system. Establishing the client's support system begins with identifying people in the client's world, and agencies that can help support and advocate for the client and assist in maintenance of the bicultural strategies learned in counseling, and by reinforcing and empowering clients in the real world. The critical task in helping clients function effectively in a culturally dissimilar environment is to help them understand the distance between their assumptions and the systems they are living in, an intervention such as Bicultural Effectiveness Training (BET) would be helpful (Szapocznik et al., 1986). BET emphasizes making cultural assumptions explicit for the client about his or her culture and the cultural environment. Lack of understanding of the larger cultural context, whether it is mainstream USA, or a host culture leads to breakdowns in communication and connection. Carrera (2013) reports that BET served as a mediator in empowering Latina/o college students, it gave them cultural knowledge and communication skills and enhanced psychological well-being.

Lafromboise, Coleman, and Gerton (1993) present an alternative model emphasizing biculturalism, and note that it is most effective, because it is comprehensive and reduces the stress and anxiety of negotiating two cultures. This model enhances bicultural competence along six dimensions: (a) knowledge of cultural beliefs and values, (b) positive attitudes toward both groups, (c) bicultural efficacy, (d) communication ability, (e) role repertoire, i.e., appropriate behavior in both settings, and (f) social groundedness, i.e., social networks in both settings. This model emphasizes that individuals who are biculturally competent, have the ability to have a satisfactory and meaningful life, both within the primary familial and cultural group, and mainstream or dominant culture, without sacrificing without having to give up their cultural identity. Lafromboise, and colleagues note that people who are biculturally competent may have higher cognitive functioning and sense of well-being than monocultural individuals. Research supports this contention, regarding cognitive functioning (Benet-Martınez, Leu, Lee, & Morris, 2002; Haritatos & Benet-Martinez, 2002), social development (Padilla, 2006), and adjustment (Lang et al., 1982; López & Contreras, 2005).

Schwartz et al. (2006) state that aspects of personal identity that are independent of cultural factors can stabilize a person in culturally inconsistent setting by reducing distress created by the acculturation experience. They used Erikson's (1980) distinction between personal and social identity as the framework for their assumptions. However, Schwartz, Montgomery, and Briones in their conceptualization separated personal identity from social identity; noting that social identity interacts with the social-cultural world and changes in acculturation occur at this level. They note that interventions at the personal identity level need to support personal identity, developmental changes, and reinforce self-efficacy, to buffer the destabilizing effects of interacting with new cultural environments; especially, if the environment is culturally unsupportive (Dahlberg, 1998). Immigrant and nondominant cultural group youth are at risk for negative outcomes in rejecting cultural contexts, and enhancing their bicultural communication and cultural knowledge and skills would be an effective intervention. This information will help youth to decide how to adapt their cultural identities, while maintaining their personal identities in dealing with unaccommodating contexts, such as poverty, lack of access to supportive social institutions, and discrimination. Their focus is on creating a smooth and positive trajectory to adulthood.

Conclusion

This chapter reviewed conceptual theories of acculturation, and the current assessments to measure acculturation. It addressed the concerns and biases inherent in acculturation assessments, especially in cross-cultural measurement. The chapter attempted to consider both immigrant and nondominant cultural groups experiences including the effect on their mental health due to discrimination, exclusion, and the stress of negotiating cultural environments with inconsistent cultural assumptions from their primary culture. Recommendations for enhancing bicultural knowledge and skills were provided. The next chapter will address issues of privilege and power, and review social justice advocacy, knowledge and skills to empower clients.

References

Adams, G. R., & Marshall, S. K. (1996). A developmental social psychology of identity: Understanding the person-in-context. *Journal of Adolescence, 19*, 429–442.

Al-Issa, I., & Tousignant, M. (Eds.). (1997). *Ethnicity, immigration, and psychopathology*. New York: Springer Science+Business Media.

American Association of Marriage and Family Therapy (AAMFT). (2012). *Code of ethics*. Alexandria, VA: American Association of Marriage and Family Therapy.

American Counseling Association (ACA). (1992). *Multicultural competencies*. Alexandria, VA: American Counseling Association.

American Psychological Association (APA). (2002). *Guidelines on multicultural education, training, research, practice, and organizational change for psychologists*. Washington, DC: American Psychological Association.

Arends-Tóth, J., & Van de Vijver, F. J. R. (2008). Family relationships among immigrants and majority members in the Netherlands. *Applied Psychology, 57*, 466–487. doi:10.1111/j.1464-0597.2008.00331.x.

Baumeister, R. F. (1986). *Identity: Cultural change and the struggle for self*. New York: Oxford University Press.

Bellah, R. N., Madsen, R., Sullivan, W. M., Swidler, A., & Tipton, S. M. (1985). *Habits of the heart: Individualism and commitment in American life*. Berkeley, CA: University of California Press.

Benet-Martınez, V., Leu, J., Lee, F., & Morris, M. (2002). Negotiating biculturalism: Cultural frame-switching in biculturals with oppositional vs., compatible cultural identities. *Journal of Cross-Cultural Psychology, 33*, 492–516.

Berry, J. W. (1980). Acculturation as varieties of adaptation. In A. Padilla (Ed.), *Acculturation: Theory, models and some new findings* (pp. 9–25). Boulder, CO: Westview.

Berry, J. W., Kim, U., Minde, T., & Mok, D. (1987). Comparative studies of acculturative stress. *International Migration Review, 21*, 491–511.

Berry, J. W. (1997). Immigration, acculturation, and adaptation. *Applied Psychology, 46*(1), 5–34. Retrieved from http://dx.doi.org/10.1111/j.1464-0597.1997.tb01087.x.

Berry, J. W. (2001). A psychology of immigration. *Journal of Social Issues, 57*, 615–631.

Berry, J. W., Kim, U., Minde, T., & Mok, D. (1987). Comparative studies of acculturative stress. *International Migration Review, 21*, 491–511.

Berry, J. W., & Sabatier, C. (2010). Acculturation, discrimination, and adaptation among second generation immigrant youth in Montreal and Paris. *International Journal of Intercultural Relations, 34*(3), 191–207.

Berry, J. W., & Sam, D. (1997). Acculturation and adaptation. In J. W. Berry, M. H. Segall, & C. Kagitçibasi (Eds.), *Handbook of cross-cultural psychology* (2nd ed., Vol. 3, pp. 291–326). Boston: Allyn & Bacon.

Bhatia, S., & Ram, A. (2001). Rethinking 'acculturation' in relation to diasporic cultures and post-colonial identities. *Human Development, 44*, 1–18.

Birman, D. (1998). Biculturalism and perceived competence of Latino immigrant adolescents. *American Journal of Community Psychology, 26*(3), 335–354.

Birman, D., & Trickett, E. J. (2001). Cultural transitions in first-generation immigrants: Acculturation of Soviet Jewish refugee adolescents and parents. *Journal of Cross-Cultural Psychology, 32*(4), 456–477.

Birman, D., Trickett, E. J., & Vinokurov, A. (2002). Acculturation and adaptation of Soviet Jewish refugee adolescents: Predictors of adjustment across life domains. *American Journal of Community Psychology, 30*(5), 585–607.

Bourhis, R. Y., Moise, L. C., Perreault, S., & Senecal, S. (1997). Towards an interactive acculturation model: A social psychological approach. *International Journal of Psychology, 32*(6), 369–386.

Byram, M., Barrett, M., Ipgrave, J., Jackson, R., & Mendez Garcia, M. (2009). *Autobiography of intercultural encounters*. Council of Europe, Language Policy Division. Retrieved from www.coe.int/lang

Carr, S. C., Marsella, A. J., & Purcell, I. (2002). Researching intercultural relations: Towards a middle way. *Asian Psychologist, 3*(1), 58–64.

Celenk, O., & Van de Vijver, F. J. (2011). Assessment of acculturation: Issues and overview of measures. *Online Readings in Psychology and Culture, 8*(1), 10.

Chun, K. M., & Akutsu, P. D. (2003). Acculturation among ethnic minority families. In K. M. Chun, P. Balls-Organista, & G. Marin (Eds.), *Acculturation: Advances in theory, measurement, and applied research* (pp. 95–119). Washington, DC: American Psychological Association.

Clance, P. R. (1985). *The impostor phenomenon: When success makes you feel like a fake*. New York: Bantam Books.

Cokley, K., McClain, S., Enciso, A., & Martinez, M. (2013). An examination of the impact of minority status stress and impostor feelings on the mental health of diverse ethnic minority college students. *Journal of Multicultural Counseling and Development, 41*(2), 82–95.

Cross, W. M. (1995). The psychology of Nigrescence: Revising the Cross model. In J. G. Ponterotto, J. M. Casas, L. A. Suzuki, & C. M. Alexander (Eds.), *Handbook of multicultural counseling* (pp. 93–122). Thousand Oaks, CA: Sage.

Cuéllar, I., Arnold, B., & Maldonado, R. (1995). Acculturation Rating Scale for Mexican Americans-II: A revision of the original ARSMA scale. *Hispanic Journal of Behavioral Sciences, 17*, 275–304.

Davidson, J. D., Pyle, R. E., & Reyes, D. V. (1995). Persistence and change in the Protestant establishment, 1930–1992. *Social Forces, 74*(1), 157–175.

Dahlberg, L. L. (1998). Youth violence in the United States: Major trends, risk factors, and prevention approaches. *American Journal of Preventive Medicine, 14*, 259–272.

de Domanico, Y. B., Crawford, I., & De Wolfe, A. S. (1994). Ethnic identity and self-concept in Mexican-American adolescents: Is bicultural identity related to stress or better adjustment? *Child and Youth Care Forum, 23*(3), 197–206.

Deardorff, D. K. (2006). The identification and assessment of intercultural competence as a student outcome of internationalization at institutions of higher education in the United States. *Journal of Studies in International Education, 10*, 241–266.

Delgado Bernal, D. (1998). Using a Chicana feminist epistemology in educational research. *Harvard Educational Review, 68*(4), 10–22.

Donà, G., & Berry, J. W. (1994). Acculturation attitudes and acculturative stress of Central American refugees. *International Journal of Psychology, 29*, 57–70.

Doucerain, M., Dere, J., & Ryder, A. G. (2013). Travels in hyper-diversity: Multiculturalism and the contextual assessment of acculturation. *International Journal of Intercultural Relations, 37*(6), 686–699.

Edgerton, R. B., & Karno, M. (1971). Mexican-American bilingualism and the perception of mental illness. *Archives of General Psychiatry, 24*(3), 286–290. doi:10.1001/archpsyc.1971.01750090092014.

Erikson, E. H. (1950). *Childhood and society*. New York: Norton.

Erikson, E. H. (1968). *Identity: Youth and crisis*. New York: Norton.

Erikson, E. H. (1980). *Identity and the life cycle: A reissue*. New York: Norton.

Erikson, E. H. (1993). *Childhood and society*. New York: Norton (Original work published 1950).

Escobar, J. I., & Vega, W. A. (2000). Mental health and immigration's AAAs: Where are we and where do we go from here? *The Journal of Nervous and Mental Disease, 188*(11), 736–740.

Esses, V. M., Jackson, L. M., & Armstrong, T. L. (1998). Intergroup competition and attitudes toward immigrants and immigration: An instrumental model of group conflict. *Journal of Social Issues, 54*(4), 699–724.

Eyou, M. L., Adair, V., & Dixon, R. (2000). Cultural identity and psychological adjustment of adolescent Chinese immigrants in New Zealand. *Journal of Adolescence, 23*(5), 531–543.

Georgas, J., & Kalantzi-Azizi, A. (1992). Value acculturation and response tendencies of biethnic adolescents. *Journal of Cross-Cultural Psychology, 23*, 228–239.

Gil, A., Wagner, E., & Vega, W. (2000). Acculturation, familism and alcohol use among Latino adolescent males: Longitudinal relations. *Journal of Community Psychology, 28*, 443–458.

Goel, M. S., McCarthy, E. P., Phillips, R. S., & Wee, C. C. (2004). Obesity among US immigrant subgroups by duration of residence. *JAMA, 292*(23), 2860–2867.

Gordon, M. M. (1964). *Assimilation in American life: The role of race, religion, and national origins*. New York: Oxford University Press.

Graves, P. L. (1967). Psychological acculturation in tri-ethnic community. *South-western Journal of Anthropology, 23*, 337–350.

Green, E. G., Deschamps, J. C., & Paez, D. (2005). Variation of individualism and collectivism within and between 20 countries a typological analysis. *Journal of Cross-Cultural Psychology, 36*(3), 321–339.

Haritatos, J., & Benet-Martinez, V. (2002). Bicultural identities: The interface of cultural, personality, and socio-cognitive processes. *Journal of Research in Personality, 36*(6), 598–606.

Helms, J. E. (1990). Toward a model of White racial identity development. In J. E. Helms (Ed.), *Black and White racial identity: Theory, research, and practice* (pp. 49–66). New York: Greenwood Press.

Henning, K., Ey, S., & Shaw, D. (1998). Perfectionism, the impostor phenomenon and psychological adjustment in medical, dental, nursing and pharmacy students. *Medical Education, 32*(5), 456–464.

Hertz, D. (1988). *How the Jews became Germans: The history of conversion and assimilation in Berlin*. New Haven, CT: Yale University Press.

Hofstede, G. (2001). *Culture's consequences. Comparing values, behaviors, institutions, and organizations across nations*. Thousand Oaks, CA: Sage.

Hunt, L. M., Schneider, S., & Comer, B. (2004). Should 'acculturation' be a variable in health research? A critical review of research on US Hispanics. *Social Science and Medicine, 59*, 973–986.

Ibrahim, F. A. (2008). *Cultural identity check list-revised.*© Denver, CO: Unpublished.

Ibrahim, F. A., & Heuer, J. R. (2013). The assessment, diagnosis, and treatment of mental disorders among Muslims. In F. A. Paniagua & A. M. Yamada (Eds.), *Handbook of multicultural mental health* (2nd ed., pp. 367–388). New York: Academic Press.

Jensen, L. A. (2003). Coming of age in a multicultural world: Globalization and adolescent cultural identity formation. *Applied Developmental Science, 7*, 189–196.

Kagitçibasi, C. (1997). Whither multiculturalism? *Applied Psychology, 46*, 44–49.

Kang, C. H. (1996). Acculturative Stress, Family Environment and the Psychological Adjustment of Korean Adolescents. Unpublished doctoral dissertation, California School of Professional Psychology.

Kim, B. S. K., & Abreu, J. M. (2001). Acculturation measurement: Theory, current instruments, and future directions. In J. G. Ponterotto, J. M. Casas, L. Suzuki, & C. M. Alexander (Eds.), *Handbook of multicultural counseling* (2nd ed., pp. 394–424). Thousand Oaks, CA: Sage.

Lafromboise, T., Coleman, H. L. K., & Gerton, J. (1993). Psychological impact of biculturalism: Evidence and theory. *Psychological Bulletin, 114*, 395–412.

LaFromboise, T. D., Trimble, J. E., & Mohatt, G. E. (1990). Counseling intervention and American Indian tradition: An integrative approach. *The Counseling Psychologist, 18*(4), 628–654.

Landrine, H., & Klonoff, E. A. (1996). *African American acculturation*. Thousand Oaks, CA: Sage.

Landrine, H., & Klonoff, E. A. (2002). *African American acculturation: Deconstructing race and reviving culture*. Thousand Oaks, CA: Sage.

Lang, J. G., Muñoz, R. F., Bernal, G., & Sorensen, J. L. (1982). Quality of life and psychological well-being in a bicultural Latino community. *Hispanic Journal of Behavioral Sciences, 4*, 433–450.

Leaper, C., & Valin, D. (1996). Predictors of Mexican-American mothers' and fathers' attitudes toward gender equality. *Hispanic Journal of Behavioral Sciences, 18*, 343–355.

Lee, C. L., & Zane, N. W. S. (Eds.). (1998). *Handbook of Asian American psychology*. Thousand Oaks, CA: Sage.

Liebkind, K. (1992). Ethnic identity: Challenging the boundaries of social psychology. In G. Breakwell (Ed.), *Social psychology of identity and the self-concept* (pp. 147–185). London: Academic.

Liebkind, K. (2001). Acculturation. In R. Brown & S. Gaether (Eds.), *Blackwell handbook of social psychology: Intergroup processes* (pp. 386–406). Oxford, England: Blackwell.

Locke, D. C. (1992). *Increasing multicultural understanding*. Newbury Park, CA: Sage.

Lonner, W. J., & Ibrahim, F. A. (2008). Assessment and appraisal in cross-cultural counseling. In P. B. Pedersen, J. Draguns, W. J. Lonner, & J. Trimble (Eds.), *Counseling across cultures* (6th ed., pp. 37–57). Thousand Oaks, CA: Sage.

López, I., & Contreras, J. (2005). The best of both worlds? Biculturality, acculturation and adjustment among young mainland Puerto Rican mothers. *Journal of Cross-Cultural Psychology, 36*, 192–208.

Marcia, J. E., Waterman, A. S., Matteson, D. R., Archer, S. L., & Orlofsky, J. L. (1993). *Ego identity: A handbook for psychosocial research*. New York: Springer.

Marin, G., Gamba, R. J., & Marin, B. V. (1992). Extreme response style and acquiescence among Hispanics: The role of acculturation and education. *Journal of Cross-Cultural Psychology, 23*, 498–509.

Marks, G., Garcia, M., & Solts, J. M. (1990). Health risk behaviors of Hispanics in the United States: Findings from the HHANES 1982–1984. *American Journal of Public Health, 80*, 20–26.

Markus, H. R., & Kitayama, S. (1991). Culture and the self: Implications for cognition, emotion, and motivation. *Psychological Review, 98*, 224–253.

Marsella, A. J., & Ring, E. (2003). Human migration and immigration: An overview. In L. L. Adler & U. P. Gielen (Eds.), *Migration: Immigration and emigration in international perspective* (pp. 3–22). Westport, CT: Praeger.

Matthews, G., & Clance, P. R. (1985). Treatment of the impostor phenomenon in psychotherapy clients. *Psychotherapy in Private Practice, 3*(1), 71–81.

Murray, C. J., & Lopez, A. D. (1996). Evidence-based health policy-lessons from the Global Burden of Disease Study. *Science, 274*(5288), 740–743.

National Association of Social Workers (NASW). (2008). *Code of ethics*. Washington, DC: National Association of Social Workers.

National Center for Education Statistics. (2013). *Public school graduates and dropouts from the common core of data: School year 2009–2010*. Retrieved from http://nces.ed.gov/pubs2013/2013309rev.pdf

Negy, C., & Woods, D. J. (1992). The importance of acculturation in understanding research with Hispanic-Americans. *Hispanic Journal of Behavioral Sciences, 14*, 224–227.

Neimeyer, R. A. (1993). An appraisal of constructivist psychotherapies. *Journal of Consulting and Clinical Psychology, 61*(2), 221.

Padilla, A. M. (1980). The role of cultural awareness and ethnic loyalty in acculturation. In A. M. Padilla (Ed.), *Acculturation: Theory, models, and some new findings* (pp. 47–84). Boulder, CO: Westview.

Padilla, A. M. (2006). Bicultural social development. *Hispanic Journal of Behavioral Sciences, 28*, 467–497.

Padilla, A. M., & Perez, W. (2003). Acculturation, social identity, and social cognition: A new perspective. *Hispanic Journal of Behavioral Sciences, 25*, 35–55.

Persky, I., & Birman, D. (2005). Ethnic identity in acculturation research: A study of multiple identities of Jewish refugees from the Former Soviet Union. *Journal of Cross-Cultural Psychology, 36*(5), 557–572.

Phalet, K., & Hagendoorn, L. (1996). Personal adjustment to acculturative transitions: The Turkish experience. *International Journal of Psychology, 31*, 131–144.

Phalet, K., Van Lotringen, C., & Entzinger, H. (2000). Islam in de multiculturele samenleving [Islam in multicultural society]. Utrecht, The Netherlands: University of Utrecht, European Research Centre on Migration and Ethnic Relations.

Phinney, J. S. (1990). Ethnic identity in adolescents and adults: Review of research. *Psychological Bulletin, 108*, 499–514.

Phinney, J. S. (1992). The multigroup ethnic identity measure. *Journal of Adolescent Research, 7*, 156–176.

Phinney, J. S., (1998, December). *Ethnic identity and acculturation*. Paper presented at the international conference on acculturation, University of San Francisco.

Phinney, J. S. (2003). Ethnic identity and acculturation. In K. M. Chun, P. B. Organista, & G. Marın (Eds.), *Acculturation: Advances in theory, measurement, and applied research* (pp. 63–82). Washington, DC: American Psychological Association.

Phinney, J. S., & Flores, J. (2002). 'Unpacking' acculturation: Aspects of acculturation as predictors of traditional sex role attitudes. *Journal of Cross-Cultural Psychology, 33*, 320–331.

Pope-Davis, D. B., Liu, W. M., Ledesma-Jones, S., & Nevitt, J. (2000). African American acculturation and Black racial identity: A preliminary investigation. *Journal of Multicultural Counseling and Development, 28*, 98–112.

Portes, A., & Zhou, M. (1993). The new second generation: Segmented assimilation and its variants. *The Annals of the American Academy of Political and Social Science, 530*, 74–96.

Poston, W. S. C. (2001). The biracial identity development model: A needed model. *Journal of Counseling and Development, 69*, 152–155.

Ramos, B. M. (2005). Acculturation and depression among Puerto Ricans in the Mainland. *Social Work Research, 29*, 95–105.

Raskin, J. D. (2002). Constructivism in psychology: Personal construct psychology, radical constructivism, and social constructionism. *American Communication Journal, 5*(3), 1–25.

Redfield, R., Linton, R., & Herskovits, M. J. (1936). Memorandum on the study of acculturation. *American Anthropologist, 38*, 149–152.

Richman, J. A., Gaviria, M., Flaherty, J. A., Birz, S., & Wintrob, R. M. (1987). The process of acculturation: Theoretical perspectives and an empirical investigation in Peru. *Social Science & Medicine, 25*(7), 839–847.

Robinson, S. L., & Goodpaster, S. K. (1991). The effects of parental alcoholism on perception of control and imposter phenomenon. *Current Psychology, 10*(1–2), 113–119.

Rogler, L. H., Cortes, D. E., & Malgady, R. G. (1991). Acculturation and mental health status among Hispanics: Convergence and new directions for research. *The American Psychologist, 46*(6), 585–597.

Rosenthal, D., Rainieri, N., & Klimdis, S. (1996). Vietnamese adolescents in Austria: Relationships between perceptions of self and parental values, intergenerational conflict, and gender dissatisfaction. *International Journal of Psychology, 31*, 81–91.

Rudmin, F. W. (2003). Critical history of the acculturation psychology of assimilation, separation, integration, and marginalization. *Review of General Psychology, 7*, 3–37. doi:10.1037/1089-2680.7.3.25.

Rudmin, F. W. (2006). *Debate in science: The case of acculturation*. Retrieved from http://www.anthroglobe.info/docs/rudminf_acculturation_061204.pdf

Rudmin, F. W., & Ahmadzadeh, V. (2001). Psychometric critique of acculturation psychology: The case of Iranian migrants in Norway. *Scandinavian Journal of Psychology, 42*, 41–56.

Rumbaut, R. G. (2005). Sites of belonging: Acculturation, discrimination, and ethnic identity among children of immigrants. In T. S. Weiner (Ed.), *Discovering successful pathways in children's development: Mixed methods in the study of childhood and family life* (pp. 111–164). Chicago: University of Chicago Press.

Sabatier, C., & Berry, J. W. (1994). Immigration et acculturation. In R. Bourhis & J. P. Leyens (Eds.), *Stirkoiypes, discrimination et relations iniergroupes*. Liege, Belgium: Mardaga.

Saxton, J. D. (2001). An introduction to cultural issues relevant to assessment with Native American youth. *The California School Psychologist, 6*, 31–38.

Schwartz, S. J. (2001). The evolution of identity: A rejoinder. *Identity: An International Journal of Theory and Research, 1*, 87–93.

Schwartz, S. J., Montgomery, M. J., & Briones, E. (2006). The role of identity in acculturation among immigrant people: Theoretical propositions, empirical questions, and applied recommendations. *Human Development, 49*, 1–30. doi:10.1159/000090300.

Searle, W., & Ward, C. (1990). The prediction of psychological and sociocultural adjustment during cross-cultural transitions. *International Journal of Intercultural Relations, 14*, 449–464.

Segall, M. H., Dasen, P. R., Berry, J. B., & Poortinga, Y. H. (1999). *Human behavior in a global perspective* (2nd ed.). Boston: Allyn & Bacon.

Serafini, T. E., & Adams, G. R. (2002). Functions of identity: Scale construction and validation. *Identity: An International Journal of Theory and Research, 2*, 361–389.

Shweder, R. A., Goodnow, J. J., Hatano, G., LeVine, R. A., Markus, H. R., & Miller, P. (2007). *The cultural psychology of development: One mind, many mentalities*. New York: Wiley. doi:10.1002/9780470147658.chpsy0113.

Smokowski, P. R., Rose, R., & Bacallao, M. L. (2008). Acculturation and Latino family processes: How cultural involvement, biculturalism, and acculturation gaps influence family dynamics. *Family Relations, 57*, 295–308. doi:10.1111/j.1741-3729.2008.00501.x.

Spitzberg, B. H., & Changnon, G. (2009). Conceptualizing intercultural competence. In D. K. Deardorff (Ed.), *The Sage handbook of intercultural competence* (pp. 2–52). Thousand Oaks, CA: Sage.

Stephan, W. G., & Stephan, C. W. (2000). An integrated threat theory of prejudice. In S. Oskamp (Ed.), *Reducing prejudice and discrimination* (pp. 23–46). Mahwah, NJ: Erlbaum.

Stephen, J., Fraser, E., & Marcia, J. E. (1992). Moratorium-achievement (Mama) cycles in lifespan identity development: Value orientations and reasoning system correlates. *Journal of Adolescence, 15*(3), 283–300.

Stone Feinstein, B. E., & Ward, C. (1990). Loneliness and psychological adjustment of sojourners: New perspectives on culture shock. In D. M. Keats, D. Munro, & L. Mann (Eds.), *Heterogeneity in cross-cultural psychology*. Lisse, The Netherlands: Swets & Zeitlinger.

Suarez-Orozco, C., & Suarez-Orozco, M. M. (2001). *Children of immigration*. Cambridge, MA: Harvard University Press.

Sue, S., Zane, N., Hall, G. C. N., & Berger, L. K. (2009). The case for cultural competency in psychotherapeutic interventions. *Annual Review of Psychology, 60*, 525.

Suinn, R., Richard-Figueora, K., Lew, S., & Vigil, P. (1987). The Suinn-Lew Asian self-identity acculturation scale: An initial report. *Educational and Psychological Measurement, 47*, 401–407.

Suleiman, R. (2002). Perception of the minority's collective identity and voting behavior: The case of the Palestinians in Israel. *Journal of Social Psychology, 142*, 753–766.

Suzuki, L. A., Ponterotto, J. G., & Meller, P. J. (Eds.). (2001). *Handbook of multicultural assessment: Clinical, psychological, and educational applications* (2nd ed.). San Francisco: Jossey-Bass.

Szapocznik, J., & Kurtines, W. M. (1980). Acculturation, biculturalism and adjustment among Cuban Americans. In A. M. Padilla (Ed.), *Acculturation: Theory, models, and some new findings* (pp. 139–159). Boulder, CO: Westview.

Szapocznik, J., Rio, A., Perez-Vidal, A., Kurtines, W., Hervis, O., & Santisteban, D. (1986). Bicultural effectiveness training (BET): An experimental test of an intervention modality for families experiencing intergenerational/intercultural conflict. *Hispanic Journal of Behavioral Sciences, 8*(4), 303–330.

Szapocznik, J., Scopetta, M. A., Kurtines, W., & Aranalde, M. D. (1978). Theory and measurement of acculturation. *Revista Interamericana de Psicologia, 12*(2), 113–130.

Tafel, H. (1981). *Human groups and social categories*. Cambridge, England: Cambridge University Press.

Tajfel, H., & Turner, J. C. (1986). The social identity theory of intergroup behavior. In S. Worchel & W. G. Austin (Eds.), *The psychology of intergroup behavior* (pp. 7–24). Chicago: Nelson Hall.

Takaki, R. T. (1979). *Iron cages: Race and culture in nineteenth-century America* (pp. 80–107). New York: Knopf.

Takaki, R. T. (1989). *Strangers from different shores: A history of Asian Americans*. Boston: Little, Brown and Company.

Tang, T. N., & Dion, K. L. (1999). Gender and acculturation in relation to traditionalism: Perceptions of self and parents among Chinese students. *Sex Roles, 41*(1–2), 17–29.

Taras, V. (2013). *Catalogue of instruments for measuring culture*. Retrieved from http://www.vtaras.com/Culture_Survey_Catalogue.pdf

Thompson, K. V., Lightfoot, N. L., Castillo, L. G., & Hurst, M. L. (2010). Influence of family perceptions of acting white on acculturative stress in African American college students. *International Journal for the Advancement of Counselling, 32*(2), 144–152.

Triandis, H. C. (1995). *Individualism & collectivism*. Boulder: Westview Press.

Triandis, H. C. (1996). The psychological measurement of cultural syndromes. *American Psychologist, 51*(4), 407.

Triandis, H. C., Kashima, Y., Shimada, E., & Villareal, M. (1986). Acculturation indices as a means of confirming cultural differences. *International Journal of Psychology, 21*, 43–70.

Trickett, E., Persky, I., & Ryerson Espino, S. R. (2002). Acculturation research: Proxies as sources of concept obfuscation. Retrieved from www.iaccp.org/sites/default/files/spetses_pdf/28_Trickett.pdf.

Trickett, E. J., Ryerson Espino, S., & Persky, I. (2006, July). *The use of proxies in acculturation research: An empirical investigation*. Paper presentation for the International Congress of the International Association for Cross-Cultural Psychology, University of Athens, Isle of Spetses, Greece.

Trimble, J. E. (2001). A quest for discovering ethnocultural themes in psychology. In J. G. Ponterotto, M. J. Casas, L. A. Suzuki, & C. M. Alexander (Eds.), *Handbook of multicultural counseling* (2nd ed., pp. 3–13). Thousand Oaks, CA: Sage.

Trinh, N. H., Rho, Y. C., Lu, F. G., & Sanders, K. M. (2009). *Handbook of mental health and acculturation in Asian American families*. New York: Springer.
Unger, J. B., Gallaher, P., Shakib, S., Ritt-Olson, A., Palmer, P. H., & Johnson, C. A. (2002). The AHIMSA acculturation scale: A new measure of acculturation for adolescents in a multicultural society. *The Journal of Early Adolescence, 22*(3), 225–251.
Van de Vijver, F. J. R., Helms-Lorenz, M., & Feltzer, M. F. (1999). Acculturation and cognitive performance of migrant children in the Netherlands. *International Journal of Psychology, 34*, 149–162.
Van de Vijver, F., & Leung, K. (1997). *Methods and data analysis of comparative research*. Boston: Allyn & Bacon.
Van de Vijver, F. J. R., & Phalet, K. (2004). Assessment in multicultural groups: The role of acculturation. *Applied Psychology: An International Review, 53*(2), 215–236.
Van der Maesen de Sombreff, P. E. A. M., & Abell, P. (2001). Interview en arbeidsproeven bij allochtone sollicitanten [Interview and sample tests with allochtonous applicants]. In N. Bleichrodt & F. J. R. Van de Vijver (Eds.), *Het gebruik van psychologische tests bij allochtonen* (pp. 157–175). Lisse, The Netherlands: Swets & Zeitlinger.
Van Oudenhoven, J. P. (2006). Immigrants. In D. L. Sam & J. W. Berry (Eds.), *The Cambridge handbook of acculturation psychology* (pp. 163–180). Cambridge, England: Cambridge University Press.
Vega, W. A., & Gil, A. G. (1998). *Drug use and ethnicity in early adolescence*. New York: Springer.
Vega, W., Kolody, B., Valle, R., & Weir, J. (1991). Social networks, social support. and their relationship to depression among immigrant Mexican women. *Human Organization, 50*, 154–162.
Verkuyten, M. (2003). Positive and negative self-esteem among ethnic minority early adolescents: Social and cultural sources and threats. *Journal of Youth and Adolescence, 32*, 267–277.
Verkuyten, M., & Kwa, G. K. (1994). Ethnic self-identification and psychological wellbeing among ethnic minority adolescents. *International Journal of Adolescence and Youth, 5*, 19–34.
Ward, C. (1996). Acculturation. In D. Landis & R. Bhagat (Eds.), *Handbook of intercultural training* (2nd ed., pp. 124–147). Thousand Oaks, CA: Sage.
Ward, C., & Kennedy, A. (1992). *The effects of acculturation strategies on psychological and sociocultural dimensions of cross-cultural adjustment*. Paper presented at the 3rd Asian Regional IACCP conference, Bangi, Malaysia.
Ward, C., & Kennedy, A. (1994). Acculturation strategies, psychological adjustment, and sociocultural competence during cross-cultural transitions. *International Journal of Intercultural Relations, 18*(3), 329–343.
Ward, C., Okura, Y., Kennedy, A., & Kojima, T. (1998). The U-curve on trial: A longitudinal study of psychological and sociocultural adjustment during cross-cultural transition. *International Journal of Intercultural Relations, 22*(3), 277–291.
Ward, C., & Rana-Deuba, A. (1999). Acculturation and adaptation revisited. *Journal of Cross-Cultural Psychology, 30*(4), 422–442. Retrieved from http://dx.doi.org/10.1177/00220221990 30004003.
Ward, C., & Searle, W. (1991). The impact of value discrepancies and cultural identity on psychological and sociocultural adjustment of sojourners. *International Journal of Intercultural Relations, 15*, 209–225.
Weaver, H. N. (1999). Indigenous people and the social work profession: Defining culturally competent services. *Social Work, 44*(3), 217–225. doi:10.1093/sw/44.3.217.
Wertsch, J. V. (1991). *Voices of the mind*. Cambridge, MA: Harvard University.
Yasuda, T., & Duan, C. (2002). Ethnic identity, acculturation, and emotional well-being among Asian American and Asian international students. *Asian Journal of Counseling, 9*(1), 1–26.
Zane, N., & Mak, W. (2003). Major approaches to the measurement of acculturation among ethnic minority populations: A content analysis and an alternative empirical strategy. In K. M. Chun, P. B. Organista, & G. Marín (Eds.), *Acculturation: Advances in theory, measurement, and applied research* (pp. 39–60). Washington, DC: American Psychological Association.
Zheng, X., Sang, D., & Wang, L. (2004). Acculturation and subjective well-being of Chinese students in Australia. *Journal of Happiness Studies, 5*(1), 57–72.

Chapter 5
Incorporating Social Justice and Advocacy in Counseling and Psychotherapy

Introduction

This chapter focuses on understanding social justice variables i.e., social class, educational level, privilege, oppression, and microaggressions, and their role in creating vulnerabilities and disempowerment for individuals (Hernandez, Carranza, & Almeida, 2010; Kimber & Delgado-Romero, 2011; Nadal et al., 2011; Owen, Tao, & Rodolfa, 2010; Sue et al., 2007; Vera & Speight, 2003). This domain is possibly the most challenging to incorporate in counseling and psychotherapy. In most cultures of the world, and specifically in the United States, it is not considered polite to ask questions about vulnerabilities. Professionals do make assumptions about people regarding their social class, race, culture, and other visible and unseen variables, and act on the assumptions unconsciously (Castro, Barrera, & Holleran Steiker, 2010; Kim & Cardemil, 2012). This chapter will include information on sensitively addressing cultural differences pertaining to gender, culture, gender, social class, religion, ability, etc., specifically to help therapists work effectively with clients. Recommendations for conducting an orientation for clients about the counseling and psychotherapy process will be included. In addition, we will consider what it means to be a social justice conscious mental health professional. Information on assessment tools that are currently available will be included. First, the concept of social justice, and its meaning for the helping professional will be addressed.

Social Justice: Meaning and Implications

Social justice pertains to the notion of a just society; inherent in the concept of social justice is the notion of challenging injustice and valuing humanity. Marsella (2013) defines social justice as "the social context, especially those societal and cultural conditions that may limit or eliminate any possibilities for individual and/

F.A. Ibrahim, J.R. Heuer, *Cultural and Social Justice Counseling*,
International and Cultural Psychology, DOI 10.1007/978-3-319-18057-1_5

or collective justice" (p. 1). Further he states "the most popular use of the term is concerned with institutional forces that fail to sustain justice" (p. 1). Social justice has been equated with the concept of equality; however, Scherlen and Robinson (2008) assert that the concept of social justice is much broader, with a focus on the concept of distributive justice. Berry (1974) notes that by equating social justice to the concept of equality, and justice, in a literal sense, has led to an emphasis on equal opportunity, and personal responsibility, which has created highly unequal societies, and it has made it difficult to achieve social justice in modern societies. Sometimes, the terms social justice and diversity, have been used interchangeably in the literature creating confusion about both concepts (Adams et al., 2013). According to Adams, although the concepts are related, they are not interchangeable. She believes that the term diversity is being used to justify the existence of inequality in society. She adds that in unequal social systems, social groups occupy unequal social locations. Therefore in unequal and unjust societies, social groups are organized in a manner that if one group has privilege, it is a disadvantage for another group. Her assertion is that social justice is about creating opportunities for all groups in a social system, regardless of race, gender, sexual orientation, national origin, religion, or disability. Deriving from the collective works of Paulo Friere (1974), Hardiman, Jackson, and Griffin (2007), and Young (1990, 2001), Adams offers the following principles for empowerment for all social groups: (a) view social identity linked to group identity, and the location of the social group versus other groups in that social system (advantaged or disadvantaged); (b) study privilege and oppression as a social construct within a sociohistorical perspective; (c) understand the meaning and scope of oppression; and (d) develop a model for empowerment and social change.

Johnson (2006) asserts that the problem is not difference, it is the social construction of difference, and the hierarchical positioning of social groups that creates difference, e.g., by providing access to opportunity for some and denying access to others. Further, he notes that the proliferation of capitalism in modern Western societies has contributed to creating hierarchical social and economic systems. Especially, since the only goal of capitalism is to make a profit at any cost, without concern about the impact on people, societies, or the environment. In such social systems having material gain as a primary goal is a motivator for people to deny and ignore human misery, to align themselves with the dominant economic system. Pinderhughes (1989) discusses the outcome of feeling different, and being treated differently. It includes alienation from self, and feeling alienated from society, it affects self-esteem, self-efficacy, and leads to low expectations and aspirations in life. These findings are consistent with the concept of internalized self-hatred (Helms, 1990; Tatum, 1992, 1997). Johnson, also addresses the fact that the way race, gender, and sexual orientation are understood and defined is socially constructed, e.g., since, the United States only recognizes two genders, intersexed babies (born with sexual characteristics of both genders) are routinely surgically altered at birth. Similarly, perceptions of homosexual behavior, as acceptable or unacceptable are socially constructed. These assumptions become the reality that people function by, without critically evaluating if the categories and hierarchies in society are acceptable ways of functioning for people in a civilized democratic society.

Social construction of difference is maintained by creating negative images of vulnerable groups, or groups less valued by the dominant group, and perpetuating the myth that there is something inherently wrong with them; resulting in violation of basic human rights of people and justifying restricting access to opportunities (Johnson, 2006; Kendall, 2013). However, as Kendall remarks, White people do not have to be good to have access to opportunities and privileges they have not earned, these are bestowed upon them. In addition, being White allows people to see themselves as having no race, and it causes distress when others point out that they do belong to a racial-cultural group. Further, Kendall notes that White women see themselves as women, relating to women of color as "sisters" sharing the same reality against the oppressor, the White male. Kendall notes that women of color do not perceive their relationship to White women as equals, based upon their social location, and the value placed on their social-cultural group. Kendall considers this White racial privilege to ignore the racial aspect, by only focusing on gender. In essence, this perspective reinforces the "supremacy of Whiteness" (p. 66).

The outcome of difference is based on the position assigned to a group, e.g., male versus female. If we review the treatment people receive based on their gender, and the worth ascribed to a gender category in the United States, we will begin to understand privilege and oppression. For example, by paying women 67 cents for every dollar a man makes for the same job, a statement is being made regarding social positioning and worth of each gender. However, we socialize women to be grateful that they have a job, and to be compliant, and not make waves, so they can retain their jobs. This makes men privileged, and women oppressed. Johnson (2006) notes that the problem with privilege is that people do not realize that they are privileged, and when confronted with this information, their response is anger or defensiveness.

Peggy McIntosh (1993) describes privilege as having access value, just because of the social group one is in, not because it is earned. Since privilege has become a loaded word in the current discourse on social justice, Blum (2008) proposes that when analyzing White privilege, the analysis should be conducted along the lines of "unearned White privilege" in Western societies, this will reduce the negative valence for the dominant group, and help in understanding the unit of analysis. Kendall (2013) asserts that White privilege is institutional, rather than personal, alluding to the set of benefits granted to those who hold positions of power in institutions, make decisions, and grant benefits to some, while ignoring others. She maintains that as a group White people keep themselves central, by silencing other groups, and by including some, and excluding others. She further notes that race in the United States is seen as a Black–White construct; viewing race from this perspective, overlooks the fact that the system in place has oppressed all people of color. Theorists consider how White privilege displays itself in discussing nondominant cultural groups: "African American and Latino/a's and other minority groups" (Blum, 2008, p. 317). This implies that the experiences of all nondominant group members are similar, such a perspective does not allow examination of the sociopolitical history and experiences of historically oppressed groups in the United States, and detracts from critical issues that need examination, to achieve the ideals of a democratic society. Lipsitz (2013) notes that there is a "possessive investment in Whiteness" it is "everywhere in US culture, but very hard to see" (p. 77). Kendall (2013) adds how much privilege White people have is determined by several factors, such as gender, sexual orientation, class, status, age, size, weight, and disability. According to her, although, all White people have privilege, it is mediated and moderated by these variables.

McIntosh (1993) provides a template for understanding privilege at two levels: (a) Unearned entitlements, and (b) unearned advantage. She identifies the first level as something everyone is entitled to in a civilized society, i.e., feeling safe, a sense of belonging where people work, and being valued for their contributions; however, when these entitlements are restricted, they become unearned advantage for the few who enjoy it. Blum (2008) expands the notion of privilege, and identifies three types: (a) being "spared injustice" privilege (p. 313); (b) "unjust enrichment" privilege (p. 312); and (c) "benefit from one's position" (p. 312). He notes these privileges are not warranted from a moral point of view, and may not be related to injustice of a disadvantaged group. Spared injustice pertains to not being subjected to unfair treatment because one is a member of an advantaged group; Unjust enrichment alludes to having opportunities because of one's membership in a valued group; the third advantage is linked to being a member of a group, and having the privilege of speaking the privileged language (linguistic privilege, i.e., membership in a less valued group, or not knowing the norms of the group, p. 313).

Blum (2008) calls the third type, a non justice-related privilege, because, although there may be discrimination against non-English speaking people because of their accents, or lack of information about the cultural norms and rules; it is an unearned privilege for mainstream cultural groups. According to Blum, it creates a moral imperative for the dominant group to acknowledge this advantage, and provide support and accommodation for people in the workplace, who do not enjoy this privilege, such as immigrants and racial-cultural minorities. In considering White privilege, it is important to consider the sociopolitical history of the United States, and the outcomes that we are confronted with today, i.e., the wealth gap between the dominant and the nondominant cultural groups, the health disparities experienced by nondominant cultural groups, including poor White people; given the changing demographics of the United States, the impact on the social capital of the United States is a critical issue because the larger percentage of the US population is not being empowered to achieve their fullest potential.

The impact of these inequities on the psychological health of the nation is unclear unless we review demographic information, and consider the current statistics on stress, mental illness, suicide rates, school violence, the drop in the work ethic, white collar crime, greed, wars, and a recession/depression every 10 years. Additionally, we must recognize the experiences of the "haves" and the "have not" in the United States, and its relationship to the gaps in access to power and resources. Another critical issue is the school-to-jail pipeline for nondominant cultural groups, and multiracial individuals, which has created the largest jail system in the civilized world, primarily because of the "War on drugs" (Alexander, 2012; Ibrahim, 2013).

Compared to the progress Europe has made on this issue, e.g., Sweden is closing prisons, as their focus has shifted to rehabilitation and lenient sentences for drug-related offenses. Interestingly, the same groups that were not allowed to access opportunities for centuries in the Unites States continue to be the oppressed as the largest population in jails. A democratic society needs to focus on the wellbeing of all, and the reduction of hierarchies based on race-culture, gender, sexual orientation, age, disability status, religion, etc., if the mission to end drug abuse is a sincere effort by the power holders. As counseling practitioners, we posit the most important issue for us is to work on multisystemic levels to bring about change and reduction in human misery and oppression. We are continually waging wars and stating that we are bringing democracy to these nations, however, we do not have democracy, but a system that encourages the same group of "haves" to intergenerationally control the legislature, even with some members of Congress having low educational attainment, or lacking the ability to do critical thinking. This has led to the enactment of laws that cut funding for the poor and disenfranchised, and send millions abroad to assist with foreign civil wars, and in financial aid, moving industry to other nations creating joblessness, and further disenfranchiment, resulting in greater social injustice in the US.

Demographics of the United States

Kendall (2013, p. 62) reported on the racial composition of the United States: "White, 64.7 %, Hispanic or Latino/a, 16.3 %, Black or African American, 12.2 %, Asian, Native-Hawaiian, or Pacific Islander, 4.6 %, and Native American or Alaskan Native, .09 %" (Kaiser Family Foundation, 2011). She compared the wealth gap by race; the White median wealth is 20 times higher than Black median wealth, and 18 times higher than Latina/o median wealth (Pew Research Center: Social and Demographic Trends, 2011). Oliver and Shapiro (2006) provide supportive evidence for the data provided by the Pew Research Center, noting that Black households have between 7 and 10 % the wealth of White households. Blum (2008) alludes to the disparity in Black and White household incomes $33,500 and $52,000 respectively (United States [US] Census Bureau, 2006), and notes that health disparities experienced by Latino/as' and Blacks are excessive compared to the experience of the White population. This lack of concern for addressing these gaps in wealth, income, and health services cannot be explained by simply labeling it White privilege (Andersen, 2003). The numbers do not provide the reasons for the disparities, the systems, and structures that have created the disparity need to be examined, to bring about change (Blum, 2008). Oliver and Shapiro (2006) provided a historical account of the wealth gap between Blacks and Whites. According to them, the reasons can be attributed to the lack of resources given to the freed slaves after emancipation in 1865, along with racial discrimination in the federal mortgage subsidizing programs for housing in the 1930s and the 1940s. Shapiro (2006) states that wealth; instead of income is the primary determinant of advancing in society, along with higher education. All the accounts of disparities in wealth, income, health, and education, show there are interconnections with race and social positioning, and brings to light the issue of racial privilege for some and disadvantage for others.

Social Justice Concerns and Advocacy in Counseling

In the last 35 years, the counseling field has been inundated with information on addressing the cultural dimension in counseling and psychotherapy. Since the report on Workforce 2000 was published (Johnson & Packer, 1987), it became apparent that the US population numbers are shifting from a primarily White European population to incorporating large numbers of Latino/a and Asian immigrants, along with the constant flux of immigrants from all parts of the world. Vera and Speight (2003) assert that the goal of multicultural efficacy for counseling psychology will not be achieved, unless strategies to respond to social justice issues are incorporated in the cultural competence paradigm. Recently there has been a surge in the counseling literature recommending incorporation of social justice principles, and operationalization of these principles in counseling and psychotherapy, education, training, and practice (Singh & Salazar, 2010). Although, counseling as a profession originated with the principles of social justice at its core, attention to these priorities changed over time (Bradley, Werth, & Hastings, 2012; Kiselica, 1999).

Counseling as a profession has held a core belief that all humans are equal and unique, and has advocated for empowering clients to achieve their fullest potential (Romano & Hage, 2000). Ratts (2009) notes that the social justice paradigm for counseling uses "social advocacy and activism as a means to address inequitable, social, political, and economic conditions that impede the academic, career, and personal/social development of individuals, families, and communities," (p. 160). Speight and Vera (2004) assert that social advocacy focuses on the attainment of justice for exploited, dominated, and marginalized people and communities.

Chang, Crethar, and Ratts (2010) note that the resurgence in the call for incorporating social justice and advocacy in counseling and psychotherapy education, training, and supervision, is intentional because oppression and inequality is rampant, and creates significant stress, leading to psychological problems. The American Counseling Association's (ACA) "Advocacy Competencies" (2003) may have been the catalyst for creating the "fifth force" in counseling, given the response from diverse counseling perspectives requiring actions to promote social justice in education, training, and practice (Blustein, 2006; Blustein, McWhirter, & Perry, 2005; Goodman et al., 2004; Ivey & Collins, 2003; Pieterse, Evans, Risner-Butner, Collins, & Mason, 2009; Ratts, 2009; Singh et al., 2010; Toporek, Gerstein, Fouad, Roysircar, & Israel, 2006; Werth, Borges, McNally, Maguire, & Britton, 2008).

The reason why there is limited response to the calls for expanding the parameters of psychology in general, and counseling and psychotherapy in particular is due to the fact that psychological thought has been dominated by the myth of rugged individualism (Jackson, 2011; Snow, 2012). We agree, along with several theorists and researchers, that counseling theory and practice has been dominated by this myth, and the socialization process in the United States reinforces it (Breton, 1995; Bronfenbrenner, 1977, 1979; Neville & Mobley, 2001; Prilleltensky, 2008; Sampson, 1988). Consequently, psychology has paid little attention to these concerns; although, there have been challenges to this thinking (Albee & George, 2000; Sampson, 1988). Social justice concerns, are at an all time high right now, given the state of the economy, joblessness, the housing crisis, and consequent homelessness; large segments of the population lives below the poverty line, suffer from health disparities, have a lower social status due to biology (gender, sexual orientation), or socialization, physical disabilities, and veteran status, and lack access to opportunities to achieve the American dream.

For the mental health professions to achieve their full potential must honor their original professional mandate and return to their roots and focus on elements that made the mental health professions unique, i.e., prevention of psychological problems, interventions to alleviate psychological suffering, understand intrapsychic and extrapsychic factors that impinge upon the lives of people, and advocate not just for the clients, but for social change. Ivey advocated for prevention and social change in the first edition of his text. Since then, several scholars have focused on systemic changes, and the importance of macrolevel interventions for reducing human suffering (Atkinson, Thompson, & Grant, 1993; Lewis, Toporek, & Ratts, 2010; Prilleltensky, 1997, 2001; Vera & Speight, 2003). The twenty-first century has seen the greatest movement among mental health professions to incorporate social justice and advocacy to work with individuals, groups, and the larger social context.

Social Justice Principles and Advocacy Competencies

The profession of social work incorporated social justice at the core of its professional standards from its inception, it is evident in the mission, vision, and goals of the National Association of Social Work (NASW, 2001). The intent of the professional association was to narrow the gap in health disparities. The Council on Social Work Education's (CSWE) Educational Policy and Accreditation Standards, and the Social Work Code of Ethics emphasizes the importance of training in cultural knowledge, and skills to enhance cultural competence and responsiveness in social work education (Negi, Bender, Furman, Fowler, & Prickett, 2010). These standards require all social work graduates to understand the mechanisms of oppression and discrimination and demonstrate the ability to practice with respect, knowledge, and skills related to client vulnerabilities (CSWE, 2008; NASW, 2001). St. Catherine University, School of Social Work (2006) adapted NASW code of Ethics to develop ten principles for social justice work practice: These include: (a) Human dignity; (b) community and the common good; (c) rights and responsibilities; (d) priority for the poor and vulnerable; (e) participation; (f) dignity of work and rights of workers; (g) solidarity; (h) stewardship; (i) governance/principle of subsidiary; and (j) promotion of peace. The principles taken together reflect what it takes to have a peaceful, democratic society.

The American Counseling Association (ACA) and the American Psychological Association (APA) have issued Multicultural Competency, and Advocacy statements (American Counseling Association (ACA), 1992, 2003) and Guidelines for Multicultural Education, Training, Research, Practice, and Organizational Change for Psychologists (American Psychological Association (APA), 2002), these statements and their code/principles of ethics, emphasize taking into account the social realities, health, and wealth disparities, and privilege, and oppression of both the therapist and the client. The American Psychiatric Association (2004) developed an action plan to reduce disparities in access to psychiatric care, and to increase cultural competence. All mental health professional associations include equity and fairness as a goal for the delivery of mental health services. Cultural sensitivity, awareness, knowledge and skills are embedded in the cultural competency statements of both the ACA and the APA (ACA, 1992; APA, 2002). In addition, state health organizations and governmental institutions all mandate sensitivity to cultural issues and incorporate issues of social equity in policy and service delivery requirements. Operationalizing social justice principles for delivery of both cultural competence and social justice in interventions is much needed, because simply telling professionals to practice from the perspective of cultural competency and social justice is not enough education and training must provide strategies to help operationalize these goals.

Marsella (2013) provides guidelines for social justice education, he notes that the principles must be incorporated in education and training across the curriculum in higher education. Further, he identifies several challenges facing societies and nations, and the individuals within them in this global era. He asserts that awareness and knowledge of "justice" should be a priority in human development and socialization processes; to help individuals confront the complexities and unpredictability of this time. Especially given the interdependence among nations, although it has created opportunities, he notes that it has also created conflicts, envy, frustration, and violence. According to Marsella personal, societal, national, and regional issues should take into consideration the fact that "justice as fairness" is usually sacrificed (2013, p. 2). He proposes a movement to socialize people living in the global era for justice, to educate individuals for social justice in any profession, and he offers the following recommendations:

1. Distribute copies of the United Nations "Universal Declaration of Human Rights" (1948) to all students and faculty at educational institutions.
2. Distribute copies of definitions of all types of justice, to all faculty and students.
3. Establish an organized programmatic effort and institutional identity embedded on the concept of justice.
4. Award a certificate or have a concentration on Justice Studies.
5. Invite at least two external speakers each year to lecture and conduct conversations on justice.
6. Position social justice art, statements, comments, poetry, and photographs at conspicuous campus locations.
7. Develop electronic materials as resources.
8. Develop community outreach programs that use "service" learning as an integrated goal.

9. Create a "justice across the curriculum" orientation for a college or university.
10. Support student and faculty projects concerned with the study or application of justice (e.g., travel, research, and teaching support).
11. Develop educational materials for justice in schools K-12.
12. Invite students upon entrance and at graduation to take a "justice" pledge: ***I pledge to explore and consider individual, social, and environmental consequences of any personal or employment actions to improve the social condition through awareness and understanding of justice.***
13. Begin each college and/or university orientation week with a statement of an institution's commitment to justice, especially the importance of using justice as an arbiter for behavior and educational development (Marsella, 2013).

Sensoy and DeAngelo (2008) agree with several of the recommendations proposed by Marsella (2013) and note that the times we live in require taking dangerous action by challenging the status quo. They note that educators must practice social justice; accepting its importance is not enough. They encourage educators to recognize that diversity, equity, and social justice, are connected. A sentiment echoed by several scholars (Jackson, 2011; King, Vigil, Herrera, Hajek, & Jones, 2007; Martin-Baro, 1994; Neville & Mobley, 2001; Vera & Speight, 2003). Sensoy and DeAngelo ask educators to recognize the importance of educating for social justice, a subject resisted by students because they do not understand its importance. They encourage their colleagues to support this difficult work, especially by learning social justice terminology, i.e., oppression, internalized dominance, and internalized oppression. They emphasize, "being for social justice necessitates basic social justice literacy" (p. 347).

David Miller (2001) argues that principles of justice must be understood contextually, with each principle finding its natural home in a different form of human interaction. Because modern societies are complex, the theory of justice must be complex, too. Lee (2007) translates social justice principles for counseling professionals and offers the following guidelines for helping professionals to make a personal commitment: (a) explore life, its meaning, and personal commitments; (b) explore personal privilege; (c) work to develop a literacy of multiculturalism; and (d) establish a personal, and social justice compass. He encourages counseling professionals to review the Universal Declaration of Human Rights (United Nations, 1948), the ACA Code of Ethics (2014), and the ACA Advocacy Competencies (2003). Two additional resources for information and guidance for developing a personal social justice ethical compass is the Counselors for Social Justice Code of Ethics and the Association for Specialists in Group Work (ASGW) Multicultural and Social Justice Competence Principles for Group Workers (Ibrahim, Dinsmore, Estrada, & D'Andrea, 2011; Singh, Merchant, Skudrzyk, & Ingene, 2012).

Vera and Speight (2003) assert that counseling psychology as a profession because of its core values of prevention and person-environment emphasis is in the best position to implement social justice initiatives. They note that it is time to reclaim the historical roots of counseling psychology (Romano & Hage, 2000; Vera, 2000). They emphasize that counseling psychology "builds on strengths, by conducting psychoeducational, and developmental interventions, and viewing people holistically, providing an advantageous position from which a meaningful synthesis of social justice and professional practice can occur" (Vera & Speight, 2003, p. 262). Goodman et al. (2004) present principles drawn from feminist and multicultural counseling to educate counseling professionals as social justice agents. They note that although there have been calls for social justice and advocacy in counseling, the principles that may facilitate the process have not been articulated. They conceptualize social justice work of counseling professionals as "scholarship and professional action designed to change societal values, structures, policies, and practices, such that disadvantaged or marginalized groups gain increased access to these tools of self-determination" (p. 795).

Operationalization of Social Justice Principles

This section will focus on: (a) knowledge and skills to be culturally responsive and become social justice advocates for clients, in individual, group, community settings; and (b) it will focus on conducting social justice work in community settings, and larger social context. Research supports the fact that most mental health professionals are unable to translate theory, and recommendations specific to cultural competence and social justice concerns to practice (Boysen & Vogel, 2008; Sue, Zane, Hall, & Berger, 2009). We agree with Yamada and Marsella (2013) that training programs must incorporate social justice and cultural responsiveness principles that can be translated into practice across the curriculum. Further, education needs to require that mental health professionals during their training conduct cultural assessments on themselves, to understand not only what they know about themselves, but also, the unconscious or unexamined aspects of their identity (Ibrahim, 2010). This will involve: cultural identity exploration, worldview, acculturation level, privilege-oppression assessments, and use of the Implicit Attitude Test to access their unexamined assumptions (Greenwald, McGhee, & Schwartz, 1998; Hays, Chang, & Decker, 2007; Ibrahim, 2007, 2008; Ibrahim & Kahn, 1984, 1987). Conducting the assessments is not enough, this should be followed by experiential activities that require discussion of these personal variables and how one feels about them, whether, one is aware of these aspects of identity or not, and develop goals to enhance their understanding of their own identity, and also an understanding of the people in their community (Ibrahim, 2010).

Lack of recognition of social justice issues in the psychological literature has impeded progress in education and training of mental health professionals. Training programs need to incorporate cultural assessments; experiential learning, critical reflection, and training that operationalize the ACA Advocacy competencies, along with the Counselors for Social Justice Ethical Code (ACA, 2003; Ibrahim et al., 2011). Further, a service learning training model that incorporates social justice and advocacy work in the community will help translate the knowledge and skills to real-world situations and will facilitate understanding about the inequities that people in lower social classes, less valued genders and cultural groups experience, and help candidates in developing programs to alleviate inequities and oppression in the community (Deeley, 2010; Fourie, 2003; Koch, Ross, Wendell, & Aleksandrova-Howell, 2014; Murray, Pope, & Rowell, 2010).

Counseling Modalities and Social Justice

This section reviews the social justice issues for individual and group counseling, and addresses social justice activism for community, society, and the global context (Pedersen, Meyer, & Hargrave, 2014). Since, other chapters have focused on the cultural, and social, dimensions, here we consider psychological interventions with an emphasis on social justice, and advocacy and activism mediated by privilege and oppression issues, as these pertain to counseling and psychotherapy, and are important in implementing cultural responsiveness and competence.

The Individual Level

Social justice counseling combines cultural responsiveness and understanding the client's cultural strengths, along with socially imposed challenges, and focuses on developing strengths, empowerment, and advocacy. It is important in social justice counseling to understand privilege and oppression assessment, and advocacy skills in counseling. Social justice approaches and practice in counseling refer to the elimination of, and actively addressing the dynamics of oppression, privilege, and "isms," through advocacy and activism (Marsella, 2006; Ratts, 2009; Speight & Vera, 2004). All social systems are a product of historical, social, cultural, and political stratifications, which have been institutionally sanctioned, along with socially constructed group hierarchies, which include race/ethnicity/culture, gender, class, sexual orientation, and ability (Cochran-Smith, 2004; Sensoy & DeAngelo, 2008). To incorporate the above mentioned assumptions and to operationalize social justice counseling assumptions, we propose some basic strategies must underlie social justice and culturally responsive counseling. These include: (a) Identification of client strengths and resources; (b) recognition of client cultural, social, and personal challenges, and contextual variables; (c) clarification of the phase of identity development as it relates to gender, culture, sexual orientation; and (d) incorporation of cultural assessment information on cultural identity, worldview, acculturation status, and privilege and oppression. Critical to the process of implementing these assumptions is the notion of psychological liberation for clients.

Both the professions of counseling psychology and social work have historically focused on social justice issues (AERA, APA, & NCME, 1999; Flynn, 1995; Gibelman, 1995). The current approaches to address oppression in individual and group counseling are feminist, liberation, multicultural, decolonization through social justice, and peace psychology and were developed to confront the status quo in the helping professions (Goodman et al., 2004; Goodman & Gorski, 2015; Ivey, 1995; Ivey, Ivey, & D'Andrea, 2011; Prilleltensky, 1989; Watkins & Shulman, 2008). These approaches address sociopolitical issues, and the effect on human lives, especially in socially stratified societies, and provide interventions to ameliorate human suffering due to biological, social, and historical factors such as race, gender, sexual orientation, etc. Psychology of liberation uses Paulo Freire's concept of critical consciousness, and applies it to counseling and psychotherapy (Freire, 1974; Ivey, 1995). It emphasizes the development of critical consciousness by focusing on the presenting problem within a social-cultural context (Ivey, 1995). Freire notes that when people become aware of their sociopolitical reality (and their place in hierarchical social systems) through reflection, and dialogue, it becomes a catalyst for attaining critical consciousness, which opens the client to learning the skills of self-advocacy. We propose that it creates the conditions for implementing social justice interventions and advocacy for clients. Young (1990) perceived social justice as a means of eliminating institutionalized domination and oppression in societies, and from a societal perspective supporting the conditions necessary for the good life.

Group Level

In group counseling, there is a need to identify both cultural and political dynamics that influence the lives of group members, and interventions must be developed to accommodate all the pertinent variables (Ibrahim, 2010). Focusing on liberation and empowerment in group counseling is critical to effect change for individuals in group counseling. This involves empowering individuals and going beyond addressing the issue the group was developed to address. The cultural assessment yields data that can assist in the process of empowering individuals on cultural, gender, sexual orientation, along with class, religion, disability, age, etc. We believe a secondary intervention enhancing the cultural, gender, sexual orientation empowerment in group work would result in psychological liberation. Group counseling is an excellent modality to address societal and systemic level oppressions; individuals in groups are able to provide empathy for conditions that they are all familiar with and support each other in working on strategies that challenge negative internalized assumptions based on negative societal attitudes that are politically instituted. Recognizing political and hierarchical assumptions institutionalized on social systems, and confronting negative self-images based on these assumptions is critical to psychological liberation.

Speight and Vera (2004) cite Bulhan (1985, p. 274) "liberation cannot only happen to one person at a time, the oppressed cannot attain liberty by individual means." Societal efforts are required to bring about change, empowerment, growth, and change. The next step is bringing about societal and structural change in social systems to support the changes accomplished in individual and group work. This echoes Prilleltensky's (2008) proposition that interventions need to move beyond remediation or amelioration of psychological problems to structural change in social systems.

Societal and Global Contexts

The critical dimension where change must take place to alleviate human suffering is at the institutional, societal, and global levels (Adams et al., 2013; Greenleaf & Willliams, 2009; Leong, Leach, Marsella, & Pickren, 2012; Vera & Speight, 2003; Watkins & Shulman, 2008; Yamada & Marsella, 2013). The institutional and societal barriers that have created the conditions for economic, and social inequities, and the imposition of western culture on cultures of the world through colonial rule, and currently through the global economy have led to psychological misery, wars, ethnic cleansings, and a host of other problems (Arnett, 2002; Diamond, 1997; Held, 1998; WHO, 2011). In the United States, the economic downturns that occur every 10 years since 1972 have decimated the middle class and created a new work force that survives on hourly wages, with no health, retirement, or vacation benefits (Anyon, 2005). In addition, historical oppressions created by segregation, and lack of access to opportunities of racial and ethnic nondominant cultural groups have wasted significant social capital and caused intergenerational trauma. Consequences of the "war on drugs" and the school-to-jail pipeline for members of the nondominant cultural groups for minor drug charges in the United States have recreated hostile living conditions for historically oppressed cultural groups (Alexander, 2012; Ibrahim, 2013). Further, the emerging crises due to global warming, Tsunamis, earthquakes, eroding coastlines, and water shortages have negative consequences for mental health (National Wild Life Federation, 2011; Pipher, 2014). Negative social, economic, and ecological conditions create severe psychological problems and mental health professionals will have to take a proactive position on these issues to live up to the goals of advocacy to ameliorate distress, beyond the therapy office, as required by the current professional mandates (ACA, 2003; APA, 2011).

Our role as identified by the social justice competencies (ACA, 2003), and ethical codes of all mental health professions is to move out of the office to focus on social justice grassroots work by educating community members about the impact of negative social conditions. Anyon (2005) notes that the only time social change has taken place in the United States was when people marched in the streets, e.g., the suffragette and civil rights movement. It is time to educate people in our communities about the negative effects of the social, economic, and ecological conditions, and move beyond blaming the victim for having psychological distress. Watkins and Shulman (2008) believe that change can happen by local regeneration and psychological theories have not provided adequate models to address the situation. Development at local levels can lead to psychological liberation and move us toward global peace. The maintenance of structural barriers such as social and cultural hierarchies will continue the cycles of human misery and psychological distress caused by oppression.

Young (2013) identified the five faces of oppression as exploitation, marginalization, powerlessness, cultural imperialism, and violence. She further notes that the presence of these five conditions is enough to consider a group oppressed. The continuing natural, economic, and social disasters maintain oppression around the world. Community engagement, and education, for local mobilization to effect change in the conditions that maintain oppression is the only path. Social justice work requires us to identify the causes of human misery, not simply empower people in therapy, but advocate for our clients and do the work to change oppressive structures.

Hays et al. (2007) emphasize that for counselors to be aware of social justice issues, i.e., privilege and oppression, is important to understand power differentials between counselor and client. Hays et al. (2007), assert that the multiple identities of clients must be given consideration in the counseling process. We believe, it needs to go beyond understanding multiple identities, to understanding structural barriers to human growth and development. Further, for global peace we need to work for social justice because until there is equity and social justice globally, there can be no peace (Pope Paul, 1972). Marsella (2006) issued a call to all counselors to "become counselors to the world, I do so with the explicit intention of informing you that the counselor's stance is the stance that fits evolution's purpose itself. As you perform your duties and you live your lives, you can be assured you are in synchrony and harmony with human nature" (p. 125). It is evident that action is needed to create global peace, as long as there is disharmony caused by structural hierarchies of poverty, racism, sexism, homophobia, etc., there cannot be peace. It is imperative that social justice activism is the key to social change, and our professional standards require us to be leaders in this domain.

Therapist Characteristics for Effective Social Justice Work

To help therapists who conduct individual and group interventions understand social justice, means developing critical thinking and reflection to understand their own socialization in the matrix of unequal relationships and its implications; to recognize mechanisms of oppression, and to develop the skills and courage to challenge these hierarchies (Cochran-Smith, 2004; Sensoy & DeAngelo, 2008). Therapists are encouraged to understand and examine their cultural identity, values, worldview, socialization processes, privilege, and oppression, emotional and psychological health, developmental history, stage of life, and strengths and challenges connected to all these variables, to ensure that they are aware of the power they wield as helping professionals. With this recognition, they can provide ethically sound, culturally responsive, and social justice-oriented service to clients.

This reflection will help in understanding the power dimension, which is a critical variable in working across cultures or working within social-hierarchical systems (Adams, Bell, & Griffin, 2007; Johnson, 2006; Pinderhughes, 1989). Incorporating social justice issues in direct service, also involves understanding and recognizing counselor assets and challenges, along with client assets and challenges and recognizing the multiple dynamics impinging upon the counselor–client relationship. Pinderhughes encouraged mental health professionals to understand the power dimension. Power issues operate in the therapeutic environment due to social-hierarchical cultural systems, causing psychological distress and severe stress for therapists, therapists in training, and clients (Frable, 1997). Recognizing and understanding the effect on both the service provider, and the client is critical to success in counseling and psychotherapy. Power operates in the counseling dyad as the level of privilege and oppression experienced by the individuals, and the distance that it creates in the therapeutic relationship, which can lead to an impasse in the therapeutic relationship (Gaztambude, 2012; Keenan, Tsand, Bogo, & George, 2005; Marsella, 2006; Owen et al., 2011).

Not understanding how power operates in counseling and the resulting impasse in counseling highlights the issue of lack of responsiveness to an intervention. In counseling this is viewed as "resistance." We urge mental health professionals to not fall prey to using resistance as the excuse for lack of progress in counseling in cross-cultural encounters, especially when race, class, gender, and sexual orientation are involved. Otani (1989) notes "resistance occurs as a result of a negative interpersonal dynamic between the counselor and the client" (p. 32). Counseling interventions falter in cross-cultural encounters when complete understanding of client concerns, life context, and privilege or oppression information is not available (Bernal & Saéz-Santiago, 2006; Ibrahim, 2003; Pinderhughes, 1989; Sue et al., 2009). We believe that a reconceptualization is needed of the concept of resistance, especially in counseling across cultures, genders, sexual orientations, social classes, age, religions, etc. Lack of progress in a counseling intervention should be seen as an opportunity for assessing the power distance between the parties, honest assessment of the counseling relationship, reconsidering the goals for the intervention with the client to address the presenting problem. Research indicates that the therapeutic relationship is the best predictor of outcome in counseling and psychotherapy (Baldwin, Wampold, & Imel, 2007; Horvath, Del Re, Fluckiger, & Symonds, 2011; Sharf, Primavera, & Diener, 2010). Several factors have been identified that can create an impasse in counseling and psychotherapy, e.g., cultural misunderstandings, ignoring or not understanding the meaning of cultural issues, religious slights, and missed opportunities to strengthen the therapeutic relationship by responding with empathy (Chang & Berk, 2009; Chang & Yoon, 2011; Vasquez, 2007). The power difference and the privilege that the therapist holds as helper has not been adequately addressed in the psychotherapy literature, along with lack of understanding of privilege and oppression issues in mainstream psychotherapy literature. This requires conducting additional explorations with clients to understand the barriers they face to make the therapeutic intervention contextually meaningful. We believe lack of understanding of the contextual variables leads to cultural oppression, as the client's context is important to understanding the possibilities that exist for resolving psychological dilemmas and mental health problems (Castillo, 1997; Dana, 1998; Lonner & Ibrahim, 2008). In addition, lack of cultural self-knowledge of the helper is a serious impediment to effective service delivery, in spite of ethical guidelines and existing competencies and recommendations by professional associations, practitioners show low understanding of their biases, although they have been exposed to cultural issues in their training and education, the need for meaningful education and training for effectiveness continues (Boysen & Vogel,

2008; Herman, 2004; Herman et al., 2007; Odegard & Vereen, 2010; Sue et al., 2009). On an optimistic note, Prilleltensky (2008) notes that the power to promote wellness, resist oppression, and foster liberation is already grounded in psychological and political dynamics. However, these two lines of research and thought have been addressed in isolation. He proposes that psychological and political power need to be integrated to lead to positive outcomes, not just in individual psychotherapy, but also to create structural change.

We agree with Sue et al. (2009) and Whaley and Davis (2007) that having specialized training in cultural and social competence is similar to having a psychological specialty, similar to other specialties such as treating anxiety disorders, or Autism Spectrum Disorders. Further, we strongly believe that cultural competence training, must incorporate training on social justice issues and advocacy, and supervised experiences, as required for other therapeutic competency areas (Ibrahim, 2010; Jun, 2010). We recommend that social justice training for mental health professionals include assessment of own and client privilege and oppressions an analysis of how class and classism are perceived and acted upon in daily life by the candidates (Ibrahim, 2010; Liu et al., 2004). In addition information about social justice challenges in society, and experiential training in exploring social justice issues is necessary to understand the depth and breadth of social problems (Adams et al., 2013; Ibrahim, 2010; Jun, 2010; Leong, Leach, & Malikiosis-Loizas, 2012). Hays, Dean, and Chang (2007) add that counselor attitudes are influenced by the social norms and may influence their work as helpers, consultants, educators, and researchers unless they are aware of their internalized and unconscious assumptions. Professionals in training need to assess their formative and summative knowledge and information on challenges that people in their social system face. In addition they need to explore various methods to understand how these challenges affect everyday life, such as being homeless, living in poverty, being a homosexual in a heterosexual world, an accomplished women and the glass ceiling, and the impact of these injustices on the individual, and the loss in social capital for society (Constantine, Hage, Kindaichi, & Bryant, 2007; Zane, 2002).

Assessment of Social Justice Concerns

Social justice assessment requires an evaluation of assets and challenges or privilege and oppression to identify the social justice issues that may create social distance between the helping professional and the client. One of the initial instruments in this domain was the *Quick Discrimination Index* (QDI; Ponterotto et al., 1995; Ponterotto, Potere, & Johansen, 2002), to assess attitudes toward racism and sexism, called the QDI. This is a 30-item inventory, it is scored on a five-point Likert scale with response options ranging from strongly agree = 1, to strongly disagree = 5. It assesses attitudes on three factors: Cognitive racial attitudes, affective racial attitudes, and cognitive gender attitudes. Higher scores indicate greater comfort and positive attitudes toward racial and gender equity. The QDI has adequate validity (face, content, construct, and criterion) and reliability, along with convergent validity, evidenced by significant correlations with Jacobsen's (1985) New Racism Scale (Ponterotto et al., 1995, 2002).

Another instrument that has been used to assess attitudes, acceptance, and comfort with culturally similar and dissimilar individuals is the Miville-Guzman Universality-Diversity Scale-Short Form (M-GUDS-S; Fuertes, Miville, Mohr, Sedlacek, & Gretchen, 2000). This is a 15-item scale with a Likert scale ranging from strongly disagree = 1, to strongly agree = 6. Higher scores indicate greater acceptance. It assesses attitudes on three factors: Relativistic Appreciation, Diversity of Contact, and Comfort with Differences. This instrument has adequate reliability and validity, as reported by Fuertes et al. (2000). Cronbach alpha coefficients for internal consistency reliability were reported as .59 for Relativistic Appreciation, .82 for Diversity of Contact, and .92 for Comfort with Differences, and .77 for the total score. The authors established criterion-related validity using data from racial-ethnic differences for the one subscale (Comfort with Differences) or the M-GUDS-S.

A newer validated instrument available is the *Privilege-Oppression Inventory* (POI: Hays et al., 2007). This inventory is composed of 39 items; it uses a six-point Likert scale (strongly disagree = 1 to strongly agree = 6). It provides scores on four factors: White Privilege Awareness, Heterosexism Awareness, Christian Privilege Awareness, and Sexism Awareness. It has a high reliability as evidenced for internal consistency (Cronbach alpha .95) and item-total correlation ranged from .26 to .70, as a result of one item with a mean correction for item-total correlation of .56. Cronbach alpha for each subscale reported: White Privilege Awareness .92, Heterosexism Awareness .81, Christian Privilege Awareness .86, and Sexism Awareness .79. Test–retest for the two administrations of the 39-item scale was established at $r = .91$, $p = .01$). In addition, the item–item correlations for the two administrations ranged from .57 to .89. All the correlations were significant at the .01 level. Convergent validity was established using the M-GUDS-S (Fuertes et al., 2000) and the QDI (Ponterotto et al., 1995, 2002). Statistically significant correlations for all the subscales of the POI were obtained using the M-GUDS-S total score. Similarly, the QDI subscales for Cognitive Racial Awareness, Affective Racial Attitudes, and Cognitive Gender subscale, yielded statistically significant correlations for all four subscales of the POI.

Primarily because clients lack power due to limited access to resources and opportunities, they could be targets of oppression (physical and psychological) and it is important that therapists commit to social justice advocacy and action (Greenleaf & Willliams, 2009). For counseling professionals, there is no choice, but to adhere to professional mandates regarding social justice as it is entrenched within cultural competence due to the despair that people have been subjected to as a result of greed, aggrandizement, and capitalism (Marsella, 2006, 2013).

References

Adams, M., Bell, L. A., & Griffin, P. (Eds.). (2007). *Teaching for diversity and social justice* (2nd ed.). New York: Routledge.

Adams, M., Blumenfeld, W. J., Castaneda, C., Hackman, H. W., Peters, M. L., & Zuniga, X. (Eds.). (2013). *Readings in diversity and social justice* (3rd ed.). New York: Routledge.

AERA, APA, & NCME. (2014). *Standards for educational and psychological testing*. Washington, DC: Author.

Albee, & George, W. (2000). The Boulder model's fatal flaw. *American Psychologist, 55*(2), 247–248.

Alexander, M. (2012). *The new Jim Crow: Mass incarceration in the age of color blindness*. New York: The New Press.

American Counseling Association (ACA). (1992). *Multicultural competencies*. Alexandria, VA: American Counseling Association.

American Counseling Association (ACA). (2003). *ACA advocacy competencies*. Alexandria, VA: American Counseling Association.

American Counseling Association (ACA). (2014). *Code of ethics*. Alexandria, VA: American Counseling Association.

American Psychological Association (APA). (2002). *Guidelines for multicultural education, training, research, practice, and organizational change for psychologists*. Washington, DC: American Psychological Association.

American Psychological Association (APA). (2011). *The guidelines for psychological practice with lesbian, gay, and bisexual clients*. Washington, DC: Author.

Andersen, M. (2003). Whitewashing race: A critical perspective on whiteness. In W. Doan & E. Bonilla-Silva (Eds.), *White out*. New York: Routledge.

Anyon, J. (2005). *Radical possibilities: Public policy, urban education, and a new social movement*. New York: Routledge.

Arnett, J. J. (2002). The psychology of globalization. *American Psychologist, 57*(10), 774–783. doi:10.1037//0003-066X.57.10.774.

Atkinson, D. R., Thompson, C. E., & Grant, S. K. (1993). A three-dimensional model for counseling racial/ethnic minorities. *The Counseling Psychologist, 21*(2), 257–277.

Baldwin, S. A., Wampold, B. E., & Imel, Z. E. (2007). Untangling the alliance–outcome correlation: Exploring the relative importance of therapist and patient variability in the alliance. *Journal of Consulting and Clinical Psychology, 75*, 842–852. doi:10.1037/0022-006X.

Bernal, G., & Saéz-Santiago, E. (2006). Culturally centered psychosocial interventions. *Journal of Community Psychology, 34*, 121–132.

Berry, J. W. (1974). Immigration, acculturation, and adaptation. *Applied Psychology: An International Review, 46*(1), 5–68.

Blum, L. (2008). White privilege: A mild critique. *Theory and Research in Education, 6*, 309–321. doi:10.1177/1477878508095586.

Blustein, D. L. (2006). *The psychology of working: A new perspective for counseling, career development, and public policy*. New York: Routledge.

Blustein, D. L., McWhirter, E. H., & Perry, J. C. (2005). Toward an emancipatory communitarian approach to vocational development theory. *The Counseling Psychologist, 33*, 141–179.

Boysen, G. A., & Vogel, D. L. (2008). The relationship between level of training, implicit bias, and multicultural competency among counselor trainees. *Training and Education in Professional Psychology, 2*, 103–110.

Bradley, J. M., Werth, J. R., & Hastings, S. L. (2012). Social justice advocacy in rural communities. *The Counseling Psychologist, 40*, 363–384.

Breton, M. (1995). The potential for social action in groups. *Social Work with Groups, 18*, 5–13.

Bronfenbrenner, U. (1977). Toward an experimental ecology of human development. *American Psychologist, 32*, 513–531.

Bronfenbrenner, U. (1979). *The ecology of human development*. Cambridge, MA: Harvard University Press.

Bulhan, H. A. (1985). *Franz Fanon and the psychology of oppression*. New York: Plenum.
Castillo, R. J. (1997). *Culture and mental illness*. Belmont, CA: Brooks/Cole.
Castro, F. G., Barrera, M. J., & Holleran Steiker, L. K. (2010). Issues and challenges in the design of culturally adapted evidence-based interventions. *Annual Review of Clinical Psychology, 6*, 213–239.
Chang, D. F., & Berk, A. (2009). Making cross-racial therapy work: A phenomenological study of clients' experiences of cross-racial therapy. *Journal of Counseling Psychology, 56*, 521–536. doi:10.1037/a0016905.
Chang, C. Y., Crethar, H. C., & Ratts, M. J. (2010). Social justice: A national imperative for counselor education and supervision. *Counselor Education & Supervision, 50*(2), 82–87.
Chang, D. F., & Yoon, P. (2011). Ethnic minority client's perceptions of the significance of race in cross-racial therapy relationships. *Psychotherapy Research, 21*, 567–582. doi:10.1080/10503307.2011.592549.
Cochran-Smith, M. (2004). Defining the outcomes of teacher education: What's social justice got to do with it. *Asia-Pacific Journal of Teacher Education, 32*(3), 193–212.
Constantine, M. G., Hage, S. M., Kindaichi, M. M., & Bryant, R. M. (2007). Social justice and multicultural issues: Implications for the practice and training of counselors and counseling psychologists. *Journal of Counseling & Development, 85*, 24–29.
Council on Social Work Accreditation (CSWE). (2008). *Educational Policy and Accreditation Standards*. Retrieved from http://www.cswe.org/CSWE/accreditation
Dana, R. H. (1998). *Understanding cultural identity in intervention and assessment*. Thousand Oaks, CA: Sage.
Deeley, S. J. (2010). Service-learning: Thinking outside the box. *Active Learning in Higher Education, 11*(1), 43–53. doi:10.1177/1469787409355870.
Diamond, J. (1997). *Guns, steel, & germs: The fates of human societies*. New York: Norton.
Flynn, J. P. (1995). Social justice in social agencies. In R. L. Edwards (Ed.), *Encyclopedia of social work* (19th ed., Vol. 1, pp. 95–100). Washington, DC: NASW Press.
Fourie, M. (2003). Beyond the ivory tower: Service learning for a sustainable community development, perspectives on higher education. *South African Journal of Higher Education, 17*(1), 31–38.
Frable, D. E. S. (1997). Gender, racial, ethnic, and class identities. *Annual Review of Psychology, 48*, 139–162.
Freire, P. (1974). *Education for critical consciousness*. New York: Continuum.
Friere, P. (1974). *Pedagogy of the oppressed*. New York: Continuum.
Fuertes, J. N., Miville, M. L., Mohr, J. J., Sedlacek, W. E., & Gretchen, D. (2000). Factor structure and short form of the Miville-Guzman Universality-Diversity Scale. *Measurement and Evaluation in Counseling and Development, 33*, 157–169.
Gaztambude, D. J. (2012). Addressing cultural impasses with rupture resolution strategies. *Professional Psychology: Research and Practice, 43*(3), 183–189. doi:10.1037/a0026911.
Gibelman, M. (1995). *What social workers do* (4th ed.). Washington, DC: NASW Press.
Goodman, R. D., & Gorski, P. C. (Eds.). (2015). *Decolonizing "multicultural" counseling through social justice*. New York: Springer.
Goodman, L. A., Liang, B., Helms, J. E., Latta, R. E., Sparks, E., & Weintraub, S. R. (2004). Training counseling psychologists as social justice agents: Feminist and multicultural principles in action. *The Counseling Psychologist, 32*, 793–837.
Greenleaf, A. T., & Willliams, J. M. (2009). Supporting social justice advocacy: A paradigm shift towards an ecological perspective. *Journal for Social Action in Counseling and Psychology, 2*(1), 1–14.
Greenwald, A. G., McGhee, D. E., & Schwartz, J. K. L. (1998). Measuring individual differences in implicit cognition: The implicit association test. *Journal of Personality and Social Psychology, 74*, 1464–1480.
Hardiman, R., Jackson, B., & Griffin, P. (2007). Conceptual foundations for social justice education. In M. Adams, L. A. Bell, & P. Griffin (Eds.), *Teaching for diversity and social justice* (2nd ed., pp. 35–66). New York: Routledge.

Hays, D. G., Chang, C. Y., & Decker, S. L. (2007). Initial development and psychometric data for the Privilege and Oppression Inventory. *Measurement and Evaluation in Counseling and Development, 40*, 66–79.

Hays, D. G., Dean, J. K., & Chang, C. Y. (2007). Addressing privilege and oppression in counselor training and practice: A qualitative analysis. *Journal of Counseling & Development, 85*, 317–324.

Held, D. (1998). Democratization and globalization. In D. Archibugi, D. Held, & M. Kohler (Eds.), *Re-imagining political community* (pp. 11–27). Stanford, CA: Stanford University Press.

Helms, J. E. (1990). *Black and white racial identity attitudes: Theory, research, and practice*. Westport, CT: Greenwood Press.

Herman, M. (2004). Forced to choose: Some determinants of racial identification in multiracial adolescents. *Child Development, 75*(3), 730–748.

Herman, K. C., Tucker, C. M., Ferdinand, L. A., Mirsu-Paun, A., Hasan, N. T., & Beato, C. (2007). Culturally sensitive healthcare and counseling psychology: An overview. *Journal of Counseling Psychology, 35*(5), 633–649.

Hernandez, P., Carranza, M., & Almeida, R. (2010). Mental health professionals' adaptive responses to microaggressions: An exploratory study. *Professional Psychology: Research and Practice, 41*(3), 202–209. doi:10.1037/a0018445.

Horvath, A. O., Del Re, A. C., Fluckiger, C., & Symonds, D. (2011). Alliance in individual psychotherapy. *Psychotherapy, 48*, 9–16. doi:10.1037/a0022186.

Ibrahim, F. A. (2003). Existential worldview theory: From inception to applications. In F. D. Harper & J. McFadden (Eds.), *Culture and counseling: New approaches* (pp. 196–208). Boston: Allyn & Bacon.

Ibrahim, F. A. (2007, September). *Understanding multiple identities in counseling: Use of the Scale to Assess Worldview© and the Cultural Identity Checklist-R©"* at the Colorado Psychological Association Society for the Advancement of Multiculturalism and Diversity (SAMD), Denver, CO.

Ibrahim, F. A. (2008). *Cultural identity check list-revised©* (CICL-R). Unpublished document, Denver, CO.

Ibrahim, F. A. (2010). Innovative teaching strategies for group work: Addressing cultural responsiveness and social justice. *Journal for Specialists in Group Work, 35*(3), 271–280. doi:10.1080/01933922.10.492900.

Ibrahim, F. A. (2013, March). *Mental illness and the "war on drugs."* Counselors for Social Justice Visioning Project for the Eighth Annual Social Justice Leadership Development Project "Visioning Process." Cincinnati, OH.

Ibrahim, F. A., Dinsmore, J., Estrada, D., & D'Andrea, M. (2011, Fall). Counselors for social justice: Ethical standards. *Journal for Social Action in Counseling and Psychology, 3*(2). Retrieved from http://jsacp.tumblr.com

Ibrahim, F. A., & Kahn, H. (1984). *Scale to assess worldviews*. Unpublished document, Storrs, CT.

Ibrahim, F. A., & Kahn, H. (1987). Assessment of worldviews. *Psychological Reports, 60*, 163–176.

Ivey, A. E., & Collins, N. M. (2003). Social justice: A long-term challenge for counseling psychology. *The Counseling Psychologist, 31*, 290–298. doi:10.1177/0011000003031003004.

Ivey, A. E., Ivey, M. B., & D'Andrea, M. (2011). *Theories of counseling and psychotheraoy: A multicultural perspective*. Thousand Oaks, CA: Sage.

Ivey, A. R. (1995). Psychotherapy as liberation. In J. G. Ponterotto, J. Casas, L. A. Suzuki, & C. M. Alexander (Eds.), *Handbook of multicultural counseling* (pp. 115–138). Thousand Oaks, CA: Sage.

Jackson, M. R. (2011). Psychology and social justice. *Peace Review, 23*(1), 69–76.

Jacobsen, C. K. (1985). Resistance to affirmative action: Self-interest or racism? *Journal of Conflict Resolution, 29*(2), 306–329. doi:10.1177/0022002785029002007.

Johnson, A. (2006). *Privilege, power, and difference*. New York: McGraw-Hill.

Johnson, W., & Packer, A. (1987). *Workforce 2000: Work and workers for the twenty-first century*. Indianapolis, IN: Hudson Institute.

Jun, H. (2010). *Social justice, multicultural counseling, and practice*. Thousand Oaks, CA: Sage.

Kaiser Family Foundation. (2011). Distribution of U.S. population by race, ethnicity, 2010 and 2050 [Online]. Retrieved July 4, 2011, from http://facts.kff.org/chart.aspx?ch=364

Keenan, E. K., Tsand, A. K. T., Bogo, M., & George, U. (2005). Micro ruptures and repairs in the beginning phase of cross-cultural psychotherapy. *Clinical Social Work Journal, 33*, 271–289. doi:10.1007/s10615-005-4944-7.

Kendall, F. E. (2013). *Understanding white privilege* (2nd ed.). New York: Routledge.

Kim, S., & Cardemil, E. (2009). Effective psychotherapy with low income clients: The importance of attending to social class. *Journal of Contemporary Psychotherapy, 39*(3), 147–212. doi:10.1007/s10879-011-9194-0.

Kimber, S., & Delgado-Romero, E. A. (2011). Sexual orientation microaggressions: The experience of lesbian, gay, bisexual, and queer clients in psychotherapy. *Journal of Counseling Psychology, 58*(2), 210–221. doi:10.1037/a002225.

King, D. W., Vigil, I. T., Herrera, A. P., Hajek, R. A., & Jones, L. A. (2007). Working toward social justice: Center for research on minority health summer workshop on health disparities. *Californian Journal of Health Promotion, 5*, 1–8.

Kiselica, M. (Ed.). (1999). *Confronting prejudice and racism during multicultural training*. Alexandria, VA: American Counseling Association.

Koch, J. M., Ross, J. B., Wendell, J., & Aleksandrova-Howell, M. (2014). Results of immersion service learning activism with peers: Anticipated and surprising. *The Counseling Psychologist, 42*, 1215–1246. doi:10.1177/0011000014535955.

Lee, C. C. (Ed.). (2007). *Counseling for social justice* (2nd ed.). Alexandria, VA: American Counseling Association.

Leong, F. T. L., Leach, M. M., & Malikiosis-Loizas, M. (2012). Internationalizing the field of counseling psychology. In F. T. L. Leong, W. E. Pickren, M. M. Leach, & A. J. Marsella (Eds.), *Internationalizing the psychology curriculum in the United States*. New York: Springer.

Leong, F. T. L., Leach, M. M., Marsella, A. J., & Pickren, W. E. (2012). Internationalizing the psychology curriculum in the USA: Meeting the challenges and opportunities of a global era. In F. T. L. Leong, W. E. Pickren, M. M. Leach, & A. J. Marsella (Eds.), *Internationalizing the psychology curriculum in the United States* (pp. 1–10). New York: Springer.

Lewis, J. A., Toporek, R. L., & Ratts, M. J. (2010). Advocacy and social justice: Entering the mainstream of the counseling profession. In M. J. Ratts, R. L. Toporek, & J. A. Lewis (Eds.), *ACA Advocacy Competencies: A social justice framework for counselors* (pp. 239–244). Alexandria, VA: American Counseling Association.

Lipsitz, G. (2013). The possessive investment in whiteness. In M. Adams, W. J. Blumenfeld, C. Castaneda, H. W. Hackman, M. L. Peters, & X. Zuniga (Eds.), *Readings in diversity and social justice* (3rd ed., pp. 77–85). New York: Routledge.

Liu, W. M., Ali, S., Soleck, G., Hopps, J., Dunston, K., & Pickett, T. (2004). Using social class in counseling psychology research. *Journal of Counseling Psychology, 51*, 3–18.

Lonner, W. J., & Ibrahim, F. A. (2008). Assessment in cross-cultural counseling. In P. B. Pedersen, J. Draguns, W. J. Lonner, & J. Trimble (Eds.), *Counseling across cultures* (6th ed., pp. 37–57). Thousand Oaks, CA: Sage.

Marsella, A. J. (2006). Justice in a global age: Becoming counselors to the world. *Counselling Psychology Quarterly, 19*(2), 121–132.

Marsella, A. J. (2013). All psychologies are indigenous psychologies: Reflections on psychology in a global era. *Psychology International, 24*(4), 5–7.

Martin-Baro, I. (1994). *Writings for a liberation psychology*. Cambridge, MA: Harvard University Press.

McIntosh, P. (1993). Examining unearned privilege. *Liberal Education, 70*(1), 61–63.

Miller, D. (2001). *Principles of social justice*. Cambridge, MA: Harvard University Press.

Murray, C. E., Pope, A. L., & Rowell, P. C. (2010). Promoting counseling students' advocacy competencies through service-learning. *Journal for Social Action in Counseling and Psychology, 2*(2), 29–47.

Nadal, K. L., Wong, Y., Issa, M. A., Meterko, V., Leon, J., & Wideman, M. (2011). Sexual orientation microaggressions: Processes and coping mechanisms for lesbian, gay, and bisexual individuals. *Journal of Counseling Psychology, 58*(2), 210–221. doi:10.1037/a0022251.

National Association of Social Workers (NASW). (2001). *Code of ethics* (Rev. ed.). Retrieved from http://www.Socialworkers.org/pubs/code/default.asp

National Wild Life Federation. (2011). *What we do to protect wild life.* Retrieved from http://www.nwf.org/What-We-Do/Protect-Wildlife.aspx.

Negi, N. J., Bender, K. A., Furman, R., Fowler, D. N., & Prickett, J. C. (2010). Enhancing self-awareness: A practical strategy to train culturally responsive social work students. *Advances in Social Work, 11*(2), 223–234.

Neville, H. A., & Mobley, M. (2001). Social identities in contexts: An ecological model of multicultural counseling psychology processes. *The Counseling Psychologist, 29*, 471–486. doi:10.1177/0011000001294001.

Odegard, M. A., & Vereen, L. G. (2010). A grounded theory of counselor educators integrating social justice into their pedagogy [Special issue]. *Counselor Education and Supervision, 50*, 130–149.

Oliver, M. L., & Shapiro, T. M. (2006). *Black wealth/white wealth: A new perspective on racial inequality* (2nd ed.). New York: Taylor & Francis.

Otani, A. (1989). Client resistance in counseling: Its theoretical rationale and taxonomic classification. *Journal of Counseling and Development, 67*(8), 458–461.

Owen, J., Imel, Z., Tao, K. W., Wampold, B., Smith, A., & Rodolfa, E. (2011). Cultural ruptures in short-term therapy: Working alliance as a mediator between clients' perceptions of microaggressions and therapy outcomes. *Counselling and Psychotherapy Research, 11*, 204–212. doi: 10.1080/14733145.2010.491551.

Owen, J., Tao, K., & Rodolfa, E. (2010). Microaggressions and women in short-term psychotherapy: Initial evidence. *The Counseling Psychologist, 38*, 923–946. doi:10.1177/0011000010376093.

Pedersen, P. J., Meyer, J. M., & Hargrave, M. (2014). Learn global; serve local-student outcomes from a community-based learning pedagogy. *Journal of Experiential Education.* doi: 10.1177/1053825914531738. (Published online May 6, 2014).

Pew Research Center: Social and Demographic Trends. (2011, July). *Wealth gaps rise to record highs between whites, blacks, and hispanics* (pp. 1–16). Retrieved from http://www.pewsocialtrends.org/2011/07/26/wealth-gaps-rise-to-record-highs-between-whites-blacks-and-hispanics

Pieterse, A. L., Evans, S. A., Risner-Butner, A., Collins, N. M., & Mason, L. B. (2009). Multicultural competence and social justice training in counseling psychology and counselor education: A review and analysis of a sample of multicultural course syllabi. *The Counseling Psychologist, 37*(1), 93–115. doi:10.1177/0011000008319986.

Pinderhughes, E. (1989). *Understanding race, ethnicity, & power: The key to efficacy in clinical practice.* New York: Free Press.

Pipher, M. (2014). *The green boat: Reviving ourselves in our capsized culture.* New York: Penguin.

Ponterotto, J. G., Burkard, A., Rieger, B. P., Grieger, I., D'Onofrio, A., Dubuisson, A., et al. (1995). Development and initial validation of the Quick Discrimination Index (QDI). *Educational and Psychological Measurement, 5S*, 1016–1031.

Ponterotto, J. G., Potere, J. C., & Johansen, S. A. (2002). The Quick Discrimination Index: Normative data and user guidelines for counseling researchers. *Journal of Multicultural Counseling and Development, 30*, 192–207.

Pope Paul VI. (1972). *Celebration for peace day.* Retrieved July 22, 2014, from http://www.Vatican.va/holyfather/paulvi/messages/peace/documents/hf_p-vi_mes_19711208_v-world-day-for-peace_en.html

Prilleltensky, I. (1989). Psychology and the status quo. *American Psychologist, 44*, 795–802.

Prilleltensky, I. (1997). Values, assumptions, and practices: Assessing the moral implications of psychological discourse action. *American Psychologist, 52*, 517–535.

Prilleltensky, I. (2001). Value-based praxis in community psychology: Moving toward Social justice and social action. *American Journal of Community Psychology, 29*(5), 747.

Prilleltensky, I. (2008). The role of power in wellness, oppression, and liberation: The promise of psychopolitical validity. *Journal of Community Psychology, 36*(2), 116–136. doi:10.1002/jcop.20225.

Ratts, M. V. (2009). Social justice counseling: Toward the development of a "fifth force" among counseling paradigms. *Journal of Humanistic Counseling Education and Development, 48*, 160–172.

Romano, J. L., & Hage, S. (2000). Prevention: A call to action. *The Counseling Psychologist, 28*, 854–856.

Sampson, E. E. (1988). The challenge of social change for psychology: Globalization and psychology's theory of the person. *American Psychologist, 44*(6), 914–921. doi:10.1037/0003-066X.44.6.914.

Scherlen, A., & Robinson, M. (2008). Open access to criminal justice scholarship: A matter of social justice. *Journal of Criminal Justice Education, 19*(1), 54–74.

School of Social Work, Graduate Catalog. (2006). *Principles of social work practice*. St. Paul, MN: St. Catherine University.

Sensoy, O., & DeAngelo, R. (2008). Developing social justice literacy: An open letter to our faculty colleagues. *Phi Delta Kappan, 90*(5), 345–352.

Shapiro, J. P. (2006). Ethics and social justice within the new DEEL: Addressing the paradox of control/democracy. *International Electronic Journal for Leadership in Learning December, 10*(32). Retrieved December 18, 2006, from www.ucalgary.ca/%7Eiejll/volume10/shapiro.htm (link is external)

Sharf, J., Primavera, L. H., & Diener, M. J. (2010). Dropout and therapeutic alliance: A meta-analysis of adult individual psychotherapy. *Psychotherapy, 47*, 637–645. doi:10.1037/a0021175.

Singh, A. A., Hofsess, C. D., Boyer, E. M., Kwong, A., Lau, A. S. M., McLain, M., et al. (2010). Social justice and counseling psychology: Listening to the voices of doctoral trainees. *The Counseling Psychologist, 38*, 766–795.

Singh, A. A., Merchant, N., Skudrzyk, B., & Ingene, D. (2012). *Association for Specialists in Group Work (ASGW): Multicultural and social justice principles for group work*. Alexandria, VA: ASGW.

Singh, A. A., & Salazar, C. F. (2010). Process and action in social justice group work: Introduction to the special issue. *Journal for Specialists in Group Work, 35*(3), 308–319.

Snow, W. H. (2012). Psychology and social justice. *Social Justice Journal, 1*, 44–46.

Speight, S. L., & Vera, E. M. (2004). A social justice agenda: Ready, or not? *The Counseling Psychologist, 32*, 109–118. doi:10.1177/0011000003260005.

Sue, D. W., Capodilupo, C. M., Torino, G. C., Bucceri, J. M., Holder, A. M. B., Nadal, K. L., et al. (2007). Racial microaggressions in everyday life: Implications for clinical practice. *American Psychologist, 62*, 271–286. doi:10.1037/0003-066X.62.4.271.

Sue, S., Zane, N., Hall, G. C. N., & Berger, L. K. (2009). The case for cultural competency in psychotherapeutic interventions. *Annual Review of Psychology, 60*, 525–548. doi:10.1146/annurev.psych.60.110707.163651.

Tatum, B. D. (1992). Talking about race, learning about racism: The application of racial identity development theory in the classroom. *Harvard Educational Review, 62*(1). Retrieved from http://isites.harvard.edu/fs/docs/icb.topic551851.files/TalkingAboutRace%20Tatum.pdf

Tatum, B. D. (1997). *Why are all the black kids sitting together in the cafeteria? And other conversations about race*. New York: Basic Books.

The American Psychiatric Association. (2004). *Reducing mental health disparities: An action plan*. Washington, DC: The American Psychiatric Association.

Toporek, R. L., Gerstein, L. H., Fouad, N. A., Roysircar, G., & Israel, T. (2006). *Handbook for social justice in counseling psychology: Leadership, vision, and action*. Thousand Oaks, CA: Sage.

United Nations. (1948). *The universal declaration of human rights*. Retrieved from http://www.un.org/en/documents/udhr/

United States (US) Census Bureau. (2006). *Income, poverty, and health insurance coverage in the United States*. Washington, DC: US Census Bureau.

Vasquez, M. J. T. (2007). Cultural difference and the therapeutic alliance: An evidence-based analysis. *American Psychologist, 62*, 875–885. doi:10.1037/0003-066X.62.8.878.

Vera, E. M. (2000). A recommitment to prevention in counseling psychology. *The Counseling Psychologist, 28*, 829–837.

Vera, E. M., & Speight, S. L. (2003). Multicultural competence, social justice, and counseling psychology: Expanding our roles. *The Counseling Psychologist, 31*, 253–272.

Watkins, M., & Shulman, H. (2008). *Toward psychologies of liberation*. New York: Palgrave Macmillan.

Werth, J. L., Jr., Borges, N. J., McNally, C. J., Maguire, C. P., & Britton, P. J. (2008). The intersections of work, health, diversity and social justice: Helping people living with HIV disease. *The Counseling Psychologist, 36*, 16–41.

Whaley, A. L., & Davis, K. E. (2007). Cultural competence and evidence based practice: A complementary perspective. *American Psychologist, 62*, 563–574. doi:10.1037/0003-066X.62.6.563.

World Health Organization (WHO). (2011). *Impact of economic crisis on world health*. Copenhagen, Denmark: WHO.

Yamada, A. M., & Marsella, A. J. (2013). Foundations: Overview of theory and models. In F. A. Paniagua & A. M. Yamada (Eds.), *Handbook of multicultural mental Health* (2nd ed., pp. 3–24). New York: Academic.

Young, I. M. (1990). *Justice and the politics of difference*. Princeton, NJ: Princeton University Press.

Young, I. M. (2001). Equality for whom? Social groups and judgments of injustice. *The Journal of Political Philosophy, 9*(1), 1–18.

Young, I. M. (2013). Five faces of oppression. In M. Adams, W. J. Blumenfeld, C. Castaneda, H. W. Hackman, M. L. Peters, & X. Zuniga (Eds.), *Readings in diversity and social justice* (3rd ed., pp. 35–45). New York: Routledge.

Zane, N. C. (2002). The glass ceiling is the floor my boss walks on: Leadership challenges in managing diversity. *The Journal of Applied Behavioral Science, 38*(3), 334–354.

Chapter 6
Immigrants: Identity Development and Counseling Issues

Introduction

A review of immigrant identity development in host culture and implications for counseling are explored in this chapter. Research literature and statistics on immigrants and refugees indicate that immigrant populations are rapidly increasing in the United States and in Western Europe (Fortuny, Chaudry, & Jargowsky, 2010; Organista, Organista, & Kurasaki, 2003). Mental health professionals will need to understand the issues and psychological changes, along with challenges faced by immigrants, to be able to provide effective mental health services (Chung, Bemak, Ortiz, & Sandoval-Perez, 2008). An important task for the helping professional is to understand the antecedent conditions that led to migration and the social-cultural conditions in the host culture. Further, similarity or dissimilarity of cultural assumptions, sociohistorical issues, and other factors may, or may not facilitate acceptance and integration. The experiences that an individual goes through in adapting to a new culture, along with their life experiences in culture of origin, influences the process of immigrant identity development in the new society (Phinney, Horenczyk, Liebkind, & Vedder, 2001). Once mental health practitioners understand the social conditions, the evolving immigrant identity, the developmental processes, and adjustment process involved in adapting to host culture, counseling strategies, and interventions can be implemented.

Identity Development

Several identity development models have been offered in the psychological literature pertaining to identity development in culture of origin, ethnicity, gender, sexual orientation, social cultural environment, and parental relationships (Chavez & Guido-DiBrito, 1999). The relationship between identity development in host

F.A. Ibrahim, J.R. Heuer, *Cultural and Social Justice Counseling*, International and Cultural Psychology, DOI 10.1007/978-3-319-18057-1_6 culture, and adaptation to a new culture is also moderated by a number of additional factors, these include: Age at time of migration, and generation of migration, along with antecedent conditions, acceptance or rejection in host culture, and the similarity of cultural assumptions between culture of origin and host culture (Phinney et al., 2001). Individuals upon migration to a new culture must adapt to new contexts, and this leads to changes in their original cultural identity. Psychological acculturation and adaptation refers to the psychological changes and eventual outcomes in a new setting (Berry, 1997). Successful acculturation implies mental and physical health, psychological satisfaction with life, high self-esteem, competent work performance, and good grades in school for younger immigrants (Liebkind, 2001). The nature of the acculturation process and the identification of factors predictive of effective cultural adaptation have been of substantial interest to researchers (e.g., Berry, 1984; Berry, Kim, Minde, & Mok, 1987; Berry, Kim, Power, Young, & Bujaki, 1989; Berry, Poortinga, Segall, & Dasen, 1992; Grossman, Wirt, & Davids, 1985; Liebkind, 1993, 1996; Nesdale, Rooney, & Smith, 1997; Nicassio, Solomon, Guest, & McCullough, 1986; Shisana & Celentano, 1985). Researchers have shown comparatively little interest on issues concerning immigrants' primary ethnic identification (i.e., their identification with their culture of origin), outside the development and maintenance of ethnic identity in immigrant adolescents, and the relationship between their ethnic identity and self-esteem, and their strategies of acculturation (e.g., Hurtado, Gurin, & Peng, 1994; Laperriere, Compere, Dkhissy, Dolce, & Fleurent, 1994; Liebkind, 1996; Nesdale & Mak, 2000; Phinney, 1989; Phinney & Alipuria, 1990; Phinney & Chavira, 1992; Phinney, Chavira, & Tate, 1992; Phinney, Chavira, & Williamson, 1992; Phinney, DuPont, Espinosa, Revill, & Sanders, 1994; Rumbaut, 2004; Saenz, Hwang, Aguirre, & Anderson, 1995; Spencer, Swanson, & Cunningham, 1992; van Oudenhoven & Eisses, 1998).

Role of Ethnic or Personal Identity

Ethnic identity is used as a theoretical framework to understand acculturation. Current thinking emphasizes that acculturation, is not a linear process of change requiring giving up one's culture of origin and assimilating into a new culture, it is instead best understood as a two-dimensional process (Berry, 1984, 1997; Lafromboise, Coleman, & Gerton, 1993). The two-dimensional models of acculturation are mostly based on the work of Berry. Researchers note that the two dominant aspects of acculturation, namely, preservation of cultural identity and adaptation to the host culture, are conceptually distinct and can vary independently (Liebkind, 2001). Given this distinction, Berry believes that two questions may help clinicians understand the processes and strategies that immigrants may use in making decisions about acculturation demands: (a) Is it important to maintain culture of origin in the new setting? (b) Is it important to develop relationships with members of the host culture? These questions determine the path people may take in adapting to a new cultural context (Nguyen et al., 1999; Phinney, 2006; Sayegh & Lasry, 1993).

Another issue that the current literature addresses is the fact that ethnic and national identities may be theoretically independent, the relationship between them varies empirically.

Schwartz, Montgomery, and Briones (2006) discuss the role of identity in acculturation. They view identity, as personal and social identity, and consider cultural identity as an aspect of personal identity. To define personal identity they use Erikson's (1968) conception of goals, values, and beliefs that a person adopts and holds. They consider social identity to have the following aspects (a) it is derived from the group one identifies with, including its self-identified ideals, mores, labels, and conventions (Erikson) and (b) the strength of this identification is exemplified by the extent to which one favors one's chosen "in group" (i.e., the group one identifies with), and the consequent distance from perceived out-groups (Tajfel & Turner, 1986). Cultural identity in this formulation is viewed as a special case of social identity (Padilla & Perez, 2003; Phinney et al., 2001) and is negotiated by the individual and the cultural context (Bhatia & Ram, 2001). Cultural identity refers to identification with the ideals of a given cultural group, which guides the attitudes, beliefs, and behaviors manifested toward one's own (and other) cultural groups (Jensen, 2003; Roberts et al., 1999).

Schwartz et al. (2006) note that acculturation leads to changes in cultural identity, and one's personal identity has the potential to anchor the individual during the transition. Their conception of acculturation is closely related to the concept of social and cultural identity (Bhatia & Ram, 2001). Further, they note that personal identity can be one's ethnic or national identity. Schwartz et al. (2006) reject the notion that there are four acculturation strategies. They use Phinney et al.'s (2001) two key dimensions of acculturation, i.e., adoption of receiving culture ideals and practices, and retention of heritage culture ideals and practices.

Integration in Host Culture

In some contexts integration into the host culture may be easier, leading to the development of a bicultural identity; whereas in other contexts it may be difficult, primarily, due to extreme cultural differences, a negative sociopolitical history or relationship between the two nations, perceived racial or religious differences, etc. (Bhatia & Ram, 2001; Phinney, 2006; Schwartz et al., 2006). Interestingly, research on developmental models of ethnic identity suggests that devaluation of one's cultural group need not result in self-derogation. Although, Phinney (1989) notes that children who are exposed to negative stereotypes about their own group may hold conflicting or negative feelings about their ethnicity. However, children are also influenced by messages received from their family and community, these may counteract the negative messages from a source that is not valued, even though it is the dominant culture (Knight, Bernal, Garza, Cota, & Ocampo, 1993). Both social psychological and developmental psychology research indicates that a strong, secure ethnic identity results in psychological well-being in the new environment. Research provides support for the idea that maintenance of a solid ethnic identity or personal identity is commonly related to psychological well-being among members of acculturating groups (Liebkind, 1996; Nesdale et al., 1997; Phinney et al., 1997; Schwartz et al., 2006). However, theory and research on acculturation also emphasizes the importance of adaptation to the new society.

As mentioned earlier, an important factor in immigrant identity development is age of migration. An important task for immigrant families is to ensure that children in these families adapt to schools in their new society. School adjustment is considered an important sociocultural and developmental task for children and adolescents (Phinney, 2006). Previously, it was assumed that immigrants would inevitably be absorbed into the receiving society, in a unilinear, unidirectional process (Gordon, 1964). However, research conducted by Berry (1974, 1980) indicates that there are two autonomous dimensions underlying the acculturation process: individuals' links to their cultures of origin and to the societies they settle in. These links manifest in a number of ways, e.g., preferences for involvement in the two cultures (termed acculturation attitudes), and in the behaviors that they participate in, e.g., their language knowledge and use, and social relationships (Berry, Phinney, & Sam, 2006).

Research on psychological adaptation to acculturation, identifies a distinction between *psychological* and *sociocultural* adaptation (Searle & Ward, 1990). Psychological adaptation alludes to internal psychological outcomes i.e., a clear sense of personal and cultural identity, good mental health, and the achievement of personal satisfaction in life and work in the new cultural context; sociocultural adaptation refers to external psychological outcomes that link individuals to their new context, including their capability to deal with daily problems, particularly in the areas of family life, work, and school. Although these two forms of adaptation are usually related empirically, researchers believe they need to be conceptually distinct due to two reasons: (a) the factors predicting these two types of adaptation are often different (Ward, 1996); and (b) psychological adaptation can best be understood within stress and psychopathology perspectives. Sociocultural adaptation is more closely linked to the social and interpersonal skills and behavior (Ward & Kennedy, 1993). An additional adaptive outcome in acculturation research pertains to *economic adaptation* (Aycan & Berry, 1996). This refers to satisfaction with work or career, and the ease with which work is obtained in the new culture (Berry, 1997).

The five main features of psychological acculturation include: (a) the acculturation experience; (b) appraisal of the experience; (c) strategies to deal with the experience; (d) immediate effects of experienced stress; and (e) long-term acculturation. These features have received many different designations in both the general and acculturation literature. There is agreement that the process of dealing with life events begins with some causal agent that places a demand on the organism (Aldwin, 1994; Lazarus, 1990, 1993). In the acculturation literature, these demands stem from the *experience* of having to deal with two cultures, and participating to various extents in both cultures. In some cases these experiences embody challenges that can improve one's life opportunities. In other cases they may seriously undermine the available life options (Berry, 1997).

Adaptation to a new setting is a multifaceted experience (Aycan & Berry, 1995) including psychological and sociocultural adaptation. There is a distinction between these two forms of adaptation that has been proposed and validated by Ward and colleagues (Searle & Ward, 1990; Ward, 1996; Ward & Kennedy, 1993). Psychological adaptation includes one's psychological and physical well-being (Schmitz, 1992). Sociocultural adaptation refers to how well acculturating individuals manage daily life in the new cultural context (Berry, 1997). Individuals begin the acculturation process with a number of personal characteristics, which include demographic and social factors. For example, one demographic variable is early biological age, and positive acculturation outcomes for adaptation to host culture. When acculturation begins prior to entry into elementary school, the process is generally smooth (Beiser et al., 1988). It is not clear why migrating before starting elementary school has a positive outcome. One hypothesis is that enculturation in culture of origin may not have been fully achieved, and therefore the individual did not have to engage in significant culture shedding to create cultural conflicts. Another reason may be that personal flexibility and adaptability is high at an earlier age. However, older youth do experience problems in adjusting to a new context particularly during adolescence (Aronowitz, 1993; Carlin, 1990; Ghuman, 1991; Sam & Berry, 1995). Quite possibly due to the adolescent developmental stage, which requires defining one's identity, and possible conflict and push-and-pull created by the demands of parents and peers, or because the problems of life transition between childhood and adulthood are compounded by cultural transitions. For example, as Phinney (1990) has noted that developmental issues of identity come to the fore at this time, and interact with questions of ethnic identity, therefore compounding the questions about one's identity. Berry's (1997) research shows that acculturation strategies have a strong relationship with positive adaptations, i.e., integration is usually the most successful; and marginalization is the least successful; assimilation and separation strategies provide intermediate success. This pattern has been found in nearly every study, and exists for all types of acculturating groups (Berry & Sam, 1996).

Berry's (1990) four modes of acculturation (integration, separation, marginalization, and assimilation) have two underlying, yet independent dimensions. The first dimension addresses the retention or letting go of native culture, and the second dimension concerns the acceptance or rejection of the dominant group. Further, Phinney (1990) notes that individuals may have independent identities with respect to their cultures of origin, and their society of settlement. This bidimensional conception has been presented frequently in the literature (e.g. Berry, 1997). This framework raises two issues: the degree to which people want to maintain their inherent culture and identity; and the degree to which people pursue involvement with the larger society. When these two issues are crossed, an acculturation area is created with four sectors within which individuals may express *how* they seek to acculturate. *Assimilation* is the path when there is little interest in maintenance of original culture combined with a preference for interacting with the larger society. *Separation* occurs when cultural maintenance is a high priority, along with avoiding involvement with host culture. *Marginalization* exists when neither cultural maintenance nor interaction with host culture is sought. *Integration* is present when both cultural maintenance and involvement with the larger society are a priority (Berry et al., 2006).

The phase of acculturation needs to be taken into account if stress and adaptation are to be understood accurately. The longer the process goes on, the greater the stress (Berry, 1997). Five models have been used to understand the process of change that occurs in transitions within, between, and among cultures, these are: Assimilation, acculturation, alternation, multiculturalism, and fusion (Lafromboise et al., 1993). Park (1928) and Stonequist (1937) propose that individuals who live at the juncture between two cultures, may consider themselves belonging to both cultures, either by being of mixed racial heritage or born in one culture and brought up in a second culture; they tend to be marginal to both cultural systems. Park suggests that marginality produces psychological conflict, a divided self, and a disjointed persona. Stonequist notes that marginality has certain social and psychological properties. The social properties include migration, racial difference, and situations in which two or more cultures share the same geographical area, with one culture maintaining a higher status than another.

Lafromboise and colleagues (1993) assert that a bicultural identity is the most adaptive, although what it means to be bicultural is interpreted differently across the psychological literature. When the contributions of each type of identity (ethnic and larger society) are included as separate variables in the analyses of well being, the results do vary (Phinney, 2006). Labeled the concept of biculturality as *double-consciousness*, or the simultaneous awareness of oneself as being a member, and an alien of two, or more cultures. This results in a "dual pattern of identification and a divided loyalty … [leading to] an ambivalent attitude" (Stonequist, 1937, p. 96).

Ethnic or personal identity and identity development as an immigrant are multifaceted processes. The Smith and Silva (2011) identifies the stages of ethnic identity development on majority/minority status in a social context. This model considers ethnic identity development as a lifelong process of differentiation and integration within the context of the boundaries of majority/minority social structures. For immigrants the boundaries could be too many, given that minority status creates an ego-dystonic ethnic identity, confusion about who they are, and where they belong, which can lead to maladaptive behavior (Smith). In general, identity development as an immigrant tends to be a difficult and complex process. The process of incorporating one's original ethnic identity into a different culture, and environment, causes confusion, and can be overwhelming for immigrants.

Phases of Development

The adaptation of immigrants is a complex phenomenon, which can vary for individuals due to several factors (Sam, 2000). This process can take individuals through several phases, requiring creative strategies to develop a cohesive identity. The following discussion presents several models that address the process of developing an integrated identity.

Ward (1996) presented a model that involves the previously mentioned psychological, and sociocultural adaptation to host culture. Ward refers to psychological adaptation as personal well-being, and good mental health; and sociocultural adaptation refers to social competence in managing daily life in an intercultural setting. Both Ward's model and the acculturation model of bicultural contact, proposed by Berry et al. (2006) emphasize) (a) the acquisition of the majority group's culture by members of the minority group, (b) a unidirectional relationship between the two cultures, and (c) assumes a hierarchical relationship between the two cultures. These two models are similar to the assimilation model proposed by Gordon (1964). The models differ on the variable of complete absorption in the host culture. The assimilation approach suggests that immigrants and their offspring, or their cultural group will ultimately become full members of the mainstream group's culture and lose identification with their culture of origin. However, Ward (1996) and Berry et al. (2006) models of acculturation models imply that the individual, while becoming a competent participant in the majority culture, will always be identified as a member of the minority culture (Lafromboise et al., 1993).

Kim (1979) proposed a model focusing on four areas of communication: intrapersonal, interpersonal, mass media, and the communication environment. In this model the level of acculturation is determined by how well a person uses various methods of communication, in the language of the majority culture. Another model of acculturation was put forth by Szapocznik and his colleagues (Szapocznik & Kurtines, 1980; Szapocznik, Kurtines, & Fernandez, 1980; Szapocznik et al., 1986; Szapocznik, Scopetta, Kurtines, & Aranalde, 1978). This model focuses on the behavior and values of immigrants, to assess the level of acculturation for an individual. The model suggests that before individuals acquire the values of the majority group, they will learn the behaviors needed to survive in a new culture. This model asserts acculturation is based on the length of time an individual is exposed to the majority culture. It also assumes that exposure to the majority culture will produce cultural competence.

Smither (1982) considers a multidimensional framework of acculturation. This is a socioanalytic approach and it considers the study of "the personality processes of the individual, which may facilitate or retard acculturation" to explain individual variation in acculturation (p. 62). Smither asserts that an individual must expand his or her role repertoire to meet the demands of the majority culture. According to the socioanalytic model, acculturation "is a function of the size of the difference between those qualities of character structure which affect role structure in the majority culture, and similar qualities of character structure in the minority culture compared to the majority role structure" (p. 64).

Several theoretical paradigms have been used to help explain both why some immigrants tend to adapt more successfully than others, and why some individual members of particular immigrant groups appear to adjust more easily to new contexts. The paradigms describe both macrolevel and microlevel forces with implications for variability in experiences of immigrant children (McCarthy, 2010). Laosa (1989) developed a *multivariate* model, which highlights the interaction of variables that mediate the stresses of migration, adaptation, adjustment, and development over time for immigrant children.

García Coll and Magnuson (1997) have argued for a positivist approach to the adaption of immigrant children. This approach focuses not just on the maladaptive behavior of children but also on "how the process of immigration can increase an individual's repertoire of coping skills, facilitate the acquisition of new and different skills, and broaden opportunities as well as worldviews (p. 105)." They combine developmental and positivist models to explain the relationship between migration, adaptation, and psychological stress. It provides a rich framework to analyze the migration experience. As Garcia-Coll and Magnuson note that:

> …Comprehensive models of immigrant children's' experiences, incorporating Laosa's model as well as the most recent developmental and contextual perspectives, provide a broad framework with which to study the adaptation and adjustment of immigrant children. There seems to be no single explanation for these differential adaptation processes and psychological outcomes. What is emerging from recent research is a need for a *multidimensional perspective* that incorporates the numerous factors that mediate the relationship between the stresses of migration, and the child's adaptation, adjustment, and development over time (p. 105).

Immigrant youth encounter different challenges than their adult counterparts. Aronowitz (1984) demonstrates that immigrant children are similar to native-born peers in schoolwork. Immigrant youth appear to understand the importance of developing a new identity in North America, and incorporating its cultural attitudes, and behaviors. They experience confusion on the issue of the degree of incorporation of their culture of origin, and the new culture they live in, into their identity (Tong, 2002; Tong & McIntyre, 1998). It is apparent that each individual must decide, consciously or not, the degree to which he/she/zir will maintain the practices of the old culture that are important to the sense of self, and adopt the ways of the new culture (Berry & Sam, 1996; Phinney, 2003). The coordination of the two cultures and languages is a complex process, involving different degrees of stress at different times during acculturation (Lupi & Tong, 2001; Tong, 1998, 2002).

A successful transition for immigrants and refugees at any age to a new culture, or country is the development of a secure cross-cultural identity that balances the values and beliefs of their home, and school cultures (Lupi & Tong, 2001; Tong, 1997, 1998, 2002). A healthy cross-cultural identity combines the values, beliefs, customs, and behavioral patterns of the two groups. Although, each individual identity will vary to an extent, in terms of how much of each culture forms the new identity; it depends on the person's experiences, needs, skills, intelligence, education, and support systems. The important aspect of this transition is that all common elements of the two cultures are perceived as symbiotic and complimentary, instead of being competitive (Tong, 1998, 2002).

Classical assimilation theory has ruled the sociological literature (McCarthy 2010, pp. 20–27). It suggests that social systems, and other settings are vital to the adaptation process of migrant groups, because they provide opportunities for significant social engagement, and participation in various social roles. These settings can be seen as activity settings and cultural support systems (O'Donnell, Tharp, & Wilson, 1993; Schwartz et al., 2006). These settings provide opportunities to spend time with the host culture, and access to resources that enables the integration of identities, and cultures into the new context. Migrant groups establish settings that create a sense of community, which, in turn, serves as a protective element for within group members, and also facilitates the adaptation process.

The Assimilation Model of immigrant identity development presents a number of subprocesses that constitute the stages of the assimilation process: (a) cultural or behavioral assimilation, (b) structural assimilation, (c) marital assimilation, (d) identificational assimilation, (e) attitudinal receptional assimilation, (f) behavioral receptional assimilation, and (g) civic assimilation (Gordon, 1964). Ruiz (1981) emphasized that the goal of the assimilation process is to achieve social acceptance from members of the host culture, as a person moves through these stages. "The underlying assumption of all assimilation models is that a member of one culture loses his or her original cultural identity as he or she obtains a new identity in a second culture" (Lafromboise et al., 1993).

The alternation model of second-culture acquisition asserts that it is possible for an individual to know and understand two different cultures. Further, it assumes that an individual can change his or her behavior to fit a particular social context. Ogbu (1990) argue "it is possible and acceptable to participate in two different cultures, or to use two different languages, perhaps for different purposes, by alternating one's behavior according to the situation" (p. 89). Ramirez (1984) alludes to the use of different problem solving, coping skills, human relational, communication, and incentive motivational styles, depending on the demands of the social context. Furthermore, the alternation model assumes that it is possible for an individual to have a sense of belonging in two cultures, without compromising his or her sense of personal identity. This model considers migrant development as a fluid process, which combines the old and new cultures into the new identity.

The multicultural model offers a pluralistic approach to understanding the relationship between two or more cultures. This model addresses the possibility of cultures maintaining distinct identities, specifically applicable to individuals from one culture working with people from another culture to achieve common national or economic interests. This model does not focus on geographic or social isolation issues, the critical factor is the multifaceted, and multidimensional institutional sharing between cultures, which sustains cultural diversity. Notes that a multicultural society emboldens all groups to (a) maintain and develop their group identities, (b) develop other-group acceptance and tolerance, (c) engage in intergroup contact and sharing, and (d) learn each other's language. While this model does not address identity development directly, it focuses on group identity, and this in turn influences how individuals acclimate, and change in a new society.

The fusion model of second-culture acquisition is a macrolevel model and represents the assumptions of the melting pot theory (Lafromboise et al., 1993). The fusion model suggests that cultures that share an economic, political, or geographic space will eventually fuse together, until they are unable to be distinguished from one another, and they will form a new culture. The sharing of institutional structures yields a new common culture. Each culture brings to the melting pot its strengths, and weaknesses, which takes on new forms as the cultures interact as equal partners. Gleason (1979) notes that cultural pluralism produces this type of change, if the various cultures share a common political entity.

Different researchers (e. g., Berry, 1984, 1997; Birman, 1998; Bulhan, 1985; Tajfel, 1981) offer models to better understand individual and community responses to intergroup interaction. Berry's (1997) model of acculturation and migrant adaptation offers four common responses to intercultural contact, i.e., integration, assimilation, separation, and marginalization. Although these models have been useful in understanding the acculturation, and adaptation processes, and outcomes for individuals, and groups, they are oversimplified, and pose problems in evaluating the dynamics of adaptation from the perspective of the dominant culture (Bhatia & Ram, 2001; Orford, 2009).

The influence of ethnic group membership on identity development, in a host culture is a complex issue studied by many researchers (Phinney, 1989). Many models of ethnic identity development share the idea that an achieved identity is the result of an identity crisis, which involved a period of exploration, leading to a commitment to an identity (Marcia, 1980). "Ethnic identity research suggests that identity changes progressively over time" (Phinney, 1989) The progressive nature of identity development suggests that minority group members begin with an acceptance of the values of the majority group culture, similar to Marcia's description of identity foreclosure, or Cross' (1991) pre-encounter phase. According to Phinney, the goal of this exploration is to arrive at an internalization of an ethnic identity, and sense of belonging to a cultural group. Understanding immigrant and refugee identity development is very important, given that it is an indicator of psychological adjustment, self-esteem, and well-being. Further, it helps in understanding mental health issues that may arise in immigrant populations.

Counseling Strategies and Psychotherapy

When immigrants experience mental health problems, in general it is related to the migration experience. A wide range of mental health problems, including grief over the loss of family and friends, familiar surroundings, and country of origin (Erikson, 1975). Further, anxiety, depression, posttraumatic stress disorder, substance abuse, and a higher prevalence of severe mental illness, and suicidal ideation have been observed among immigrant populations in the United States (American Psychological Association (APA), 2002; Desjarlais, Eisenberg, Good, & Kleinman, 1995; Duldulao, Takeuchi, & Hong, 2009).

Assessment of these issues is difficult given that the classic tools of psychology—normed psychological tests and psychological batteries—have a long history of misuse, particularly with nondominant ethnic, and diverse cultural populations (Dana, 2005; Lonner & Ibrahim, 2008; Strickland, 2000). The assessment tools used in psychology and mental health assessments are not normed on the culturally and linguistically different immigrant, and refugee populations (Suzuki, Kugler, &

Aguiar, 2005). The challenge for mental health professionals is to appropriately assess immigrants and linguistically diverse populations without relying on psychological tests and batteries. Inability to do this effectively results in: (a) placement in special education (Lesaux, 2006; Solano-Flores, 2008); (b) inaccurate ability, achievement, and aptitude evaluation (Menken, 2008; Solano-Flores, 2008); and (c) misuse of clinical assessment and diagnostic measures (APA, 2002, Lonner & Ibrahim, 2008; Suzuki, Ponterotto, & Meller, 2008).

For culturally appropriate psychological assessments, mental health professionals need to have an indepth knowledge about a specific culture, its languages, idioms, metaphors, etc., gained through continuous, intentional, and active participation with the culture of the group. Appropriate multicultural assessment requires that practitioners "arrive at an accurate, sound, and comprehensive description of the client's psychological presentation" (Ridley, Tracy, Pruitt-Stephens, Wimsatt, & Beard, 2008, p. 27). This can occur if data is available on historical, familial, economic, social, and community issues for the community under study (APA, 2002; Lonner & Ibrahim, 2008). Barriers to arriving at an accurate identification of psychological issues exist, these include sociocultural, contextual-structural, and clinical-procedural barriers. *Social-cultural barriers* encompass differences in symptom expression e.g., somatic symptoms (Alegría et al., 2008; Lonner & Ibrahim, 2008). Further, conflicting views about the cause i.e., attributions, and ways of coping with psychological problems (Atkinson, 2004; Koss-Chioino, 2000). *Contextual-structural barriers* refer to lack of access to appropriate and culturally sensitive mental health services (Lazear, Pires, Isaacs, Chaulk, & Huang, 2008; Wu, Kviz, & Miller, 2009). Additionally, lack of knowledge of available and existing mental health services (Garcia & Saewyc, 2007), and a shortage of racial/ethnic minority mental health workers, and persons trained to work with racial/ethnic minority persons, and older culturally diverse populations (APA, 2009), lack of access to trained interpreters, and lack of resources for accessing services (Rodríguez, Valentine, Son, & Muhammad, 2009). *Clinical-procedural* indicate the lack of culturally relevent and sensitive services (Lonner & Ibrahim, 2008; Maton, Kohout, Wicherski, Leary, & Vinokurov, 2006); "clinician bias" (Maton et al., 2006), communication problems related to language differences and cultural distinctions (Kim et al., 2011), misdiagnosis of presenting issues (Olfson et al., 2002), failure to assess cultural and linguistic constructs and appropriateness of tests for targeted populations (Dana, 2005; Kwan, Gong, & Younnjung, 2010; Suzuki et al., 2008), lack of attention to culturally entrenched expressions of resilience (Tummala-Narra, 2007), and failure to use the most effective mental health interventions e.g., evidence-based interventions adapted for use with nondominant, and immigrant populations (APA; McNeill & Cervantes, 2008).

While research on evidence-based treatments is needed to address the utility of interventions with immigrants, clinicians and researchers can benefit from using practice-based evidence that provides important lessons in culturally competent interventions (Birman et al., 2008). To increase the accessibility and efficacy of services, clinicians and practitioners should be following these guiding principles: (a) Conduct a multilevel cultural assessment (Ibrahim & Heuer, 2013a, 2013b;

Lonner & Ibrahim, 2008); (b) use an ecological perspective to create and guide interventions (Bronfenbrenner & Morris, 2006); (c) combine and integrate evidence-based practice with practice-based evidence (Birman et al., 2008); (d) provide culturally competent and responsive treatment (APA, 2002; Birman et al., 2005; Ibrahim & Heuer, 2013a; Marmol, 2003; Nastasi, Moore, & Varjas, 2004; Pedersen, 2003; Vera, Vila, & Alegría, 2003); (e) partner with community-based groups (Birman et al., 2008; Casas, Pavelski, Furlong, & Zanglis, 2001); and incorporate social justice principles in providing service (APA; Crethar, Torres Rivera, & Nash, 2008; Ibrahim & Heuer, 2013b).

Erik Erikson's (1975) fascination with identity, especially cultural identity, and life-span development provided an important path to understanding the dilemmas faced by immigrants. As an immigrant, he introduced the psychohistorical paradigm. This paradigm provides a guide for clinical work with immigrants. It takes a qualitative approach to identify the chronology of events in the life of an immigrant, i.e., family history. The clinician acts as both a historian and mental health service provider in this intervention that emphasizes the interactions between the inner selves of clients, their families, and the social contexts in which they live. This approach helps in identifying the conscious and unconscious stories of families (Erikson, 1975). This psychohistorical approach, focuses on the client's narrative, and brings the themes of identity conflict, acculturative stress, loss and grief, homesickness, guilt, and other emotions to the surface. Through an exploration of family history, reasons for migration, and an analysis of expectations of life in host culture, several issues can be identified.

Neville and Mobley (2001) identified the ecological systems framework offered by Bronfenbrenner (1979) as a useful framework for contextualizing cross-cultural counseling processes. Bronfenbrenner's ecological model includes four subsystems that he maintains are interrelated, and influence human behavior, these include: The *macrosystem*—the ideological aspect of a social system that influences the culture, traditions, norms, and values; the *microsystem*, focuses on interpersonal interactions of individuals in a family, at work, and in a community; the *mesosystem* considers the interactions between different subsystems; and finally the *exosystem* refers to the connections between subsystems that have an indirect effect on individuals. Neville and Mobley note that "ecological models operate from the assumption that human behavior is multiply determined, by a series of dynamic interactions between social systems. Individual psychological adjustment is thus dependent on who, or what, he or she interacts with on a daily basis, as well as those systems that structure an individual's day-to-day realities" (p. 472). An ecological framework is useful in understanding the multiple influences impinging upon immigrants, and the impact they have on an individual who comes from one macrosystem, and now resides in another macrosystem. One key component of this transition is stress that immigrants feel as they negotiate social subsystems, and the contrary demands of each macrosystem (culture of origin and host culture). Using an ecological perspective can facilitate understanding of the stressors, and assist clinicians in providing effective therapeutic services. Additionally, clinicians will consider concepts such as acculturation, transition, change, and identity, relevant to working with immigrants. To conduct culturally responsive therapeutic interventions, clinicians will need to assess their own self-awareness, cultural identity, acculturation to the norms of the dominant culture, privilege and oppression, emotional intelligence, cultural knowledge, critical thinking, and culturally relevant practices, as these are the processes that will lead to effective and ethical delivery of counseling services (Gamst & Liang, 2013; Ibrahim & Heuer, 2013b; Lonner & Ibrahim, 2008).

The concept of worldview, cultural values, and social justice are the foundation for multicultural counseling literature (American Multicultural Counseling Association (AMCD)/American Counseling Association (ACA), 1992; Ibrahim, 2010; Ibrahim & Dykeman, 2011; Lonner & Ibrahim, 2008). Often, the multicultural and social justice literature considers a culture-specific worldview, suggesting that all persons who have a specific cultural heritage share a similar worldview (Sue & Sue, 2013). Although individuals from the same cultural heritage may share some values, and traditions, there tends to be significant differences among people within a cultural group. Sundberg (1981) noted that research shows that the variations within a cultural group, tend to be greater than the differences between groups.

The Multilevel Model (MLM; Bemak et al., 2003) is a culturally sensitive model based on social justice theory and human rights principles to provide culturally sensitive, and effective services to immigrants, and refugees. A brief description of MLM follows: The MLM incorporates the AMCD/ACA multicultural (1992) and advocacy competencies (ACA, 2003), and is unique in that it incorporates both social justice and cultural competence principles, i.e., advocacy, consultation, attention to human rights issues, social justice concerns, indigenous healing practices, social networking, and heightened cultural responsiveness. It requires understanding of the cultural, historical, sociopolitical, and help-seeking behaviors of immigrant clients. Also the impact of pre- and post-migration experiences must be taken into consideration. It encourages professionals to have an expert level understanding of the racial and ethnic identity of the client, and of themselves, as well as, knowledge about the contextual, political, and social variables, including acceptance or rejection of immigrants, factors that can have a positive or negative effect on their mental health, and their acculturation process (Schwartz et al., 2006). Bemak et al. and Bemak (1989) highlight important issues that can impede the therapeutic process, such as falling prey to political countertransference, and the psychological recoil effect, that can occur when immigrants and refugees have strong traumatic reactions, as a result of witnessing others being harmed (Bemak & Chung, 2008).

Bemak and Chung (2003, 2008) also provide a comprehensive five-level intervention program, this include: *Level 1*: *Mental health education*. This includes psycho-educational interventions to help clients understand the counseling process, and what to expect in counseling; *Level 2*: *Individual, group, and family counseling interventions*; *Level 3*: *Cultural empowerment*. Providing assistance and support to immigrant clients and their families, to master the new culture, information about the host culture, and social skills for the host context; *Level 4*: *Integration of traditional and western healing practices*. Employing the client's own traditional healing practices and working with traditional healers, along with incorporating relevant counseling practices from a western perspective; and *Level 5: Social justice and human rights issues*. This includes an emphasis on promoting fair and equal treatment, using advocacy approaches to help negotiate numerous political, social, and systemic obstacles resulting from migration. The MLM model is a comprehensive intervention to work with immigrant populations, it incorporates culturally responsive counseling, and social justice practices, with respect for the client's cultural identity, basic human rights, and offers cultural empowerment, along with traditional healing practices (Bemak & Chung, 1998; Chung, Bemak, & Grabosky, 2011).

Challenges for Immigrant Populations

In working with immigrant and refugee populations it is important for professionals to recognize the politically charged atmosphere that currently exists in the United States regarding immigrants (Kira, Lewandowski, Chiodo, & Ibrahim, 2014). In addition, mental health professionals need to know the effect of immigration policies, pre-migration experiences, post-migration challenges, and the various forms of racism and discrimination and the impact on the mental health of immigrant and refugee clients (Bigelow, 2010; Sue & Capodilupo, 2008). It is clear that mental health professionals cannot provide professional services to immigrants without considering the multidimensional factors associated with immigrant populations (Kira et al., 2014).

The following section highlights several major issues that need to be taken into account when working with immigrants: (a) Negative perceptions of immigrants that are created by the media, and the unpredictable changes in terrorist alert levels that produce constant reminders of 9/11. These media messages have heightened concerns about immigrants and refugees, resulting in the current culture of fear regarding immigrants in the United States (Kira et al., 2014). Counselors who work with immigrants need to be aware of the ways in which this culture of fear adversely affects immigrant populations. It is critical that counselors understand these issues when developing counseling interventions to help promote immigrants' psychological well-being from a multicultural/social justice perspective. It is also important to be aware of the ways in which counselors are vulnerable to engaging in the culture of fear, which may lead to unconscious prejudicial and racist thinking about immigrant groups (Bemak et al., 2003).

Schwartz et al. (2006) identified several challenges faced by immigrants, which can deter the process of developing a positive immigrant identity and adaptation to host culture, these challenges include: (a) socioeconomic disadvantage (Phillips & Pittman, 2003). This refers to the fact, that immigrants usually occupy lower socioeconomic levels than the host culture, this lowers the immigrants ability to interface with the dominant culture, or to access opportunities, it can lead to several negative outcomes (Vazsonyi & Killias, 2001); (b) differences in cultural orientation between immigrants and the receiving society (Côté, 1993). This results in exclusion and lack of access to resources. Research shows that people with similar cultural orientation are much more accepted, and formal and informal sources within a culture are more willing to offer them support; (c) there is a lack of social-institutional support for identity development in host culture (Côté, 2000). This is the result of the individualistic assumptions of Western cultures, and people from collectivistic cultures are expected to adapt on their own, and it retards the process of identity development and adaptation in Western settings; and (d) ethnicity-related barriers, i.e., ethnically different people have a harder time getting acceptance in host cultures (Schwartz, 2005). Negative experiences related to nondominant status in host culture can restrict access to opportunities, even when an immigrant has the necessary knowledge and skills (Suárez-Orozco & Suárez-Orozco, 2001). Schwartz et al. (2006) note that research must focus on studying these issues and their impact on positive identity development in host culture.

Working with immigrant populations can lead to ethical concerns in service delivery. Counselors are increasingly likely to encounter immigrant clients who have cultures that are dissimilar to the norms of host society. In addition immigrants may not understand the legal statutes of the host culture (Nicassio et al., 1987). Such situations require counselors to think carefully about their response prior to implementing multicultural/social justice counseling interventions with immigrants. Mental health professionals will need to incorporate increased flexibility and critical consciousness into their professional repertoire. An example of a cultural misunderstanding that may lead to a report to Child Protective Services is a case of coining (Amshel & Caruso, 2000). By law, all health professionals are required to report signs of physical and/or child abuse. The practice of coining is a Far East Asian healing method that may leave bruises on a person's body. Health professionals working with immigrants from Far East Asia have occasionally misinterpreted such bruises as evidence of child and/or elder abuse, and notified authorities when, in effect, the bruises actually resulted from coining, a cultural healing practice. Instead of assuming that abuse has occurred, mental health professionals need to conduct a comprehensive cultural assessment of such cases to determine whether the bruises were actually the result of abuse. It is important to approach work with immigrants keeping all these factors in mind, to provide services that are culturally sensitive, and with a flexible attitude to understand situations that may be confusing, to avoid cultural misunderstandings that can lead to severe consequences for immigrant families.

Mental health professionals working with immigrant clients are encouraged to be prepared to use a broad range of helping strategies. This includes being an advocate and learning to question and challenge policies, regulations, rules, and systems that negatively affect the mental health of immigrants. The recent changes in professional guidelines of mental health professional associations require mental health professionals to attend to cultural variables, and to incorporate social justice strategies of advocacy, empowerment, i.e., going beyond traditional counseling strategies and incorporating liberation perspectives (Goodman et al., 2004; Kiselica & Robinson, 2001; Martin-Baró, 1994; Tate, Rivera, Brown, & Skaistis, 2013; Vera & Speight, 2003).

Recommendations for Interventions for Positive Immigrant Identity Development

Considering all the issues that immigrants confront on entering a new culture, it is important to have systems and policies in place that would facilitate a positive sense of self, and a strong bicultural identity in the host culture. Segal and Mayadas (2005) provide some useful recommendation for counseling interventions with immigrants, these include: (a) Helping professionals must know and understand the culture of origin of the client, and understand the immigration experience, the reasons that led to the decision to migrate, and the strengths, and resources clients possess; (b) recognize, and understand what has been lost in migrating to a new culture, familiar places, people, family, friends, cultural traditions and rituals, and allow for a grieving process; (c) recognize that several experiences in the United States as a result of migration, are confusing and bewildering for the newcomers, and their traditional support systems are no longer available. Finally, (d) they emphasize that the stress of relocation is immense, and strategies to cope with the daily stressors, along with discrimination, and exclusion due to phenotype, skin color, or accents, are needed. They emphasize that it is important to educate newcomers about the social and political systems, laws, healthcare options, and daily living and occupational issues that confront immigrants. Finally, they note that self-disclosure and openness to understanding immigrants and refugees are essential in developing and maintaining a positive therapeutic relationship.

Schwartz et al. (2006) recommend the following as important interventions to promote healthy adjustment and positive identity development: (a) alleviation of cultural identity confusion, for individuals from "ideologically-based, diaporic, or enclave groups, or those with multiple heritage cultures" (p. 22); (b) advocacy for the creation of social institutions to ease the transition, by providing language, cultural information, an orientation to host culture; and; (c) for immigrants confronted with negative socioeconomic conditions, to work within the negative conditions to help them develop a positive sense of self and identity.

These recommendations focus on lowering the stressors created by adaptation to a host culture. Some critical issues in these formulations are: (a) attention to the push-and-pull of heritage culture, and host culture assumptions; (b) successful acculturation would rest on individuals learning how to cope with criticism from people from their heritage culture, accusing them of abandoning their culture, and recognizing that successful adaptation can only happen if they opt for a bicultural personal and social identity. Mental health professionals can help in this process by working to empower individuals to develop a bicultural identity; a much needed ingredient for successful adaptation to the host culture. There are negative consequences for immigrants who are not able to develop an integrated personal and social identity, and this confusion can be transmitted to the next generation (Shields & Behrman, 2004; Szapocznik et al., 1986).

Some populations have been overlooked in the acculturation literature as most analyses focus on specific cultural groups rather than gender (male, female, intersex, and transgender), age, and sexual orientation issues (Gay, Lesbian, and Bisexual [GLB]) within cultural groups (Buschr, 2011; Koyabashi & Prus, 2012; Yakusko & Morgan-Consoli, 2014). Another group that until recently did not get much attention includes undocumented immigrants (Fong & Earner 2007). With regard to age, the focus has been on youth and children, and their integration and healthy personal, social, and cultural identity development, because they are seen as the social capital of the host society (Côté, 1996). Acculturating families, including grandparents, parents, youth, and children should be the focus because family dysfunction can affect all the generations in a household, and reduce the possibility of healthy integration to host culture (Fong, 2004). Older immigrant adults are possibly the most vulnerable, since they are unable to establish a bicultural identity, especially if migration took place after the age of retirement and they have no opportunity to reestablish support systems, and are completely dependent on the family for all their support and needs. Portes and Rumbaut (2006) report on the high suicide rates of older immigrants from Asia. Older immigrants face several health challenges, and tend to have less economic resources, and a longer life expectancy than US-born older adults. They also tend to suffer from isolation and loneliness (Singh & Hiatt, 2006; Treas & Mazumdar, 2002; Weeks & Cuellar, 1983).

Some research exists on immigrant women and the challenges they face (Berger, 2004; Espín, 2006; Hondagneu-Sotelo, 1994; Kelly, 2009; Lee & Bell-Scott, 2009; Marsella & Ring, 2003; Miller & Chandler, 2002; Perilla, 1999). It identifies the needs of women from rigid, fundamental religious, and/or patriarchal systems, and the challenges they face in developing a coherent bicultural identity in Western cultures (Aziz, 2011a, 2011b; Bhuyan, Mell, Senturia, Sullivan, & Shiu-Thornton, 2005; Darvishpour, 2002; Merali, 2008). Research also suggests that the adaptation processes experienced by women, differs from the experiences of men, youth, and older adults. The current literature shows that the largest research base on acculturation has focused on youth and children, with an emphasis on integration in host cultures (Schwartz et al., 2006).

The migration experiences of GLB and transgendered individuals have not been very encouraging due to difficulties in getting immigration status, lack of recognition of binational marriages, lack of acceptance of marital status, inability to adopt or provide foster care, lack of provision for healthcare, job insecurity, and lack of support for housing. On the surface, there are no legal limits on transgender migration (Buschr, 2011; Catholic Bridge, 2009; Koyabashi & Prus, 2012; National Center for Transgendered Equality [NCTE], 2011). NCTE recommends that US Federal Immigration Policies need to endorse the Yogyakarta Principles on the application of international human rights law, in relation to sexual orientation and gender identity expression, and include a definition for gender identity and expression. Further, NCTE notes that Congress needs to pass the "Uniting American Families Act" to facilitate the unification of transgendered couples. The most vulnerable group of undocumented immigrants are LGBT individuals, and it is reported that they suffer the greatest discrimination and abuse both in country of origin and in host cultures (Burns, Garcia, & Wolgin, 2013; Jeanty & Tobin, 2013; NCTE, 2013).

Creating institutional support through government policies and agencies helps in the adaptation process (Fielding & Anderson, 2008; Teram & White, 1993). It serves as a buffer against discrimination and exclusion because immigrants are exposed to supportive helpers, who can provide assistance and information to help negotiate the culture, and it can help create a positive and safe environment. Fielding & Anderson recommend building collective resilience, which encompasses both community and individual resilience for immigrants and refugees. Further, they note that collective resilience is enhanced by community protective factors, which include: (a) Social support by involving volunteer, professional, and community support; (b) empowerment results from public participation, communal responsibility, and communal action; and (c) community coping is both problem and emotion-focused. They emphasize that "collective resilience is built when there is community to keep hope alive; to discuss and manage big problems; to celebrate important occasions; to hold ceremonies which need to be performed in a community with others who share values" (p. 24). Creating these collectives through group counseling would facilitate adaptation in a new culture.

Without funding or adequate governmental support it is not possible for immigrants to establish themselves and develop a positive sense of self in the new cultural system. It is obvious that none of the Western cultures provide adequate support, although, they allow migration to their countries (Teram & White, 1993). If support is provided it is veiled in so much bureaucratic language that the constituents who are supposed to receive the services, and support cannot understand what is offered, however, limited. This is a social justice issue that counselors and mental health professionals can assist in, by identifying the lack of services, and advocate for their clients. It is important to recognize that mental health professionals need to educate their communities, and start grass roots movements to bring about social change, by publicizing the need of the immigrant and refugee communities to social and political systems who take responsibility for accepting immigrants.

Conclusion

This chapter reviews issues immigrants face due to migration. One key variable, i.e., the development of a strong ethnic (or personal and social identity) is explored, along with how racism, exclusion, and lack of support and services, can negatively affect the process of adaptation to host culture. Models of adaptation are presented along with counseling interventions from the literature. Finally, within immigrant populations, overlooked populations and their needs are presented, along with actions needed for social justice interventions for immigrants.

References

Aldwin, C. (1994). *Stress, coping and development*. New York: Guilford Press.
Alegría, M., Canino, G., Shrout, P., Woo, M., Duan, N., Vila, D., et al. (2008). Prevalence of mental illness in immigrant and non-immigrant U.S. Latino groups. *American Journal of Psychiatry, 165*, 359–369.
American Counseling Association (ACA). (2003). *Advocacy competencies*. Alexandria, VA: American Counseling Association.
American Multicultural Counseling Association (AMCD)/American Counseling Association (ACA). (1992). *Multicultural competencies*. Alexandria, VA: American Counseling Association.
American Psychological Association. (2002). *APA guidelines on multicultural education, training, research, practice, and organizational change for psychologists*. Retrieved from http://www.apa.org/pi/oema/resources/policy/multicultural-guidelines.aspx
American Psychological Association. (2009). *Health disparities and the mental/behavioral health workforce*. Retrieved from http://www.apa.org/about/gr/issues/workforce/disparity.aspx
Amshel, C., & Caruso, D. (2000). Vietnamese 'coining': A burn case report and literature review. *Journal of Burn Care and Rehabilitation, 21*(2), 112–114.
Aronowitz, M. (1984). The social and emotional adjustment of immigrant children: A review of the literature. *International Migration Review, 18*(2), 237–257.
Aronowitz, M. (1992). Adjustment of immigrant children as a function of parental attitudes to change. *International Migration Review, 26*, 86–110.
Atkinson, D. R. (2004). Current issues and future directions in counseling ethnic minorities. In D. R. Atkinson (Ed.), *Counseling American minorities* (pp. 354–367). New York: McGraw-Hill.
Aycan, Z., & Berry, J. W. (1995). *Cross-cultural adaptation as a multifaceted phenomenon*. Paper presented at 4th European Congress of Psychology, Athens.
Aycan, Z., & Berry, J. W. (1996). Impact of employment-related experiences on immigrants' well-being and adaptation to Canada. *Canadian Journal of Behavioral Science, 28*, 240–251.
Aziz, N. (2011a). What self-immolation means to Afghan women. *Peace Review: A Journal of Social Justice, 23*(1), 45–51.
Aziz, N. (2011b). The psychological and human rights condition of Afghan women. In J. Heath & A. Zahedi (Eds.), *Land of the unconquerable: The lives of contemporary Afghan women*. Berkeley, CA: University of California Press.
Beiser, M., Barwick, C., Berry, J. W., da Costa, G., Fantino, A., Ganesan, S., et al. (1988). *Menial health issues affecting immigrants and refugees*. Ottawa, ON: Health and Welfare Canada.
Bemak, F. (1989). Cross-cultural family therapy with Southeast Asian refugees. *Journal of Strategic and Systemic Therapies, 8*(1), 22–27.
Bemak, F., & Chung, R. C. Y. (1998). Vietnamese Amerasians: Predictors of distress and self-destructive behavior. *Journal of Counseling & Development, 76*(4), 452–458.
Bemak, F., & Chung, R. C. Y. (2008). New professional roles and advocacy strategies for school counselors: A multicultural/social justice perspective to move beyond the nice counselor syndrome. *Journal of Counseling & Development, 86*(3), 372–381.
Bemak, F., Chung, R. C. Y., & Pedersen, P. (2003). *Counseling refugees: A psychosocial approach to innovative multicultural interventions* (Vol. 40). Westport, CT: Greenwood Publishing Group.
Berger, R. (2004). *Immigrant women tell their stories*. New York: The Haworth Press.
Berry, J. W. (1974). Psychological aspects of cultural pluralism. *Culture Learning, 2*, 17–22.
Berry, J. W. (1980). Acculturation as varieties of adaptation. In A. Padilla (Ed.), *Acculturation: Theory, models and some new findings* (pp. 9–25). Boulder, CO: Westview.
Berry, J. W. (1984). Multicultural policy in Canada: A social psychological analysis. *Canadian Journal of Behavioural Science/Revue Canadienne des Sciences du Comportement, 16*(4), 353.
Berry, J. W. (1990). Psychology of acculturation. In J. Berman (Ed.), *Nebraska symposium on motivation* (Vol. 37, pp. 201–234). Lincoln, NE: University of Nebraska Press.

Berry, J. (1997). Immigration, acculturation, and adaption. *Applied Psychology: An international Review, 46*(1), 5–68.

Berry, J. W., Kim, U., Minde, T., & Mok, D. (1987). Comparative studies of acculturative stress. *International Migration Review, 21*, 491–511.

Berry, J. W., Kim, U., Power, S., Young, M., & Bujaki, M. (1989). Acculturation attitudes in plural societies. *Applied Psychology: An International Review, 38*, 185–206.

Berry, J. W., & Sam, D. (1996). Acculturation and adaptation. In J. W. Berry, M. H. Segall, & C. Kagitcibasi (Eds.), *Handbook of cross-cultural psychology. Vol. 3. Social behavior and applications* (pp. 291–326). Boston: Allyn & Bacon.

Berry, J. W., Phinney, J. S., & Sam, D. L. (2006). Immigrant youth: Acculturation, identity and adaptation. *Applied Psychology: An International Review, 55*(3), 303–332.

Berry, J. W., Poortinga, Y. H., Segall, M. H., & Dasen, P. R. (1992). *Cross-cultural psychology: Research and applications*. Cambridge, England: Cambridge University Press.

Bhatia, S., & Ram, A. (2001). Rethinking 'acculturation' in relation to diasporic cultures and postcolonial identities. *Human Development, 44*, 1–18.

Bhuyan, R., Mell, M., Senturia, K., Sullivan, M., & Shiu-Thornton, S. (2005). "Women must endure according to their karma": Cambodian immigrant women talk about domestic violence. *Journal of Interpersonal Violence, 20*, 902–921.

Bigelow, M. H. (2010). The policies and politics of educating refugee adolescents. *Language Learning, 60*(Suppl 1), 119–145.

Birman, D. (1998). Biculturalism and perceived competence of Latino immigrant adolescents. *American Journal of Community Psychology, 26*, 335–354.

Birman, D., Beehler, S., Harris, E. M., Everson, M. L., Batia, K., Liautaud, J., et al. (2008). International Family Adult and Child Enhancement Services (FACES): A community-based comprehensive services model for refugee children in resettlement. *American Journal of Orthopsychiatry, 78*, 121–132. doi:10.1037/0002-9432.78.1.121.

Birman, D., Ho, J., Pulley, E., Batia, K., Everson, M. L., Ellis, H., et al. (2005). *Mental health interventions for refugee children in resettlement* (White Paper II). Chicago: National Child Traumatic Stress Network, Refugee Trauma Task Force. Retrieved from http://www.nctsnet.org/nctsn_assets/pdfs/materials_for_applicants/MH_Interventions_for_Refugee_Children.pdf

Bronfenbrenner, U. (1979). *The ecology of human development*. Cambridge, MA: Harvard University Press.

Bronfenbrenner, U., & Morris, P. A. (2006). The bioecological model of human development. In W. Damon & R. M. Lerner (Eds.), *Handbook of child psychology* (6th ed., Vol. 1, pp. 793–828). Hoboken, NJ: Wiley.

Bulhan, H. A. (1985). *Franz Fanon and the psychology of oppression*. New York: Plenum.

Burns, C., Garcia, A., & Wolgin, P. E. (2013, March). *Living in dual shadows: LGBT undocumented immigrants*. Washington, DC: Center for American Progress. Retrieved from http://www.americanprogress.org/issues/immigration/report/2013/03/08/55674/living-in-dual-shadows/

Buschr, D. (2011). Unequal in exile: Gender equality, sexual identity, and refugee status. *Amsterdam Law Forum, 3*(2), 92–102.

Carlin, J. (1990). Refugee and immigrant populations at special risk: Women, children and the elderly. In W. H. Holtzman & T. Bornemann (Eds.), *Mental health of immigrants and refugees*. Austin, TX: Hogg Foundation for Mental Health.

Casas, J. M., Pavelski, R., Furlong, M. J., & Zanglis, I. (2001). Advent of systems of care: Practice, research perspective, and policy implications. In J. G. Ponterotto, J. M. Casas, L. A. Suzuki, & C. M. Alexander (Eds.), *Handbook of multicultural counseling* (2nd ed., pp. 189–221). Thousand Oaks, CA: Sage.

Catholic Bridge. (2009). *Human rights complaint*. Retrieved from http://catholicbridge.com/downloads/human_rights_complaint.pdf

Chavez, A. F., & Guido-DiBrito, F. (1999). Racial and ethnic identity and development. *New Directions for Adult and Continuing Education, 1999*(84), 39–47.

Chung, R. C. Y., Bemak, F., & Grabosky, T. K. (2011). Multicultural-social justice leadership strategies: Counseling and advocacy with immigrants. *Journal for Social Action in Counseling and Psychology, 3*(1), 57–69.

Chung, R. C. Y., Bemak, F., Ortiz, D. P., & Sandoval-Perez, P. A. (2008). Promoting the mental health of immigrants: A multicultural/social justice perspective. *Journal of Counseling & Development, 86*(3), 310–317.

Côté, J. E. (1993). Foundations of a psychoanalytic social psychology: Neo-Eriksonian propositions regarding the relationship between psychic structure and social institutions. *Developmental Review, 13*, 31–53.

Côté, J. E. (1996). Sociological perspectives on identity development: The culture-identity link and identity capital. *Journal of Adolescence, 19*, 419–430.

Côté, J. E. (2000). *Arrested adulthood: The changing nature of maturity and identity*. New York: New York University Press.

Crethar, H., Torres Rivera, E., & Nash, S. (2008). In search of common threads: Linking multicultural, feminist, and social justice counseling paradigms. *Journal of Counseling & Development, 86*, 269–278. doi:10.1002/j.1556-6678.2008.tb00509.x.

Cross, W. E., Jr. (1991). *Shades of black: Diversity in African-American identity*. Philadelphia: Temple University Press.

Dana, R. H. (2005). *Multicultural assessment: Principles, applications, and examples*. Mahwah, NJ: Lawrence Erlbaum.

Darvishpour, M. (2002). Immigrant women challenge the role of men: how the changing power relationship within Iranian families in Sweden intensifies family conflicts after immigration. *Journal of Comparative Family Studies, 33*, 270–296.

Desjarlais, R., Eisenberg, L., Good, B., & Kleinman, A. (1995). *World mental health: Problems and priorities in low-income countries*. New York: Oxford University Press.

Duldulao, A. A., Takeuchi, D. T., & Hong, S. (2009). Correlates of suicidal behaviors among Asian Americans. *Archives of Suicide Research, 13*, 277–290. doi:10.1080/13811110903044567.

Erikson, E. H. (1968). *Identity: Youth and crisis*. New York: Norton.

Erikson, E. H. (1975). *Life history and the historical moment*. New York: Norton.

Espín, O. M. (2006). Gender, sexuality, language, and migration. In R. Mahalingam (Ed.), *Cultural psychology of immigrants* (pp. 241–258). Mahwah, NJ: Lawrence Erlbaum.

Fielding, A., & Anderson, J. (2008). *Working with refugee communities to build collective communities*. Perth, WA: Association for Services to Torture and Trauma Survivors.

Fong, R. (Ed.). (2004). *Culturally competent practice with immigrant and refugee children and families*. New York: Guilford Press.

Fong, R., & Earner, I. (2007). Multiple traumas of undocumented immigrants crisis reenactment play therapy, case example of Ximena, age 12. In N. B. Webb (Ed.), *Play therapy with children in crisis* (3rd ed., pp. 408–425). New York: Guilford Press.

Fortuny, K., Chaudry, A., & Jargowsky, P. (2010). *Immigration trends in metropolitan America, 1980–2007*. Washington, DC: The Urban Institute. Retrieved from http://www.urban.org/publications/412273.html

Gamst, G. C., & Liang, C. T. H. (2013). A review and critique of multicultural competence measures: Toward a social justice-oriented health service delivery model. In F. A. Paniagua & A.-M. Yamada (Eds.), *Handbook of multicultural mental health* (2nd ed., pp. 547–570). New York: Academic Press.

Garcia, C. M., & Saewyc, E. M. (2007). Perceptions of mental health among recently immigrated Mexican adolescents. *Issues in Mental Health Nursing, 28*, 37–54. doi:10.1080/01612840600996257.

García Coll, C., & Magnuson, K. (1997). The psychological experience of immigration: A developmental perspective. In A. Booth, A. C. Crouter, & N. Landale (Eds.), *Immigration and the family* (pp. 91–132). Mahwah, NJ: Lawrence Erlbaum.

Ghuman, P. A. S. (1991). Best or worst of two worlds? A study of Asian adolescents. *Educational Review, 33*, 121–132.

Gleason, P. (1979). Confusion compounded: The melting pot in the 1960's and 1970's. *Ethnicity, 6*(1), 10–20.

Goodman, L. A., Liang, B., Helms, J. E., Latta, R. E., Sparks, E., & Weintraub, S. R. (2004). Training counseling psychologists as social justice agents: Feminist and multicultural principles in action. *The Counseling Psychologist, 32*, 793–837. doi:10.1177/0011000004268802.

Gordon, M. M. (1964). *Assimilation in American life. The role of race, religion and national origins*. New York: Oxford. University Press.

Grossman, B., Wirt, T., & Davids, A. (1985). Self-esteem, ethnic identity, and behavioral adjustment among Anglo and Chicano adolescents in West Texas. *Journal of Adolescence, 8*, 57–68.

Hondagneu-Sotelo, P. (1994). *Gendered transitions: Mexican experiences of immigration*. Berkeley, CA: University of California Press.

Hurtado, A., Gurin, P., & Peng, T. (1994). Social identities: A framework for studying the adaptations of immigrants and ethnics: The adaptations of Mexicans in the United States. *Social Problems, 41*, 129–151.

Ibrahim, F. A. (2010). Innovative teaching strategies for group work: Addressing cultural responsiveness and social justice. *Journal for Specialists in Group Work, 35*(3), 271–280.

Ibrahim, F. A., & Dykeman, C. (2011). Muslim-Americans: Cultural and spiritual assessment for counseling. *Journal of Counseling and Development, 89*, 387–396.

Ibrahim, F. A., & Heuer, J. R. (2013a). The assessment, diagnosis, and treatment of mental disorders among Muslims. In F. A. Paniagua & A.-M. Yamada (Eds.), *Handbook of multicultural mental health* (2nd ed., pp. 367–388). New York: Academic Press.

Ibrahim, F. A., & Heuer, J. R. (2013b, August). *Social justice and cultural responsiveness in counseling: Using cultural assessments*. Presentation at the American Psychological Association Annual Conference, Honolulu, HI.

Jeanty, J., & Tobin, H. J. (2013). Our moment for reform: *Immigration and transgender people*. Washington, DC: National Center for Transgender Equality. Retrieved from https://www.documentcloud.org/documents/801544-cir-en-1.html.

Jensen, L. A. (2003). Coming of age in a multicultural world: Globalization and adolescent cultural identity formation. *Applied Developmental Science, 7*, 189–196.

Kelly, U. A. (2009). "I'm a mother first": The influence of mothering in the decision-making processes of battered immigrant Latino women. *Research in Nursing and Health, 32*(3), 286–297.

Kim, Y. Y. (1979). Toward an interactive theory of communication-acculturation. *Communication Yearbook, 3*, 435–453.

Kim, G., Loi, C. X. A., Chiriboga, D. A., Jang, Y., Parmelee, P., & Allen, R. S. (2011). Limited English proficiency as a barrier to mental health service use: A study of Latino and Asian immigrants with psychiatric disorders. *Journal of Psychiatric Research, 45*, 104–110. doi:10.1016/j.jpsychires.2010.04.031.

Kira, I. A., Lewandowski, L., Chiodo, L., & Ibrahim, A. (2014). Advances in systemic trauma theory: Traumatogenic dynamics and consequences of backlash as a multisystemic trauma on Iraqi refugees. *Psychology, 5*, 389–412. Retrieved from http://www.scirp.org/journal/psych, http://dx.doi.org/10.4236/psych.2014.55050

Kiselica, M. S., & Robinson, M. (2001). Bringing advocacy counseling to life: The history, issues, and human dramas of social justice work in counseling. *Journal of Counseling and Development, 79*(4), 387–398.

Knight, G., Bernal, M., Garza, C., Cota, M., & Ocampo, K. (1993). Family socialization and the ethnic identity of Mexican-American children. *Journal of Cross-Cultural Psychology, 24*, 99–114.

Koss-Chioino, J. D. (2000). Traditional and folk approaches among ethnic minorities. In J. F. Aponte & J. Wohl (Eds.), *Psychological intervention and cultural diversity* (pp. 149–166). Needham Heights, MA: Allyn & Bacon.

Koyabashi, K. M., & Prus, S. G. (2012). Examining the gender, ethnicity, and age dimensions of healthy immigrant effect: Factors in the development of equitable health policy. *International Journal for Equity in Health, 11*(8). doi:10.1186/1475-9276-11:8. Retrieved from http://www.equityhealthj.com/content/11/1/8

Kwan, K. K., Gong, Y., & Younnjung, M. (2010). Language, translation, and validity in the adaptation of psychological tests for multicultural counseling. In J. G. Ponterotto, J. M. Casas, L. Suzuki, & C. M. Alexander (Eds.), *Handbook of multicultural counseling* (3rd ed., pp. 397–412). Thousand Oaks, CA: Sage.

Lafromboise, T., Coleman, H. L., & Gerton, J. (1993). Psychological impact of biculturalism: Evidence and theory. *Psychological Bulletin, 114*, 395–412.

Laosa, L. (1989). Psychosocial stress, coping, and development of Hispanic immigrant Children. *ETS Research Report Series, 1989*(2), 1–50.

Laperriere, A., Compere, L., Dkhissy, M., Dolce, R., & Fleurent, N. (1994). Mutual perceptions and interethnic strategies among French, Italian and Haitian adolescents of a multi-ethnic school in Montreal. *Journal of Adolescent Research, 9*, 193–217.

Lazarus, R. S. (1990). Theory-based stress measurement. *Psychological Inquiry, I*, 3–13.

Lazarus, R. S. (1993). From psychological stress to the emotions: A history of changing outlooks. *Annual Review of Psychology, 44*, 1–21.

Lazear, K. J., Pires, S., Isaacs, M., Chaulk, P., & Huang, L. (2008). Depression among low-income women of color: Qualitative findings from cross-cultural focus groups. *Journal of Immigrant Minority Health, 10*, 127–133. doi:10.1007/s10903-007-9062-x.

Lee, Y. M., & Bell-Scott, P. (2009). Korean immigrant women's journey from abused wives to self-reliant women. *Women & Therapy, 32*(4), 377–392. doi:10.1080/02703140903153435.

Lesaux, N. K. (2006). Building consensus: Future directions for research on English language learners at risk for learning difficulties. *Teachers College Record, 108*, 2406–2438. doi:10.1111/j.1467-9620.2006.00787.x.

Liebkind, K. (1993). Self-reported ethnic identity, depression, and anxiety among youth Vietnamese refugees, and their parents. *Journal of Refugee Studies, 6*, 25–39.

Liebkind, K. A. (1996). Acculturation and stress: Vietnamese refugees in Finland. *Journal of Cross-Cultural Psychology, 27*, 161–180. doi:10.1177/0022022196272002.

Liebkind, K. (2001). Acculturation. In R. Brown & S. Gaertner (Eds.), *Blackwell handbook of social psychology: Intergroup processes* (pp. 386–406). Oxford, England: Blackwell.

Lonner, W. J., & Ibrahim, F. A. (2008). Assessment in cross-cultural counseling. In P. B. Pedersen, J. G. Draguns, W. J. Lonner, & J. E. Trimble (Eds.), *Counseling across cultures* (6th ed., pp. 37–57). Thousand Oaks, CA: Sage.

Lupi, M., & Tong, V. (2001). Reflecting on personal interaction style to promote successful cross-cultural school-home partnerships. *Preventing School Failure, 45*(4), 162–166.

Marcia, J. E. (1980). Identity in adolescence. In J. Adelson (Ed.), *Handbook of adolescent psychology* (pp. 159–187). New York: Wiley.

Marmol, L. (2003). The ethical practice of psychology: Ethnic, racial, and cultural issues. In G. Bernal, J. E. Trimble, A. K. Burlew, & F. T. L. Leong (Eds.), *Handbook of racial and ethnic minority psychology* (pp. 167–176). Thousand Oaks, CA: Sage.

Marsella, A. J., & Ring, E. (2003). Human migration and immigration: An overview. In L. L. Adler & U. P. Gielen (Eds.), *Migration: Immigration and emigration in international perspective* (pp. 3–22). Westport, CT: Praeger.

Martin-Baró, I. (1994). *Writings for a liberation psychology*. Cambridge, MA: Harvard University Press.

Maton, K. I., Kohout, J. L., Wicherski, M., Leary, G. E., & Vinokurov, A. (2006). Minority students of color and the psychology graduate pipeline: Disquieting and encouraging trends: 1989–2003. *American Psychologist, 61*, 117–131. doi:10.1037/0003- 066X.61.2.117.

McCarthy, K. (2010). *Adaptation of immigrant children to the United States: A review of the literature (Working paper #98-03)*. New York: Center for Research on Child Wellbeing/Columbia University.

McNeill, B., & Cervantes, J. M. (2008). *Latina/o healing practices: Mestizo and indigenous perspectives*. New York: Routledge.

Menken, K. (2008). *English language learners left behind: Standardized testing as language policy*. Clevedon, England: Multilingual Matters.

Merali, N. (2008). Theoretical frameworks for studying female marriage migrants. *Psychology of Women Quarterly, 32*(3), 281–289. doi:10.1111/j.1471-6402.2008.00436.x.

Miller, A. M., & Chandler, P. J. (2002). Acculturation, resilience, and depression in midlife women from the former Soviet Union. *Nursing Research, 51*, 26–32.

Nastasi, B. K., Moore, R. B., & Varjas, K. M. (2004). *School-based mental health services: Creating comprehensive and culturally specific programs*. Washington, DC: American Psychological Association.

National Center for Transgendered Equality. (2011). *Immigration*. Retrieved from http://transequality.org/Issues/immigration.html

National Center for Transgender Equality. (2013). Our moment for reform: Immigration and transgender people. Retrieved from http://equalityfederation.org/blog/201310/speaking-out-undocumented-transgender-people.

Nesdale, D., Rooney, R., & Smith, L. (1997). Migrant ethnic identity and psychological distress. *Journal of Cross-Cultural Psychology, 28*(5), 569–588.

Nesdale, D., & Mak, A. (2000). *Immigrant acculturation attitudes and host country identification*. Griffith University.

Neville, H. A., & Mobley, M. (2001). Social identities in contexts: An ecological model of multicultural counseling psychology process. *The Counseling Psychologist, 29*, 471–485. doi:10.1177/0011000001294001.

Nguyen, H., Messe, L., & Stollak, G. (1999). Toward a more complex understanding of acculturation and adjustment: Cultural involvement and psychosocial functioning in Vietnamese youth. *Journal of Cross-Cultural Psychology, 30*, 5–31.

Nicassio, P. M., Solomon, G. S., Guest, S. S., & McCullough, J. E. (1986). Emigration stress and language proficiency as correlates of depression in a sample of Southeast Asian refugees. *International Journal of Social Psychiatry, 32*, 22–28.

Nicassio, P. M., Solomon, G. S., Guest, S. S., & McCullough, J. E. (1987). Emigration stress and language proficiency as correlates of depression in a sample of Southeast Asian refugees. *Pacific/Asian American Research Center Review, 6*, 10–13.

O'Donnell, C. R., Tharp, R. G., & Wilson, K. (1993). Activity settings as the unit if analysis: A theoretical basis for community intervention and development. *American Journal of Community Psychology, 21*(4), 501–520.

Ogbu, J. (1990). Cultural models. Identity and literacy. In J. Stigler, R. Shweder, & G. Herdt (Eds.), *Culrural psychology: Essays on comparative human development* (pp. 520–541). New York: Cambridge University Press.

Olfson, M., Lewis-Fernandez, R., Weissman, M. M., Feder, A., Gameroff, M. J., Pilowsky, D., et al. (2002). Psychotic symptoms in an urban general medicine practice. *American Journal of Psychiatry, 159*, 1412–1419. doi:10.1176/appi. ajp.159.8.1412.

Orford, J. (2009). Empowering family and friends: A new approach to the secondary prevention of addiction. *Drug and Alcohol Review, 13*, 417–429.

Organista, P. B., Organista, K. C., & Kurasaki, K. (2003). Overview of the relationship between acculturation and ethnic minority mental health. In K. M. Chun, P. B. Organista, & G. Marin (Eds.), *Acculturation: Advances in theory, measurement, and applied research* (pp. 139–161). Washington, DC: American Psychological Association.

Padilla, A. M., & Perez, W. (2003). Acculturation, social identity, and social cognition: A new perspective. *Hispanic Journal of Behavioral Sciences, 25*, 35–55.

Park, R. E. (1928). Human migration and the marginal man. *American Journal of Sociology, 33*, 881–893.

Pedersen, P. B. (2003). Cross-cultural counseling: Developing culture-centered interactions. In G. Bernal, J. E. Trimble, A. K. Burlew, & F. T. L. Leong (Eds.), *Handbook of racial and ethnic minority psychology* (pp. 167–176). Thousand Oaks, CA: Sage.

Perilla, J. L. (1999). Domestic violence as a human rights issue: The case of immigrant Latinos. *Hispanic Journal of Behavioral Sciences, 21*, 107–133.

Phillips, T. M., & Pittman, J. F. (2003). Identity processes in poor adolescents: Exploring the linkages between economic disadvantage and the primary task of adolescence. *Identity, 3*, 115–129.

Phinney, J. S. (1989). Stages of ethnic identity development in minority group adolescents. *Journal of Early Adolescence, 9*, 34–49.

Phinney, J. S. (1990). Ethnic identity in adolescents and adults: a review of research. *Psychological Bulletin, 108*(3), 499–514.

Phinney, J. S. (2003). Ethnic identity and acculturation. In K. M. Chun, P. B. Organista, & G. Marin (Eds.), *Acculturation: Advances in theory, measurement, and applied research* (pp. 63–81). Washington, DC: APA Books.

Phinney, J. S. (2006). Ethnic identity exploration in emerging adulthood. In J. J. Arnett & J. L. Tanner (Eds.), *Emerging adults in America: Coming of age in the 21st century* (pp. 117–134). Washington, DC: American Psychological Association.

Phinney, J. S., & Alipuria, L. (1990). Ethnic identity in college students from four ethnic groups. *Journal of Adolescence, 13*, 171–183.

Phinney, J., Cantu, C., & Kurtz, D. (1997). Ethnic and American identity as predictors of self-esteem among African American, Latino, and White adolescents. *Journal of Research on Adolescence, 26*, 165–185.

Phinney, J. S., & Chavira, V. (1992). Ethnic identity and self-esteem: An exploratory longitudinal study. *Journal of Adolescence, 15*, 271–281.

Phinney, J. S., Chavira, V., & Tate, J. D. (1992). The effect of ethnic threat on ethnic self-concept and own group ratings. *Journal of Social Psychology, 133*, 469–478.

Phinney, J. S., Chavira, V., & Williamson, L. (1992). Acculturation attitudes and self-esteem among high school and college students. *Youth and Society, 23*, 299–312.

Phinney, J. S., DuPont, S., Espinosa, C., Revill, J., & Sanders, K. (1994). Ethnic identity and American identification among ethnic minority youths. In A. M. Boury, F. J. R. van de Vijver, P. Boski, & P. Schmitz (Eds.), *Journeys into cross-cultural psychology* (pp. 167–183). Lisse, The Netherlands: Swets & Zeitlinger.

Phinney, J. S., Horenczyk, G., Liebkind, K., & Vedder, P. (2001). Ethnic identity, immigration, and wellbeing: An interactional perspective. *Journal of Social Issues, 57*, 493–510.

Portes, A., & Rumbaut, R. G. (2006). *Immigrant America: A portrait*. Berkeley, CA: University of California Press.

Ramirez, M. (1984). Assessing and understanding biculturalism-multiculturalism in Mexican-American adults. In J. L. Martinez & R. H. Mendoza (Eds.), *Chicano psychology* (2nd ed., pp. 77–94). New York: Academic Press.

Ridley, C. R., Tracy, M. L., Pruitt-Stephens, L., Wimsatt, M. K., & Beard, J. (2008). Multicultural assessment validity: The preeminent ethical issue in psychological assessment. In L. A. Suzuki & J. G. Ponterotto (Eds.), *Handbook of multicultural assessment: Clinical, psychological, and educational applications* (3rd ed., pp. 22–33). San Francisco, CA: Wiley.

Roberts, R. E., Phinney, J. S., Masse, L. C., Chen, Y. R., Roberts, C. R., & Romero, A. (1999). The structure of ethnic identity in young adolescents from diverse ethnocultural groups. *Journal of Early Adolescence, 19*, 301–322.

Rodríguez, M., Valentine, J. M., Son, J. B., & Muhammad, M. (2009). Intimate partner violence and barriers to mental health care for ethnically diverse populations of women. *Trauma, Violence & Abuse, 10*, 358–374. doi:10.1177/1524838009339756.

Ruiz, R. (1981). *The territory (Motion picture)*. Lisbon, Portugal: Orion Films.

Rumbaut, R. G. (2004). Ages, life stages, and generational cohorts: Decomposing the immigrant. *International Migration Review, 38*(3), 1160–1205.

Saenz, R., Hwang, S. S., Aguirre, B. E., & Anderson, R. N. (1995). Persistence and change in Asian identity among children of intermarried couples. *Sociological Perspectives, 38*, 175–194.

Sam, D. L. (2000). Psychological adaptation of adolescents with immigrant backgrounds. *Journal of Social Psychology, 140*, 5–25.

Sam, D. L., & Berry, J. W. (1995). Acculturative stress among young immigrants in Norway. *Scandinavian Journal of Psychology, 36*, 10–24.

Sayegh, L., & Lasry, J.-C. (1993). Immigrants' adaptation in Canada: Assimilation, acculturation, and orthogonal identification. *Canadian Psychology, 34*(1), 98–109.

Schmitz, P. (1992). Immigrant mental and physical health. *Psychology and Developing Societies, 4*, 117–131.

Searle, W., & Ward, C. (1990). The prediction of psychological and sociocultural adjustment during cross-cultural transitions. *International Journal of Intercultural Relations, 14*, 449–464.
Schwartz, S. J. (2005). A new identity for identity research: Recommendations for expanding and refocusing the identity literature. *Journal of Adolescent Research, 20*, 293–308.
Schwartz, S. J., Montgomery, M. J., & Briones, E. (2006). The role of identity in acculturation among immigrant people: Theoretical propositions, empirical questions, and applied recommendations. *Human Development, 49*, 1–30.
Segal, U. A., & Mayadas, N. S. (2005). Assessment of issues facing immigrant and refugee families. *Child Welfare, 84*(5), 563–583.
Shields, M. K., & Behrman, R. E. (2004). Children of immigrant families: Analysis and recommendations. *Children of Immigrant Families, 14*(2), 4–15.
Shisana, O., & Celentano, D. D. (1985). Depressive symptomatology among Namibian adolescent refugees. *Social Science & Medicine, 21*(11), 1251–1257.
Singh, G. K., & Hiatt, R. A. (2006). Trends and disparities in socioeconomic and behavioral characteristics, life expectancy, and cause-specific mortality of native-born and foreign-born populations in the United States, 1979–2003.". *International Journal of Epidemiology, 35*(4), 903–919.
Smith, T. B., & Silva, L. (2011). Ethnic identity and personal well-being of people of color: A meta-analysis. All Faculty Publications. Paper 88. Retrieved from http://scholarsarchive.byu.edu/facpub/88.
Smither, R. (1982). Human migration and the acculturation of minorities. *Human Relations, 35*, 57–68.
Solano-Flores, G. (2008). Who is given tests in what language by whom, when and where? The need for probabilistic views of language in the testing of English language learners. *Educational Researcher, 37*, 189–199. doi:10.3102/0013189X08319569.
Spencer, M. B., Swanson, D. P., & Cunningham, M. (1992). Ethnicity, ethnic identity, and competence formation: Adolescent transition and cultural transformation. *Journal of Negro Education, 60*, 366–387.
Strickland, B. R. (2000). Misassumptions, misadventures, and the misuse of psychology. *American Psychologist, 55*, 331–338. doi:10.1037/0003-066X.55.3.331.
Stonequist, E. V. (1937). *The marginal man: A study in personality and culture conflict*. New York: Scribner/Simon & Schuster.
Suárez-Orozco, C., & Suárez-Orozco, M. M. (2001). *Children of immigration*. Cambridge, MA: Harvard University Press.
Sue, D. W., & Capodilupo, C. M. (2008). Racial, gender, and sexual orientation microaggressions: Implications for counseling and psychotherapy. In D. W. Sue & D. Sue (Eds.), *Counseling the culturally diverse: Theory and practice* (5th ed., pp. 105–130). Hoboken, NJ: Wiley.
Sue, D. W., & Sue, D. (2013). *Counseling the culturally diverse: Theory and practice* (6th ed.). Hoboken, NJ: Wiley.
Sundberg, N. D. (1981). Cross-cultural counseling and psychotherapy: A research overview. In A. J. Marsella & P. B. Pedersen (Eds.), *Cross-cultural counseling and psychotherapy*. New York: Pergamon Press.
Suzuki, L. A., Kugler, J. F., & Aguiar, L. J. (2005). Assessment practices in racial-cultural psychology. In R. T. Carter (Ed.), *Training and practice* (Vol. 2, pp. 297–315). Hoboken, NJ: Wiley.
Suzuki, L. A., Ponterotto, J. G., & Meller, P. J. (Eds.). (2008). *Handbook of multicultural assessment: Clinical, psychological, and educational applications* (3rd ed.). San Francisco, CA: Jossey-Bass.
Szapocznik, J., Santisteban, D., Rio, A., Perez-Vidal, A., Kurtines, W. M., & Hervis, O. E. (1986). Bicultural effectiveness training (BET): An intervention modality for families experiencing intergenerational/intercultural conflict. *Hispanic Journal of Behavioral Sciences, 6*, 303–330.
Szapocznik, J., Kurtines, W. M., & Fernandez, T. (1980). Bicultural involvement and adjustment in Hispanic American youths. *International Journal of Intercultural Relations, 4*, 353–365.
Szapocznik, J., & Kurtines, W. M. (1980). Acculturation, biculturalism and adjustment among Cuban Americans. In A. M. Padilla (Ed.), *Acculturation: Theory, models, and some new findings* (pp. 139–159). Boulder, CO: Westview.

Szapocznik, J., Scopetta, M. A., Kurtines, W., & Aranalde, M. D. (1978). Theory and measurement of acculturation. *Revista Interamericana de Psicologia, 12*(2), 113–130.

Tajfel, H. (1981). *Human groups and social categories*. Cambridge, UK: Cambridge University Press.

Tajfel, H., & Turner, J. C. (1986). The social identity theory of intergroup behavior. In S. Worchel & W. G. Austin (Eds.), *The psychology of intergroup behavior* (pp. 7–24). Chicago: Nelson Hall.

Tate, K. A., Rivera, E. T., Brown, E., & Skaistis, L. (2013). Foundations for liberation: Social justice, liberation, and counseling psychology. *Interamerican Journal of Psychology, 47*(3), 373–382.

Teram, E., & White, H. (1993). The bureaucratic disentitlement of clients: Strategies to address the bureaucratic disentitlement of clients from cultural minority clients. *Canadian Journal of Community Mental Health, 12*(2), 59–70.

Tong, V. (1997). The relationship between first and second languages and culture: Finding a cross-cultural identity. *NYSABE Journal, 12*, 43–61.

Tong, V. (1998). Helping LEP students learn to belong in a new culture. *Reclaiming Children and Youth, 7*(3), 161–164.

Tong, V. M. (2002). Amy's story: The development of an ESL student's cross-cultural identity. *Beyond Behavior, Spring*, 19–22.

Tong, V., & Mclntyre, T. (1998). Cultural and linguistic factors impacting on the education of youngsters with emotional and behavioral disorders. *Perceptions, 32*(3), 9–12.

Treas, J., & Mazumdar, S. (2002). Older people in America's immigrant families: Dilemmas of dependence, integration, and isolation. *Journal of Aging Studies, 16*(3), 243–258.

Tummala-Narra, P. (2007). Conceptualizing trauma and resilience across diverse contexts: A multicultural perspective. *Journal of Aggression, Maltreatment, and Trauma, 14*(1–2), 33–53. doi:10.1300/J146v14n01_03.

van Oudenhoven, J. P., & Eisses, A. M. (1998). Integration and assimilation of Moroccan immigrants in Israel and The Netherlands. *International Journal of Intercultural Relations, 22*(3), 293–307.

Vazsonyi, A. T., & Killias, M. (2001). Immigration and crime among youth in Switzerland. *Criminal Justice and Behavior, 28*, 329–366.

Vera, E. M., & Speight, S. L. (2003). Multicultural competence, social justice, and counseling psychology: Expanding our roles. *The Counseling Psychologist, 31*(3), 253–272.

Vera, E. M., Vila, D., & Alegría, M. (2003). Cognitive-behavioral therapy: Concepts, issues, and strategies for practice with racial/ethnic minorities. In G. Bernal, J. Trimble, A. Burlew, & F. T. L. Leong (Eds.), *Handbook of racial and ethnic minority psychology* (pp. 1–18). Thousand Oaks, CA: Sage.

Ward, C. (1996). Acculturation. In D. Landis & R. Bhagat (Eds.), *Handbook of intercultural training* (2nd ed., pp. 124–147). Thousand Oaks, CA: Sage.

Ward, C., & Kennedy, A. (1993). Psychological and socio-cultural adjustment during cross-cultural transitions: A comparison of secondary students overseas and at home. *International Journal of Psychology, 28*(2), 129–147.

Weeks, J. R., & Cuellar, J. B. (1983). Isolation of older persons: The influence of immigration and length of residence. *Research on Aging, 5*(3), 369–388.

Wu, M. C., Kviz, F. J., & Miller, A. M. (2009). Identifying individual and contextual barriers to seeking mental health services among Korean American immigrant women. *Issues in Mental Health Nursing, 30*, 78–85. doi:10.1080/01612840802595204.

Yakusko, O., & Morgan-Consoli, M. L. (2014). Gendered stories of adaptation and resistance: A feminist multiple case study of immigrant women. *International Journal for the Advancement of Counseling, 36*, 70–83. doi:10.1007/s10447-013-9191-y.

Chapter 7
Refugees: Adaptation and Psychological Interventions

This chapter focuses on refugees, their psychological health, and counseling needs. In reviewing the psychological literature, we realized that although, refugees are eventually considered immigrants, placing both populations in the same chapter would be a disservice to refugees, as their premigration experiences, including the traumas experienced, and lack of desire to migrate, along with post-migration challenges demand a separate chapter. Our focus is on psychological adjustment as mental health professionals, and we will consider factors that are critical to psychological adaptation and well-being of refugees.

Who Are Refugees?

The United Nations High Commission for Refugees (UNHCR), defines a refugee as a person (child and adult) who is residing outside their country and cannot return due to a well-founded fear of persecution because of their race, religion, nationality, political opinion, sexual orientation, or membership in a particular social group (United Nations High Commission for Refugees [UNHCR], 2011a, 2011b). This is one of the most traumatized and tortured populations in the world, and their premigration experiences range from persecution, isolation, physical mutilation, slave labor, starvation, beatings, rapes, threats, mock executions conflict, persecution, hostility, to political and religious upheaval (Clarke & Borders, 2014). Further, a large number of refugees come to Western countries, usually affected by civil and ethnic wars (Dujmic, 2013). There are also large refugee populations, known as "urban refugees" who have fled their countries to avoid religious or ethnic persecution, and their lived experiences are different from refugees who lived in camps and were allocated to Western settings (Thomas, Roberts, Luitel, Upadhaya, & Tpi, 2011). Many third-world countries did not sign the agreement on the UNHCR policy on refugee protection and solutions in urban areas, because they did not have the resources to assist urban refugees, as is the case in Nepal (UNHCR, 2009a, 2011a, 2011b).

F.A. Ibrahim, J.R. Heuer, *Cultural and Social Justice Counseling*,
International and Cultural Psychology, DOI 10.1007/978-3-319-18057-1_7

This makes these populations with no means of earning or government support, or health services vulnerable to exploitation.

Some vulnerable populations were denied asylum or refugee status by receiving nations. The UNHCR (2009b) issued additional guidance on accepting gay, lesbian, bisexual (GLB), and intersex and transgendered (IT) refugees. The rationale of the Refugee Convention on sexual orientation and gender identity is that people should be allowed to live their lives free from the fear of serious harm coming to them as a result of being from a protected class (UNHCR, 2011a, 2011b). Several nations who are signatories on the UN convention have not accepted GLBIT populations, UK finally changed its guidelines in 2010, and the United States and several European countries have not fully accepted these guidelines, especially for transgendered populations (Büscher & de Beer, 2011; LaViolette, 2013; UNHCR, 2009a, 2009b).

The UNHCR (2011) also issued guidance on providing asylum to women who were psychologically and physically abused. Hardly any research has focused on the experiences of violence throughout the lifespan, or the physical and mental health consequences among immigrant and refugee women (Guruge, Roche, & Catallo, 2012). Guruge et al. (2012) further note that women coming from highly oppressive and patriarchal societies face serious physical and mental health consequences. Further, there is considerable evidence that women and girls who become refugees are subjected to violence from family members, and from people in the host culture, combined with what they already suffered in their own country (Blanck, 2000; Cianciarulo & David, 2009; Guruge, Tiwari, & Lucea, 2010; Hossain, Zimmerman, Abas, Light, & Watts, 2010; Menjívar & Salcido, 2002; Watts & Zimmerman, 2002; Zimmerman et al., 2006).

Women from Africa, Asia, the Middle East, and South America live in highly oppressive, and patriarchal societies, where they are considered chattel and are physically and psychologically abused by parents, brothers, and spouses (Aziz, 2011a, 2011b; Blanck, 2000; Mason et al., 2008). If their country is unable or unwilling to provide protection, the next step is to seek asylum in a country that will. However, in narrowly interpreting the UNHCR ruling, most countries did not see the relevance of domestic violence fitting in the guidelines, primarily the "social group" criteria was always used as a specific category to deny asylum to "gender refugees" (Blanck, 2000; Cianciarulo & David, 2009; Ibrahim, personal communication, 2014).

Pumariega, Rothe, and Pumariega (2005) note that the last three decades have seen a significant increase in refugees from around the world due to wars, famines, political, civil, and ethnic conflicts, these events have considerably increased the number of refugees worldwide. UNHCR (2000) reports that one in 135 people alive in the world is a refugee. The United States has received some of the refugees from these conflicts, however, given the number of problems that have led to people being forced out of their own countries. A sizable number of people have arrived in the United States as refugees, due to political and economic crises. Mental health professionals in the United States need to understand that with the arrival of refugees and immigrants, the social structure of the nation is changed, and unless the new arrivals are provided the services they need, the consequences for the US economy, and its well-being would be compromised. Since, immigrants or refugees, and their offspring become part of the social capital of a nation, not providing services for integration into the culture, or attending to traumas experienced en route or prior to arriving in the host culture can have serious consequences. Pumariega (2003) notes that the numerical majority in the US population in the next several decades will be immigrants and their offspring.

Several scholars have argued against considering refugees, similar to immigrants, considering the challenges they have faced, and continue to deal with, and its effect on the process of acculturation and adaptation to a new culture (Mosselson, 2006). According to the UN guidelines, after a year of residence in a country of relocation, a refugee is classified an immigrant. The classification of immigrants as refugees has had a deleterious effect on research funding, and on support for possible psychological interventions for refugees (Ahearn & Athey, 1991; Mosselson, 2006). The objection to considering refugees the same as immigrants is primarily due to the fact that the process of acculturation, and adaptation to host culture varies for refugees from immigrants due to: (a) the trauma and suffering they have experienced prior to arrival, (b) the fact that they did not choose to migrate, but were forced by circumstances that propelled them out of their world, into a very different country, and (c) becoming a refugee means loss of social support systems, familial ties, familiar physical environments, and language. The process of negotiating a new identity in a foreign setting and the challenges of relocation can be facilitated by social, cultural, and psychological interventions (American Psychological Association [APA], 2009). However, first, the mental health practitioner needs to understand the myriad of issues that refugees confront. One of the primary concerns for a mental health professional is to consider the identity development process and how refugees understand their situation, and the goals for seeking professional psychological assistance. In addition, the psychological literature notes a lack of support for refugees and immigrants to help them adapt to their new settings, especially, because of the number of issues that refugees confront during and after the transition to a host culture (APA, 2009; Porter & Haslam, 2005; Smith & Halbert, 2013).

Mosselson (2006) notes that despite the large influx of refugees in the United States, research has not considered their experiences, needs, and possible outcomes of the acculturation process. Further, she notes that ethnic studies and psychology are the two fields that have studied immigrants and refugees; each field has studied different aspects in researching refugee experiences. For example, ethnic studies consider only cultural aspects, without understanding the developmental processes involved, or subjective experiences of refugees; and psychology has overlooked cultural issues in identity development (Mosselson, 2006). Other disciplines focus on identity, however the emphases vary, e.g., anthropology views identity as a group phenomenon, with an emphasis on the group; similarly sociology views identity as a macropolitical concept (Campbell & Rew, 1999). Similar to immigrants, the adaptation of refugees is also influenced by the politics and perceptions of the culture they are entering, and the reception they receive in host cultures (Mosselson, 2006;

Schwartz, Montgomery, & Briones, 2006). Further, Kaprielian-Churchill and Churchill (1994) note that another similarity relates to both groups is that on arrival they are confronted with the language and culture of a new land, and must learn to adapt to the norms of a new society, and modify previously held assumptions and adapt to a new social-cultural system. Erdogan (2012) notes that refugees are at greater risk of identity distress and crisis, and research has not addressed this variable, nor has it considered how identity resolution affects the acculturation process.

Identity Development of Refugees

In lifespan theory, a critical life task is the development of a coherent identity (Erikson, 1980). Erikson's (1968) theory considers identity development as the most significant task and challenge of life. Although, identity development is considered to be an important task of middle adolescence to early adulthood, current research has posited that identity is redefined and reconstructed throughout the lifespan as individuals interact with their sociocultural world (McSpadden & Moussa, 1993). Further, migration, or traumatic departure from home culture constitutes a major psychohistorical moment (Erikson) that requires reintegration of identity and follows a similar path to identity development as posited for adolescence. Since an individual's identity status is closely related to psychological adjustment, and influences all the experiences an individual goes through, it makes sense to consider that identity would be integrally connected to the traumatic events of becoming a refugee, dislocation, and acculturation to the final location (Erdogan, 2012; Fadjukoff, Pulkkinen, & Kokko, 2005).

Luyckx, Schwartz, Soenens, Vansteenkiste, and Goosens (2010) note that research literature documents the positive association between identity commitments, and psychological well-being. Shultheiss and Blustein (1994) consider identity development as a core therapeutic issue for adolescents, however, we believe that due to the losses involved in becoming a refugee, an individual's identity is thrown into a state of disequilibrium, along with the ensuing settlement issues in host culture, identity reintegration is needed. Research notes that post-migration experiences include: loneliness, financial, and health issues, and concerns relating to the transition and adaptation to new cultural and educational contexts (Boman & Edwards, 1984; Clinton-Davis & Fassil, 1992; Kopinak, 1998; Pittaway, Muli, & Shteir, 2009; Wilkinson, 2002).

In psychological interventions with refugees, we propose that a primary task along with focusing on the presenting problem is to assess the status of identity development and to assist with the integration of identity, i.e., empowering the client's primary personal, and social-cultural identity (gender, age, primary social-cultural and ethnic values, beliefs and assumptions, etc.), along with focusing on building a strong social-cultural identity in host culture, i.e., bicultural identity or integration as the goal of acculturation (Berry, 1980, 1997; Erdogan, 2012; Schwartz et al., 2006).

Developing a secure integrated identity requires the ability to process the experiences an individual has lived through, and working through the traumatic events, and finally coming to a place of comfort with the current social and cultural conditions (O'Brien & Epstein, 1988). Luyckx et al. (2010) have identified motivational and meditational factors that facilitate identity commitments. They used antecedent variables proposed by Deci and Ryan (1985), i.e., three causality or motivational orientations (autonomous, controlled, or impersonal orientations), and mediating variables such as identity integration (O'Brien & Epstein, 1988) to study the identity commitment and adjustment pathways. Luyckx et al. (2010), primarily applied Marcia's (1966) model of identity development, which conceptualizes identity development on two dimensions: exploration and commitment. Luyckx Schwartz, Soenens, et al., expanded Marcia's model to subsume two processes for identity commitment, instead of one outcome as identified by Marcia, i.e., commitment-making and identification with commitment, this perspective takes a process-approach to identity commitment (Luyckx, Goossens, Soenens, & Beyers, 2006). Both these processes can be very helpful in working with refugees who present a distressed or confused identity. Luyckx et al. (2010), recommend focusing on the underlying processes to understand the relationship of psychological adjustment to identity commitment.

Refugees from nonwestern cultures, and now residing in a Western context would find it useful to be exposed to a multicultural identity development model. Chavez and Guido-DeBrito (1999) note that for visible and legally defined minority groups, it is important to develop a racial-ethnic identity within the framework of individual and collective identity. Birman, Persky, and Chan (2010) posit that cultural groups with complex identities cannot be studied only considering ethnic and national identity, because they may also have a religion, or the ethnicity of a subculture within their larger cultural system, and this needs to be taken into account. For example Russian Jews, ethnic Taiwanese, or Somali Bantu among others, who are negotiating several national and cultural identities. Further, Sneed, Schwartz, and Cross (2006) contend that the experiences of non-White immigrants or refugees have not been adequately addressed in the psychological literature. They also note that the experiences of acculturation of nondominant cultural groups are not adequately explored or understood in the psychological literature, since current research literature is based on mostly White or the dominant cultural perspectives of communities studied (Sneed et al., 2006).

There are several social identity development models have been proposed following Erikson's (1980) conception, mostly pertaining to ethnic identity (Phinney, 1989), racial identity (Cross, 1995; Helms, 1990, 1995), multiracial identity (Poston, 1990; Root, 1990), gender identity (O'Neil, Egan, Owen, & Murray, 1993; Ossana, Helms, & Leonard, 1992), sexual orientation identity development models (Cass, 1979; McCarn & Fassinger, 1996), and occupational identity theory, which included religious beliefs and political ideology (Marcia, 1966). Sneed et al. (2006) propose it is time to bring all these models together to make them relevant to a specific individual. Further, it will help in creating coherence in the psychological literature and research. Further, they note there is significant similarity in the previous models and recommend identity development theory needs to be broadened to encompass all the various identity-related variables and domains. We believe that Ibrahim's (1990, 1999) conception of cultural identity and worldview incorporates all the dimensions that need to be considered to comprehend the multidimensional identity of an individual. Although, this is not a stage model, popular in multicultural psychology, it allows for several combinations and permutations of identity variables to help identify the key variables critical to the presenting problem. Stage models that present identity development in terms of statuses or stages have been strongly criticized for two primary reasons. First, the statuses operate at least somewhat independently within a variety of content domains, and often a person may be in one status in Domain A, but in a different status in Domain B (Goosens, 2001). Ibrahim's cultural identity model helps in focusing on the specific dimensions involved and is useful in a therapy and resolution context. Her conceptualization takes an ecological perspective, and provides dimensions that identify key variables from the socialization process that define a mature identity (Fig. 7.1).

We conceptualize cultural identity and worldview at the core of all the identities and contexts a person resides in, and the influence of all the identity variables (gender, sexuality, ethnicity, family influences, religion and/or spirituality) surrounding cultural identity and worldview will vary, depending on life experiences, and status

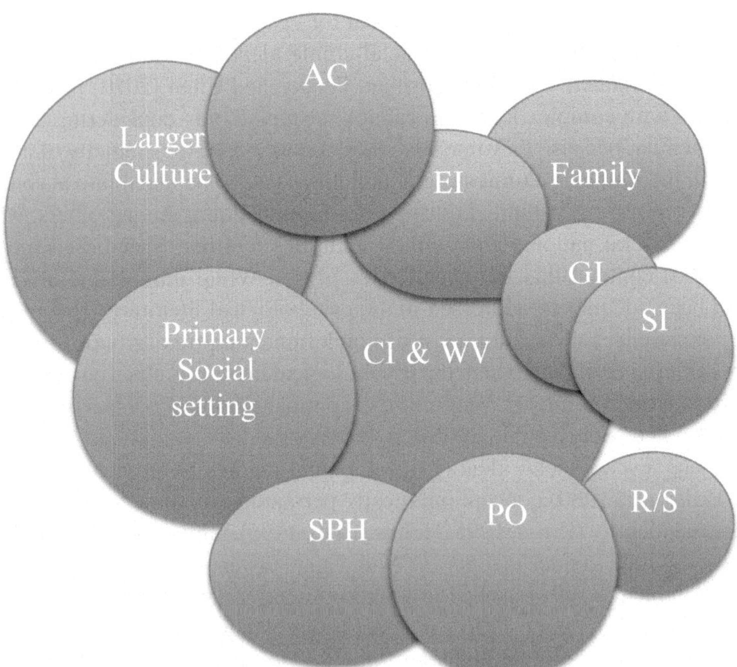

Fig. 7.1 The multidimensionality of cultural identity. *AC* acculturation, *CI* cultural identity, *EI* ethnic identity, *GI* gender identity, *PO* privilege and oppression, *R/S* religion/spirituality, *SI* sexual identity, *SPH* sociopolitical history, *WV* world view

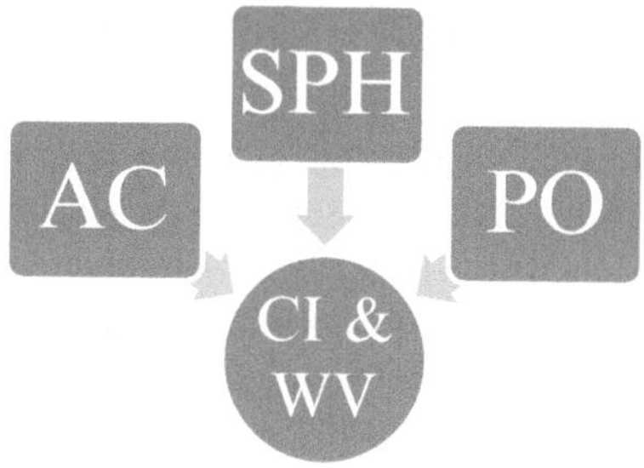

Fig. 7.2 Refugee cultural identity

in the primary and larger social setting, especially privilege and oppression. Ultimately, acculturation and development of an integrated identity will depend on how the refugee is received and integrated into the ongoing social system, and the support, services, etc., that are provided to assist with adaptation.

For refugees it may be critical to consider their cultural identity in relationship to three critical variables, sociopolitical history (SPH); including the traumatic journey to host culture, and what they are facing in the host culture), its effect on their worldview (WV: beliefs, values, assumptions, including spirituality/religion), and their status determined by privilege and oppression in the host culture (dominant group member, or nondominant group member, educated/uneducated, skilled/unskilled/professional, importance of ethnicity, similarity/dissimilarity to host culture, language proficiency, etc.). Based on the findings in the research literature all these variables influence the integration of identity in host culture. The diagram in Fig. 7.2 identifies the primacy of the identified variables.

The task of identity development in host culture involves taking all the experiences that affect these three key variables, the experiences can be transformative and positive, or negative, due to unmet needs, rejection by host culture due to ethnicity/culture, accent, etc., and lead to identity confusion (Schwartz, 2001). Identity confusion results in constant shifting of beliefs, assumptions, role, goals, and life planning (Luyckx, Goossens, Soenens, Beyers, & Vansteenkiste, 2005). Kroger and Marcia (2011) identify a structured and coherent sense of identity as an important aspect of psychosocial and relational identity. Erikson (1968) conceptualized identity development at the intersection of an individual and his/her social environment. This intersection determines the adjustment to host culture depending on how refugees are received in the country that has offered to provide a safe haven.

Psychosocial adjustment and familial connectedness are also critical in understanding adjustment to host culture. Considering Attachment Theory, the sense of belonging and positive connections to primary caregivers is also relevant in understanding adjustment after trauma, relocation, and adjustment to a new setting (Bowlby, 1982). Erikson's (1968) key concept of trust vs. mistrust is very relevant to the way refugees will adapt and adjust as this provides an internal model of self in relationship to others (Bowlby, 1973). Bowlby (1982) notes that the earliest sense of acceptance is identified by being considered lovable or not, and the attachment bond within which this sense is created, leads to a positive sense of self, and it characterizes how a person conducts her/him/zir over the lifespan.

Trauma and Its Impact on Refugees

Trauma as a result of being uprooted and moved to other settings is inevitable (Dana, 2005; Marsella, 2005; Wilson, 2007). According to the Substance Abuse and Mental Health Services Administration's (SAMSHA) Trauma and Justice Strategic Initiative "trauma results from an event, series of events, or set of circumstances that is experienced by an individual as physically or emotionally harmful or threatening and that has lasting adverse effects on the individual's functioning and physical, social, emotional, or spiritual wellbeing" SAMSHA, 2012, p. 2). There are several levels and types of trauma (SAMSHA, 2014). Understanding the meaning, the effect, and the outcome of a traumatic event resides within the cultural identity of an individual. It is important to recognize that the Western conceptualization of trauma and posttraumatic stress is not universal, and should not be applied across cultures/subcultures. Dana (2007) notes that "psychopathology is not an inevitable aftermath of trauma, refugee distress is frequently translated into psychopathology for conformity with Western health/mental health care resources. Follow-up studies generally suggest progress toward adaptation in host societies over time for acculturated and settled ethnic minorities" (p. 91). To be culturally responsive, it is important to allow the client to describe the traumatic event, it's meaning, and affect on an individual. Wilson (2007) notes that "culture shapes the way that individuals form Trauma Complexes after a traumatic experience and, once formed, articulate with other psychic complexities" p. 12).

Although a person's traumatic experience does not meet the criteria established for trauma-related disorders, it is important to look for prolonged reactions to trauma that may help in determining the lasting effects of experiences related to refugee status. These include: psychological problems (mood disorders, substance use, inability to sleep), and physical disorders (arthritis, headaches, chronic pain, etc.), also culturally expressed symptoms such as somatization, trance states, and dissociation (SAMSHA, 2014; Wilson, 2007). The issue is to recognize that these responses to trauma are culturally defined adaptations, and therefore treatment needs to incorporate culturally approved interventions, and the key to this information is also with the individual. Involving the client in the goals and processes that would lead to resolution can have a beneficial effect because the resolution would resonate with the client's cultural assumptions, and be meaningful and culture-specific for the client. Symptoms related to trauma and its aftermath are an adaptive, culturally defined, response to a situation that was psychologically, physically, and emotionally overwhelming. According to SAMSHA (2014), from a trauma-informed perspective, the trauma-related symptoms are a person's most resilient attempt to cope with the experience. However, these responses may have worked in the past, but depending on the severity of the event, they may not work in a different situation. SAMSHA's trauma-informed treatment protocol requires mental health professionals to focus on resilience, rather than pathology, and offer services with this mindset. It is important to recognize that responses to trauma are not abnormal per se, but normal responses to an abnormal situation (SAMSHA). This perception helps professionals to initiate treatment from a strength-based, and hopeful perspective.

The psychological literature notes that there are no universal measures of trauma, or cross-cultural standardized psychological treatment protocol, or psychopharmacological agents that work across cultures available for trauma resolution (Dana, 2005; Friedman, 2001; Wilson, 2007). However, studies have identified some antidepressants that have proven efficacious in reducing depression across cultures (Lin, Poland, Anderson, & Lesser, 1996). Dana (2007) identifies several assessment objectives, domains, and healing and adaptation outcomes; however, he notes that the range of resources to facilitate growth, strengths, and resilience, with attention to cultural values and assumptions of clients is limited. He advocates for a positive psychology stance focusing on holistic health, which includes: (a) core adaptation and restoration of psychosocial meaning systems, (b) posttraumatic growth, stimulating direct coping strategies with trauma, (c) strength, teaching problem-solving skills and competencies, (d) resilience, enhancing protective factors, (e) well-being, emphasizing physical, mental, and spiritual balance, and (f) salutogenesis, i.e., provide generalized resistance resources. Although, assessment measures are lacking to assess all these domains, it is important that these perspectives form the bedrock for initiating work with refugees.

In conducting interventions as early as the initial encounter with refugee populations, it important to use care to not re-traumatize the client. Refugees with vulnerable identities who have also suffered from a traumatic event, or multiple traumas, can easily be re-traumatized when they are asked to revisit the event, or when they see images that remind them of the trauma in the agency, or the therapist's office, or if they are treated in a manner (not allowed to make decisions, forced to have physical exams, before they are ready that remind them of the original trauma) (Drozdek & Wilson, 2007; SAMSHA, 2014). SAMSHA (2014) offers the following advice for avoiding retraumatization:

- Anticipate and be sensitive to the needs of clients who have experienced trauma regarding program policies and procedures in the treatment setting that might trigger memories of trauma, such as lack of privacy, feeling pushed to take psychotropic medications, perceiving that they have limited choices within the program or in the selection of the program, and so forth.
- Attend to clients' experiences. Ignoring clients' behavioral and emotional reactions to having their traumatic memories triggered is more likely to increase these responses than decrease them.
- Develop an individual coping plan in anticipation of triggers that the individual is likely to experience in treatment based on her/his/zir history.
- Rehearse routinely the coping strategies highlighted in the coping plan. If the client does not practice strategies prior to being triggered, the likelihood of being able to use them effectively upon triggering is lessened. For example, it is far easier to practice grounding exercises in the absence of severe fear than to wait for that moment when the client is reexperiencing an aspect of a traumatic event (Najavits, 2002).
- Recognize that clinical and programmatic efforts to control or contain behavior in treatment can cause traumatic stress reactions, particularly for trauma survivors for whom being trapped was part of the trauma experience.

- Listen for the specific trigger that seems to be driving the client's reaction. It will typically help both the counselor and client understand the behavior and normalize the traumatic stress reactions.
- Make sure that staff and other clients do not shame the trauma survivor for his or her behavior, such as through teasing or joking about the situation.
- Respond with consistency. The client should not get conflicting information or responses from different staff members; this includes information and responses given by administrators.
- Having clients undress in the presence of others.
- Inconsistently enforcing rules and allowing chaos in the treatment environment.
- Imposing agency policies or rules without exceptions or an opportunity for clients to question them.
- Enforcing new restrictions within the program without staff–client communication.
- Limiting access to services for ethnically diverse populations.
- Accepting agency dysfunction, including lack of consistent, competent leadership (pp. 45–46).

Implications for Counseling Refugees

A primary consideration in working with refugees is the practitioner's recognition of own strengths and challenges as a culturally responsive, trauma-informed therapist. It is important for helpers assess their own ability to understand the cultural idioms of health, and wellness of the varied cultures of the world to work, in essence, take the "not knowing" stance and allow the client to educate them about what the trauma means to the individual, and what in the culture of origin, and would help from a cultural perspective. Brown (2008) offers the following recommendations for cultural competence in working with trauma survivors, counselors' knowledge of: (a) whether the client is a survivor of cultural trauma (e.g., genocide, war, government oppression, torture, terrorism); (b) how to use cultural brokers (i.e., authorities within the culture who can help interpret cultural patterns and serve as liaisons to those outside the culture); (c) how trauma is viewed by an individual's sociocultural support network; (d) how to differentiate PTSD, trauma-related symptoms, and other mental disorders in the culture.

Using cultural assessments to understand own and client's cultural identity, worldview, acculturation status, and privilege and oppression would be an excellent starting point. Training in the Multicultural Assessment Intervention Process (MAIP) Model (Dana, Gamst, Rogers, & Der-Karabetian, 2006) would help in focusing on key cultural variables for positive clinical outcomes. This model includes the following variables: client-provider ethnic/cultural match, client acculturation status, client ethnic identity, and service provider's self-perceived cultural competence.

Engagement in therapy can be challenging with trauma survivors, Mahalik (2001), recommends the standard method of handling clients' lack of engagement is exploring it with them, by clarifying the situation through discussion with them, and reinterpreting (e.g., from "can't" to "won't" to "willing"), and working through the situation toward progress. Another recommended approach to engagement in therapy is motivational interviewing and enhancement techniques (TIP 35, *Enhancing motivation for change in substance abuse treatment* (Center for Substance Abuse Treatment [CSAT], 1999). Abrahams et al. (2010) offered a Trauma-Informed Competencies Checklist for professionals:

Trauma Awareness

1. Know and understand the difference between trauma-informed and trauma-specific services.
2. Recognize and understand the difference between different types of trauma and abuse including: physical, emotional, sexual abuse, domestic violence, experiences of war, natural disasters, and community violence.
3. Understand the different effects that various kinds of trauma have on human development and the development of psychological, and substance use issues.
4. Understand how protective factors, such as strong emotional connections and nonjudgmental people, and individual resilience can prevent and ameliorate the negative impact trauma has on both human development and the development of psychological and substance use issues.
5. Understand the importance of ensuring the physical and emotional safety of clients.
6. Understand the importance of not engaging in behaviors, such as confrontation of substance use or the seemingly unhealthy client behaviors, that might activate trauma symptoms or acute stress reactions.
7. Demonstrate knowledge of how trauma affects diverse people throughout their lifespan and with different mental health problems, cognitive and physical disabilities, and substance use issues.
8. Demonstrate knowledge of the impact of trauma in diverse cultures with regard to the meanings various cultures attach to trauma and the attitudes they have regarding behavioral health treatment.
9. Demonstrates knowledge of a variety of ways clients express stress reactions both behaviorally, and psychologically/emotionally.

Counseling Skills

1. Expedite client-directed choice and demonstrate a willingness to work within mutually empowering power structure in the therapeutic relationship.
2. Maintain clarity of roles and boundaries in the therapeutic relationship.
3. Demonstrate competence in screening and assessment of trauma history (within bounds of his or her licensing and scope of practice), including knowledge and practice with specific screening tools.

4. Shows competence in screening, and assessment of substance use disorders (within the bounds of his or her licensing and scope of practice), including knowledge of, and practice with specific screening tools.
5. Demonstrates an ability to identify client strengths, coping resources, and resilience.
6. Facilitates collaborative treatment and recovery planning with an emphasis on personal choice and a focus on clients' goals and knowledge of what has previously worked for them.
7. Respects clients' ways of managing stress reactions, while supporting and facilitating taking risks to acquire different coping skills that are consistent with clients' values and preferred identity and way of being in the world.
8. Demonstrates knowledge and skill in general trauma-informed counseling strategies, including but not limited to, grounding techniques that manage dissociative experiences, cognitive-behavioral tools that focus on both anxiety reduction and distress tolerance that reduce hyperarousal.
9. Identifies signs of secondary trauma reactions and takes steps to engage in appropriate self-care activities that lessen the impact of these reactions on clinical work with clients.
10. Recognize when the needs of clients are beyond his or her scope of practice and/or when clients' trauma material activates persistent secondary trauma or countertransference reactions that cannot be resolved in clinical supervision; makes appropriate referrals to other behavioral health professionals (pp. 5–7).

This checklist is helpful for professionals to understand the boundaries and parameters within which trauma-informed professionals must function.

Treatment Modalities

Cross-cultural treatment of traumatized refugees is complicated and difficult, because of values and expectations of treatment, along with language issues, makes the task of providing services challenging (Kinsie, 1988). Kinsie notes that it is a difficult task to provide services for clients with PTSD, depression, and other psychiatric disorders within a cultural context, and it becomes much more complex when dealing with traumatized refugees. Trauma-informed treatment interventions are designed for two specific phases of treatment, (a) immediately after a traumatic event, and (b) interventions that are provided once the immediate crisis has been addressed. Najavits (2007) notes that trauma-specific therapies vary in their objectives and approaches. They can be present-focused (providing coping skills, psychoeducation, and skills for better functioning), or past-focused (the trauma story to understand the impact of the trauma, experiencing emotions that could not be experienced in the past due to the overwhelming nature of the trauma, helping clients through the trauma to enhance present-day functioning). Both present- and past-focused interventions can also be used concurrently, depending on the type of trauma and its after effects. The specific therapy selected depends on the goals of treatment and the outcomes sought. Many of the therapies can be used for both individual and group interventions. All trauma-informed treatment modalities require training and supervision for safe and effective interventions (SAMSHA, 2014).

Although several treatments exist for trauma-informed interventions, there are hardly any treatments available that have been empirically tested for refugees (Kinzie, 2007; National Center for PTSD, 2014). Crumlish and O'Rourke (2010) conducted a systematic review of treatments for PTSD among refugees. They report that no treatment was firmly supported, but there was support for narrative exposure therapy and cognitive-behavioral therapy. They recommend that future research needs to focus on developing and evaluating treatments developed within the cultural norms of refugees, and the cultural understanding of trauma and its treatment. Kinzie provided a report on one case based on psychological and psychopharmacological intervention. Recommendations for treatment include: Group counseling for refugees who have had similar traumatic experiences (Yule, 2000); psychosocial interventions for strengthening the community and providing support to large groups, using psychoeducational approaches, and management of therapeutic activity centers (De Jong, Scholte, Koeter, & Hart, 2000); and targeting psychosocial risk factors for enhancing treatments (Mollica, Cui, McInnes, & Massagli, 2002).

The Harvard Program in Refugee Trauma (HPRT) (2014) focuses on the importance of involving refugees in their own recovery. They focus on identifying strengths and resilience, and use these to produce positive outcomes for therapeutic outcomes. They encourage work, altruistic behavior, and spirituality to maximize positive outcomes. The importance of the refugee's family and community is emphasized, and the interventions are contextualized within the family and community. The norms of the culture are honored, and the staff is specifically educated to honor cultural norms and traditions. The program addresses all the basic, psychosocial, and cultural needs of refugees, e.g., English language education, job skills, housing, citizenship, etc.

Once trauma resolution is achieved, identity development in host culture can proceed, with similar approaches that are employed with immigrants. In the interim, it is critical that a strength-based approach is used to help refugees start the rebuilding process by recognizing their strengths and resilience, and providing coping strategies. Additionally, attending to addressing basic needs, langauge acquisition and skills is important, as these are empowering and boost self-esteem.

Summary

Refugees tend to be highly traumatized and endure significant suffering and trauma prior to leaving their country. After relocation, they are subjected to several more traumatic experiences during the relocation process and the final placement in a host country. The challenges to providing services for refugees exist due to lack of understanding of their cultural contexts, cultural beliefs about trauma and its resolution. Traditional psychotherapy has not developed the cultural flexibility to accommodate the needs of traumatized refugees. However, the last 30 years have shown a significant increase in the education and training of counseling psychologists and counselors to enhance cultural awareness, knowledge and skills. The critical variable of understanding the cultural context, and cultural norms about mental illness and treatment in cultures of the world has been the challenge in providing appropriate services to refugees. It is critical that the client is involved in developing the treatment (goals and plan), and encouraged to be a mutual partner in the process of healing and recovery for mental health services to provide meaningful interventions that will lead to positive outcomes for refugees. Identity development in host culture, and acculturation cannot be fully addressed, without resolution of the trauma and posttraumatic effects of relocation. Therefore the primary task for therapists is to focus on resolving the trauma and providing coping strategies, along with attending to basic needs such as housing, acquisition of language and job skills.

References

Abrahams, I. A., Ali, O., Davidson, L., Evans, A. C., King, J. K., Poplawski, P., et al. (2010). *Philadelphia behavioral health services transformation: Practice guidelines for recovery and resilience oriented treatment*. Philadelphia, PA: Department of Behavioral Health and Intellectual Disability Services.

Ahearn, F. L., Jr., & Athey, J. L. (Eds.). (1991). *Refugee children: Theory, research, and services*. Baltimore, MD: The Johns Hopkins University Press.

American Psychological Association. (2009). *Working with refugee children and families: An update for health professionals*. Washington, DC: Author.

Aziz, N. (2011a). The psychological and human rights condition of Afghan women. In J. Heath & A. Zahedi (Eds.), *Land of the unconquerable: The lives of Contemporary Afghan Women* (pp. 244–290). Berkeley, CA: University of California Press.

Aziz, N. (2011b). What self-immolation means to Afghan women. *Journal of Social Justice, 23*, 45–51.

Berry, J. W. (1980). Acculturation as varieties of adaptation. In A. Padilla (Ed.), *Acculturation: Theory, models and some new findings* (pp. 9–25). Boulder, CO: Westview.

Berry, J. W. (1997). Immigration, acculturation, and adaptation. *Applied Psychology, 46*(1), 5–34. Retrieved from http://dx.doi.org/10.1111/j.1464-0597.1997.tb01087.x.

Birman, D., Persky, I., & Chan, W. Y. (2010). Multiple identities of Jewish immigrant adolescents from the former Soviet Union: An exploration of salience and impact of ethnic identity. *International Journal of Behavioral Development, 34*, 193–205.

Blanck, A. (2000). Domestic violence as a basis for asylum status: A human rights based approach. *Women's Rights Law Reporter, 22*(1), 47–58.

Boman, B., & Edwards, M. (1984). The Indochinese refugee: An overview. *Australian and New Zealand Journal of Psychiatry, 18*(1), 40–52.

Bowlby, J. (1973). *Attachment and loss: Vol. 2. Separation: Anxiety and anger*. New York: Basic Books.

Bowlby, J. (1982). *Attachment and loss: Vol. 1. Attachment* (2nd ed.). New York: Basic Books. (Original work published 1969)

Brown, L. S. (2008). Feminist therapy. In J. L. Lebow (Ed.), *Twenty-first century psychotherapies: Contemporary approaches to theory and practice* (pp. 277–306). Hoboken, NJ: Wiley.

Büscher, B., & de Beer, E. (2011). The contemporary paradox of long-term planning for social-ecological change and its effects on the discourse-practice divide: Evidence from Southern Africa. *Journal of Environmental Planning and Management, 54*(3), 301–318.

Campbell, J. R., & Rew, A. (1999). *Identity and affect: Experiences of identity in a globalizing world*. London: Pluto Press.

Cass, V. C. (1979). Homosexual identity formation: A theoretical model. *Journal of Homosexuality, 4*, 219–235.

Center for Substance Abuse Treatment. (1999). *Enhancing motivation for change in substance abuse treatment*. Treatment Improvement Protocol (TIP) Series 35. HHS Publication No. (SMA) 99-3354. Rockville, MD: Substance Abuse and Mental Health Services Administration.

Chavez, A. F., & Guido-DeBrito, F. (1999). Racial and ethnic identity development. *New Directions for Adult and Continuing Education, 1999*(84), 39–47.

Cianciarulo, M. S., & David, C. (2009). Pulling the trigger: Separation violence as a basis for refugee protection for battered women. *American University Law Review, 59*(2), 337–384.

Clarke, L. K., & Borders, L. D. (2014). "You got to apply seriousness": A phenomenological inquiry of Liberian refugees' coping. *Journal of Counseling & Development, 92*, 294–303. doi:10.1002/j.1556-6676.2014.00157.x.

Clinton-Davis, L., & Fassil, Y. (1992). Health and social problems of refugees. *Social Science & Medicine, 35*(4), 507–551.

Cross, W. E., Jr. (1995). The psychology of Nigrescence: Revising the Cross model. In J. G. Ponterotto, J. M. Casas, L. A. Suzuki, & C. M. Alexander (Eds.), *Handbook of multicultural counseling* (pp. 93–122). Thousand Oaks, CA: Sage.

Crumlish, N., & O'Rourke, K. (2010). A systematic review of treatments for post-traumatic stress disorder among refugees and asylum-seekers. *The Journal of Nervous and Mental Disease, 198*(4), 237–251. http://www.ncbi.nlm.nih.gov/pubmed/20386252.

Dana, R. H. (2005). *Handbook of cross-cultural and multicultural personality assessment*. Matwah, NJ: Lawrence Erlbaum.

Dana, R. J. (2007). Refugee assessment practices and cultural competency training. In J. P. Wilson & C. C. So-Kum Tang (Eds.), *Cross-cultural assessment of psychological trauma and PTSD* (pp. 91–112). New York: Springer.

Dana, R. H., Gamst, G., Rogers, R., & Der-Karabetian, A. (2006). Addressing mental health disparities: A preliminary test of the Multicultural Assessment Intervention Process (MAIP) model. In E. V. Metrosa (Ed.), *Racial and ethnic disparities in health and healthcare* (pp. 131–147). New York: Nova.

Deci, E. L., & Ryan, R. M. (1985). The General Causality Orientation Scale: Self determination in personality. *Journal of Research in Personality, 19*, 109–134.

De Jong, J. P., Scholte, W. F., Koeter, M. W. J., & Hart, A. A. (2000). The prevalence of mental health problems in Rwandan and Burundese refugee camps. *Acta Psychiatrica Scandinavica, 102*, 171–177.

Drozdek, B., & Wilson, J. P. (2007). Wrestling with ghosts from the past in exile: Assessing trauma in exile seekers. In J. P. Wilson & C. C. So-Kum Tang (Eds.), *Cross-cultural assessment of psychological trauma and PTSD* (pp. 113–134). New York: Springer.

Dujmic, S. (2013). *Counseling refugees: Risk and resilience*. Retrieved from http://counsellingbc.com/article/counselling-refugees-risk-and-resilience

Erdogan, S. (2012). *Identity formation and acculturation: The case of Karen refugees in London*. Unpublished doctoral dissertation, The University of Western Ontario, London.

Erikson, E. (1968). *Identity, youth and crisis*. New York: Norton.

Erikson, E. H. (1980). *Identity and the life cycle*. New York: W.W. Norton.

Fadjukoff, P., Pulkkinen, L., & Kokko, K. (2005). Identity processes in adulthood: Diverging domains. *Identity: An International Journal of Theory and Research, 5*, 1–20.

Friedman, M. J. (2001). Allostatic versus empirical perspectives on pharmacotherapy. In J. P. Wilson, M. J. Friedman, & J. D. Lindy (Eds.), *Treating psychological trauma and PTSD* (pp. 94–125). New York: Guilford Press.

Goosens, L. (2001). Global versus domain-specific statuses in identity research: A comparison of two self-report measures. *Journal of Adolescence, 12*, 681–699.

Guruge, S., Roche, B., & Catallo, C. (2012). Violence against women: An exploration of the physical and mental health trends among immigrant and refugee women in Canada. *Nursing Research and Practice*. Retrieved from http://dx.doi.org/10.1155/2012/434592

Guruge, S., Tiwari, A., & Lucea, M. B. (2010). International perspectives on family violence. In J. Humphreys & J. Campbell (Eds.), *Family violence and nursing practice* (2nd ed.). New York: Springer.

Harvard Program in Refugee Trauma (HPRT). (2014). Retrieved from http://hprt-cambridge.org/about/.

Helms, J. E. (1990). Toward a model of White racial identity development. In J. E. Helms (Ed.), *Black and White racial identity: Theory, research, and practice* (pp. 49–66). New York: Greenwood Press.

Helms, J. E. (1995). An update of Helms's White and people of color racial identity models. In J. G. Ponterotto, J. M. Casas, L. A. Suzuki, & C. M. Alexander (Eds.), *Handbook of multicultural counseling* (pp. 181–198). Thousand Oaks, CA: Sage.

Hossain, M., Zimmerman, C., Abas, M., Light, M., & Watts, C. (2010). The relationship of trauma to mental disorders among trafficked and sexually exploited girls and women. *American Journal of Public Health, 100*(12), 2442–2449.

Ibrahim, F. A. (1990). *Cultural identity check list©* (CICL). Storrs, CT. Unpublished document.

Ibrahim, F. A. (1999). Transcultural counseling: Existential world view theory and cultural identity: Transcultural applications. In J. McFadden (Ed.), *Transcultural counseling* (2nd ed., pp. 23–57). Alexandria, VA: ACA Press.

Kaprielian-Churchill, I., & Churchill, S. (1994). *The pulse of the world: Refugees in our schools*. Toronto, ON: OISE Press.

Kinsie, J. D. (1988). The psychiatric effects of massive trauma on Cambodian refugees. In J. P. Wilson, Z. Harel, & B. Kahana (Eds.), *Human adaptation to extreme stress* (pp. 305–319). New York: Plenum Press.

Kinzie, J. (2007). High-impact practices boost learning, involved parents no problem. *National Survey of Student Engagement Annual Report*. Bloomington, IN: Indiana University Center for Postsecondary Research.

Kopinak, J. (1998). *Bosnian refugees in Canada: Trauma, resettlement and health in temporal perspective*. Master's thesis. University of Toronto.

Kroger, J., & Marcia, J. E. (2011). The identity statuses: Origins, meanings, and interpretations. In S. J. Schwartz et al. (Eds.), *Handbook of identity theory and research*. New York: Springer.

LaViolette, A. (2013). *It could happen to anyone: Why battered women stay* (3rd ed.). Thousand Oaks, CA: Sage.

Lin, K. L., Poland, R. E., Anderson, D., & Lesser, I. M. (1996). Ethnopharmacology and the treatment of PTSD. In A. J. Marsella, M. J. Friedman, E. T. Gerrity, & R. M. Scurfield (Eds.), *Ethnocultural aspects of posttraumatic stress disorder* (pp. 505–529). Washington, DC: American Psychological Association.

Luyckx, K., Goossens, L., Soenens, B., & Beyers, W. (2006). Unpacking commitment and exploration: Validation of an integrative model of adolescent identity formation. *Journal of Adolescence, 29*, 361–378.

Luyckx, K., Goossens, L., Soenens, B., Beyers, W., & Vansteenkiste, M. (2005). Identity statuses based on 4 rather than 2 identity dimensions: Extending and refining Marcia's paradigm. *Journal of Youth and Adolescence, 34*(6), 605–618. doi:10.1007/s10964-005-8949-x.

Luyckx, K., Schwartz, S. J., Soenens, B., Vansteenkiste, M., & Goosens, L. (2010). The path from identity commitments to adjustment: Motivational and mediating mechanisms. *Journal of Counseling and Development, 88*, 52–60.

Mahalik, J. R. (2001). Cognitive therapy for men. In G. R. Brooks & G. E. Good (Eds.), *The new handbook of psychotherapy and counseling with men: A comprehensive guide to settings, problems, and treatment approaches* (pp. 544–564). San Francisco: Jossey-Bass.

Marcia, J. E. (1966). Development and validation of ego identity status. *Journal of Personality and Social Psychology, 5*, 551–558.

Marsella, A. J. (2005). Rethinking the 'talking cures' in a global era. *Contemporary Psychology, 50*(45), 2–12.

Mason, R., Hyman, I., Berman, H., Guruge, S., Kanagaratnam, P., & Manuel, L. (2008). Violence is an international language: Tamil women's perceptions of intimate partner violence. *Violence Against Women, 14*(12), 1397–1412.

McCarn, S. R., & Fassinger, R. E. (1996). Revisioning sexual minority identity formation: A new model of lesbian identity and its implications for counseling and research. *The Counseling Psychologist, 24*, 508–534. doi:10.1177/0011000096243011.

McSpadden, L. A., & Moussa, H. (1993). I have a name: The gender dynamics in asylum and resettlement of Ethiopian and Eritrean refugees in North America. In G. Buijs (Ed.), *Migrant women*. Oxford, England: Berghahn Boo.

Menjívar, C., & Salcido, O. (2002). Immigrant women and domestic violence: Common experiences in different countries. *Gender and Society, 16*(6), 898–920.

Mollica, R. F., Cui, X., McInnes, K., & Massagli, M. P. (2002). Science-based policy for psychosocial interventions in refugee camps: A Cambodian example. *Journal of Nervous and Mental Disease, 190*(3), 158–166.

Mosselson, J. (2006). *Roots & routes: Bosnian adolescent refugees in New York City*. New York: Peter Lang.

Najavits, L. M. (2002). *Seeking safety: A treatment manual for PTSD and substance abuse*. New York: Guilford Press.

Najavits, L. M. (2007). Psychosocial treatments for posttraumatic stress disorder. In P. E. Nathan & E. M. Gorman (Eds.), *A guide to treatments that work* (3rd ed., pp. 513–530). New York: Oxford Press.

National Center for PTSD. (2014). Retrieved from http://www.ptsd.va.gov/.

O'Brien, E. J., & Epstein, S. (1988). *The multidimensional self-esteem inventory (MSEI): Professional manual*. Odessa, FL: Psychological Assessment Resources.

O'Neil, J. M., Egan, J., Owen, S. V., & Murray, V. M. (1993). The gender role journey measure: Scale development and psychometric evaluation. *Sex Roles, 28*, 167–185.

Ossana, S. M., Helms, J. E., & Leonard, M. M. (1992). Do "womanist" identity attitudes influence college women's self-esteem and perceptions of environmental bias? *Journal of Counseling & Development, 70*, 402–408.

Phinney, J. (1989). Stages of ethnic identity development in minority group adolescents. *Journal of Early Adolescence, 9*, 34–49.

Pittaway, E., Muli, C., & Shteir, S. (2009). I have a voice-hear me: Findings of an Australian study examining the resettlement and integration experience of refugees and migrants from the Horn of Africa in Australia. *Refuge, 26*(2), 133–146.

Porter, M., & Haslam, N. (2005). Predisplacement and postdisplacement factors associated with mental health of refugees and internally displaced persons: A meta-analysis. *Journal of the American Medical Association, 294*(5), 602–612.

Poston, W. S. C. (1990). The biracial identity development model: A needed addition. *Journal of Counseling and Development, 69*, 152–155.

Pumariega, A. J. (2003). Cultural competence in systems of care for children's mental health. In A. J. Pumariega & N. C. Winters (Eds.), *Handbook of community systems of care: The new child & adolescent community psychiatry* (pp. 82–106). San Francisco: Jossey Bass.

Pumariega, A. J., Rothe, E., & Pumariega, J. B. (2005). Mental health of immigrants and refugees. *Community Mental Health Journal, 41*(5), 581–597. doi:10.1007/s10597-005-6363-1.

Root, M. P. P. (1990). Resolving 'Other' Status: Identity development of biracial individuals. *Women and Therapy, 9*, 185–205.

Schwartz, S. J. (2001). The evolution of Eriksonian and neo-Eriksonian identity theory and research: A review and integration. *Identity: An International Journal of Theory and Research, 1*, 7–58.

Schwartz, S. J., Montgomery, M. J., & Briones, E. (2006). The role of identity in acculturation among immigrant people: Theoretical propositions, empirical questions, and applied recommendations. *Human Development, 49*, 1–30. doi:10.1159/000090300.

Shultheiss, D. P., & Blustein, D. L. (1994). Contributions of family relationship factors to the identity formation process. *Journal of Counseling & Development, 73*, 159–166.

Smith, C., & Halbert, K. (2013, December). *"They look like paper": Refugee students' experiencing and constructing 'the social' at a Queensland High School*. Paper presented at the Australian Association for Research in Education, Adelaide, Australia.

Sneed, J. R., Schwartz, S. J., & Cross, W. E. (2006). A multicultural critique of identity status theory and research: A call for integration. *Identity: An International Journal of Theory and Research, 6*(1), 61–84.

Substance Abuse and Mental Health Services Administration (SAMSHA). (2012). *Behavioral Health, United States*, (HHS Publication No. [SMA] 13–4797). Rockville, MD: Substance Abuse and Mental Health Services Administration.

Substance Abuse and Mental Health Services Administration (SAMSHA). (2014). *A treatment improvement protocol: Trauma-informed care in behavioral health services, TIP 57*. Rockville, MD: US Department of Health and Human Services.

Thomas, F. C., Roberts, B., Luitel, N. P., Upadhaya, N., & Tpi, W. A. (2011). Resilience of refugees displaced in the developing world: A qualitative analysis of strengths and struggles of urban refugees in Nepal. *Conflict and Health, 5*, 20. doi:10.1186/1752-1505-5-20. Retrieved from http://www.conflictandhealth.com/content/5/1/20

United Nations High Commission on Refugees (UNHCR). (2000). *World refugee statistics*. Retrieved from http://www.mfa.by/eng/org.htm

United Nations High Commissioner for Refugees (UNHCR). (2009a). *UNHCR policy on refugee protection and solutions in urban areas*. Retrieved June 21, 2014, from http://www.unhcr.org/refworld/docid/4ab8e7f72.html

United Nations High Commissioner for Refugees (UNHCR). (2009b). *Guidelines on International Protection No. 9: Claims to refugee status based on sexual orientation and/or gender identity within the context of article 1A(2) of the 1951 convention and/or its 1967 protocol relating to the status of refugees*. Retrieved August 13, 2014, from http://www.refworld.org/docid/50348afc2.html

United Nations High Commissioner for Refugees (UNHCR). (2011a). *UNHCR country operations profile-Nepal*. Retrieved September 7, 2011, from http://www.unhcr.org/pages/49e487856.html

United Nations High Commissioner for Refugees (UNHCR). (2011b). *Handbook and guidelines on procedures and criteria for determining refugee status under the 1951 convention and the 1967 protocol relating to the status of refugees*. Retrieved May 21, 2013, from www.refworld.org/docid/4f33c8d92.html

Watts, C., & Zimmerman, C. (2002). Violence against women: Global scope and magnitude. *The Lancet, 359*(9313), 1232–1237.

Wilkinson, L. (2002). Factors influencing the academic success of refugee youth in Canada. *Journal of Youth Studies, 5*(2), 173–193.

Wilson, J. P. (2007). The lens of culture: Theoretical and conceptual perspectives in the assessment of psychological trauma and PTSD. In J. P. Wilson & C. C. So-Kum Tang (Eds.), *Cross-cultural assessment of psychological trauma and PTSD* (pp. 3–30). New York: Springer.

Yule, W. (2000). From pogroms to "ethnic cleansing": Meeting the needs of war affected children. *Journal of Child Psychology & Psychiatry, 41*(6), 695–702.

Zimmerman, C., Hossain, M., Yun, K., Roche, B., Morison, L., & Watts, C. (2006). *Stolen smiles: The physical and psychological health consequences of women and adolescents trafficked in Europe*. London: The London School of Hygiene and Tropical Medicine.

Chapter 8
Application of Social Justice and Cultural Responsiveness Strategies: Using Cultural Assessments in Counseling and Psychotherapy

Introduction

The importance of broaching cultural issues with clients has been addressed in the counseling and psychotherapy literature (Arnold, 2010; Cardemil & Battle, 2003; Chang & Yoon, 2011; Day-Vines et al., 2007; Ibrahim & Heuer, 2013; Ibrahim, Ohnishi, & Wilson, 1994; Zegley, 2007; Zhang & Burkard, 2008). However, concrete approaches to understanding a clients experience, culture, values, etc., are unclear, beyond a recommendation to address these issues. Broaching the cultural dimension by seeking to conduct cultural assessments is a process that helps in bringing cultural issues into the counseling process (Ibrahim, 2010; Ibrahim & Heuer, 2013). The rapidly changing demographic profile of the United States requires that clinicians acquire knowledge and skills to identify cultural dimensions of the counseling encounter, i.e., the helpers and client cultural identity, and cultural context, before proceeding with setting goals and process for counseling (Ibrahim, 1999, 2003). This chapter will have an introductory section identifying the process for conducting assessments on cultural variables, and incorporating them in interventions and in the second section case studies highlighting how cultural assessments were used to help design interventions, and the evaluation of the interventions will be presented.

Process for Conducting Cultural Assessments

We recommend two approaches for incorporating the cultural assessments into the counseling process: (1) integrated into the initial interview; and (2) giving the paper-pencil tests and inventories to the client and having the client complete the information and bring it in to the second session. Reviewing the results on the tests and inventories can corroborate the information provided by the client in the initial

F.A. Ibrahim, J.R. Heuer, *Cultural and Social Justice Counseling*,
International and Cultural Psychology, DOI 10.1007/978-3-319-18057-1_8

interview. Further, where there are discrepancies, these can be explored with the client to clarify the client's perception of his or her cultural identity, worldview (beliefs, values, and assumptions), perception of the acculturation level, and privilege and oppression status.

In the first approach to conducting cultural assessments, we recommend integrating the cultural assessments into the initial interview, and subsequent sessions. The Cultural Identity Check List-Revised© (CICL-R; Ibrahim, 2008) is the starting point for gathering client information. It is easy to integrate the questions within the initial interview with clients. As part of the process of identifying the presenting problem, the antecedent variables and the consequent variables and effect on the client's life, it is important to incorporate this information within the context of client's culture, cultural identity, gender, sexual orientation, age, religion or spirituality, and ability/disability issues. The CICL-R can be used as a backdrop for the therapist, to understand the client's presenting problem within her/his/zir cultural identity and cultural context (culture, acculturation level, privilege, and oppression status). This especially works well for clients who are not comfortable with paper-pencil inventories. In addition it makes the process of collecting client information, perception of the presenting problem, and how it is affecting the client's life much more organic, and natural.

The second approach works well with people who have been educated with a college education, as they are more comfortable with paper–pencil assessments. Further, it is useful with clients who want to save time, and want an immediate response to their presenting problem. Once the assessments are completed, it is important to review them prior to discussing them in the session, to be prepared for exploring the presenting problem within the client's cultural identity, and cultural context. Using either approach, the cultural assessments can help in: (a) identifying the client's cultural identity and worldview, and personal identity variables (Ibrahim, 1999, 2003); (b) identify clients' acculturation level, privilege and oppression, which in combination with vulnerable aspects of cultural identity, help identify external stressors, and variables that constitute extrapsychic variables (Ibrahim & Heuer, 2013).

Cultural Information: Application in Counseling

The identification of core values and assumptions (worldview), and cultural identity helps in understanding the level of stress caused by the presenting problem on the client's life, primarily, in the three areas of cultural identity (noted at the end of the CICL-R), it is critical to understanding the cultural identity variables that are implicated, and the distress experienced. This question on the CICL-R pertains to the link between the presenting problem and the link with core identity dimensions of a client. In addition, acculturation level, privilege and oppression status evaluations are helpful in making a determination of whether the presenting problem is linked to intrapsychic (biological, neurological, or psychological issues) or extrapsychic (environmental constraints, due to societal biases toward less valued culture or ethnicity, gender, sexual orientation, age, religion/spirituality, or disability status) factors. The assessments provide an in-depth understanding of the client's identity, her/his/zir place in the world and life context, and what options are available to resolving the presenting problem. These cultural assessments reduce the chance of imposing interventions on clients' that may not be effective given the cultural identity, worldview, acculturation level, privilege, and oppression status of clients.' Further, when there is congruence between a helper and the client in understanding the client, trust increases, and the therapeutic relationship is enhanced (Arnold, 2010; Chang & Yoon, 2011; Dana, 2008; Ibrahim, 1999; Zegley, 2007).

The ability to explore these variables with clients helps in determining the socio-cultural context, and real life options available to clients. This process also helps balance the interpersonal, cultural, and sociopolitical (contextual) aspects of the client's world (Rosenberger, 2014; Tosone, 2004). It conveys respect and solidifies the therapeutic relationship, as the client experiences the therapist affirming her/his/zir reality, and clients feel understood and accepted (Baker Miller, 2012; Cornish, Schreier, Nadkarni, Metzger, & Rodolfa, 2010; Zegley, 2007).

Implications for Psychological Interventions

Using cultural assessments to begin the counseling process ensures that the client's reality (personal, interpersonal, and sociopolitical issues) has been encountered, and the outcome in counseling and psychotherapy will be relevant and meaningful for the client. The underlying assumption in our approach assumes that the clinicians have the ability: (a) to be authentic; (b) to connect with the client with empathy; (c) to establish a mutual relationship, and engage in co-construction of meaning; (d) to approach the client from a "not knowing" perspective; (e) to identify and affirm the client's strengths; (f) to understand the dynamics of the dyadic relationship, as mutually supportive encounters, where the relationship is the key to success; (g) to engage in collaborative goal setting; (h) to evaluate the effectiveness of the intervention; and (i) to be able to recognize limits of own knowledge and skills, as they pertain to clinical issues, cultural responsiveness, and privilege and oppression issues.

Being Authentic

To be authentic in cross-cultural encounters requires a clear idea about one's own cultural identity, worldview, acculturation level to mainstream culture, privilege and oppression. Understanding one's own biases allows us to be honest about our biases and misconceptions about others. Owning the limits of our knowledge and skills is also critically important in working across cultures. This will also help in making amends, or apologizing when assumptions are made about clients in therapy resulting in "ruptures" that negatively affect the therapeutic alliance (Gaztambide, 2012). Cardemil and Battle (2003) recommend suspending "preconceptions about clients' race/ethnicity and that of their family members" (p. 279). They note that race/ethnicity of clients' is not usually obvious, and it is also important to broach the subject early on, to reduce the chance of making errors of judgment. Cardemil and Battle note they broach the subject of race/ethnicity by asking:

> Often, I ask my clients about their racial and ethnic background because it helps me have a better understanding of who they are. Is that something you'd feel comfortable talking about? (p. 279).

Relational counseling and psychotherapy encourages helpers to openly discuss issues of "bias, core beliefs, adaptive, and maladaptive coping, projections and introjections, historical forces, and especially important in diversity practice, current sociopolitical realities" as natural subjects to explore in a therapeutic relationship (Rosenberger, 2014, p. 4)

Connecting with the Client with Empathy

To connect with the client with empathy, is complicated in cross-cultural counseling, it requires understanding how to be empathic in a culturally responsive manner. This requires understanding the client's cultural context well enough to be culturally intentional, i.e., to respond with an understanding of the culture and the client's context, and to be able to allude to it with a culturally specific reference. Ivey, Pedersen, & Ivey (2008) recommend being culturally intentional, i.e., generating adequate responses with reference to the specific culture and context of the client. Culturally empathic responses relate to responding with empathy, i.e., with an understanding of the client's culture, and what the issue means to the client, and to convey this understanding to the client (Ivey et al., 2008).

Mutual Relationship and Co-construction

Establishing a mutual relationship requires the counseling process to be bidirectional, where no one holds more power or value than another. Both the therapist and the client have their areas of expertise, the therapist on knowledge and skills for effective and ethical practice, and the client on his or her subjective reality (Rosenberger, 2014). Mutuality in counseling derives from the feminist theory of counseling, and it also predicates co-construction of goals in counseling, to establish realistic solutions to the dilemmas clients bring to counseling (Baker Miller, 2012). Castillo (1997) emphasizes that clients know the solution to the issues they bring to counseling, they are simply not able to resolve the dilemma, but need help in finding the path to resolution. Therapists with their training in clinical knowledge and skills, can facilitate self-reflection, and create openness to possibilities, to explore positive outcomes for clients.

The Not-Knowing Perspective

The "not knowing" perspective implies that clinicians are not defensive about what they do not know, and take the position that clients are the experts on their world and issues, and allows clients to educate them about the cultural meaning of the issues they are confronted with, and the possible resolutions that will work in their social-cultural contexts (Rosenberger, 2014). This stance also helps clients' feel in charge of their issues, and their knowledge about their world, boosting their self-confidence and empowering them to be active participants in the therapy process.

Identify and Affirm the Client Strengths

Using a positive psychology approach by identifying strengths of clients' to empower them to take charge of the problem resolution process is critically important (Maslow, 1987; Seligman, Steen, Park, & Peterson, 2005). Empowered individuals are better able to generate positive outcomes to resolve the issues they are wrestling with, and to move toward independence, by recognizing their own potential and ability to understand their own cultural and social world. This process facilitates therapy and produces resolutions that are meaningful and culturally sensitive.

Dynamics of a Dyadic Relationship and Collaborative Goal Setting

Recognize the dynamics of the dyadic relationship, as mutually supportive encounters, where the relationship is the key to success. As noted in previous chapters, finding common ground in values, socialization processes, acculturation, privilege and oppression can help create a *shared worldview*, and enhance the counseling relationship. Mutuality in cross-cultural counseling relationships requires treating the other as an equal and involving them in the process of counseling by developing counseling goals as a collaborative process. This is an essential requirement for cross-cultural encounters, client trust, and engagement in counseling will be enhanced. Further as noted throughout the text, since clinicians cannot always have full understanding of everyone's culture, socialization process, primary and secondary cultural affiliations, without client involvement in the goals setting process, the intervention can go awry (Ibrahim, 2003; Ibrahim & Heuer, 2013).

Evaluate the Effectiveness of the Intervention

Evaluating the efficacy of counseling interventions is critical for ethical practice (Miller, Hubble, Chow, & Seidal, 2013). Research on psychotherapy evaluation has focused on three main areas: efficacy, effectiveness, and efficiency (Howard, Krasner, & Saunders, 1999). Efficacy evaluation pertains to assessing the usefulness of psychotherapy with large samples under experimental conditions. Effectiveness of psychotherapy studies consider the delivery of psychotherapy in clinical settings. Efficiency studies focus on progress in psychotherapy of individual clients (Howard et al., 1999). The last 25 years research on the efficacy of psychotherapy with large samples has not provided information on the usefulness of one type of therapy over another. However based on over 1,000 studies, it is evident that psychotherapy works (Howard et al., 1999; Howard, Moras, Brill, Martinovich, & Lutz, 1996).

For clinicians the question is client progress and amelioration of distress. Getting feedback from the client on the efficacy of the interventions is helpful for therapists. It helps clinicians' in identifying what worked and why, and in refining interventions to best meet the needs of their diverse clients. Kazdin (2006) recommends that during the goals development phase, clinicians must think about strategies for assessment of the treatment goals. Evaluation of counseling interventions can be accomplished with a repeated measures approach.

Stiles, Gordon, and Lani (2002) developed a *Session Evaluation Questionnaire Form-5* (SEQ-Form-5) to evaluate the effectiveness of each session. According to the authors' counseling sessions can be judged to be good or bad, i.e., having depth (powerful and valuable or weak and worthless), have a "smoothness" quality (relaxed and comfortable, or tense and distressing) (Stiles, 1980; Stiles et al., 1994; Stiles & Snow, 1984; Stiles, Tupler, & Carpenter, 1982). The SEQ has two additional dimensions, these are: participants' post session mood, positivity and arousal (Stiles & Snow, 1984; Stiles et al., 1994). The SEQ-Form-5 has been used to evaluate individual, group counseling, and encounter groups, along with family therapy sessions, and supervision sessions (Stiles et al., 2002). The SEQ-Form-5 is empirically validated and has adequate reliability across all three indices: internal consistency measured by coefficient alpha is .90 for depth and .93 for smoothness (Reynolds et al., 1996).

Recognize Limits of Cultural Competence

Finally, cultural responsiveness, competence, and social justice efficacy is essential for clinicians to provide effective counseling and psychotherapy. There is great variability in training models for cultural competence across mental health education and training programs (Dana, 2008; LaFromboise & Foster, 1992; Lopez & Rogers, 2007; Marsella & Pedersen, 2004; Mollen, Ridley, & Hill, 2003; Ponterotto, 1996; Suarez-Balcazar, Durlak, & Smith, 1994; Sue, Zane, Hall, & Berger, 2009). Boysen and Vogel (2008) conducted research to assess if therapists who had training in multicultural counseling and felt they were competent has any negative implicit biases, and they showed that training and education on cultural competence does not seem to address implicit biases. Although, there is considerable information available on cultural competence, there is not much research that shows that the available models are effective, or useful. Specifically, training needs to address implicit bias and help therapists in confronting the underlying biases that they may not be aware of in everyday life, but may surface in working with vulnerable clients. We recommend that mental health professionals reflect on their own cultural identity, worldview, acculturation level, privilege and oppression, and work on identifying and understanding their own implicit bias (https://implicit.harvard.edu/implicit/). Training programs may want to incorporate experiential learning to explore cultural differences and the all dimensions of diversity, i.e., ethnicity, gender, sexual orientation. Developing cultural awareness, knowledge and skills is a developmental process over the professional lifespan (Leong, Leach, & Malikiosos-Loizos, 2012).

Research has shown that the therapeutic relationship is enhanced, and clients report satisfaction when the therapist is culturally competent (i.e., aware of own cultural identity and worldview, culturally sensitive, responsive, and uses worldview assessment to understand the client's core values), clients' reported satisfaction with the interventions and the therapist (Cunningham-Warburton, 1988; Sadlak, 1986). Although these two studies are dated, given the myriad of concerns identified by researchers it is critical that we continue to identify the most effective process to enhance cultural competence and responsiveness among mental health professionals.

The case studies included in this chapter include professionals who have examined their cultural identity, worldview, acculturation level, privilege and oppression. Some have also taken the Implicit Attitudes Test (IAT; Greenwald, Nosek, & Banaji, 2003; https://implicit.harvard.edu/implicit/). These cases are examples that incorporate the client's cultural identity, and use the results of the cultural assessments to develop interventions. These cases also provide reflections by some of the mental health professionals on their own cultural identity, and on interventions that worked and did not work. Mostly self-report of the client was used to assess success or satisfaction with counseling, and the professional's clinical judgment to evaluate the effectiveness of the interventions.

Case 1: Counseling a Native American Client

Aimee Aron-Reno

Introduction

The following is an assessment and intervention strategy for Frank Wapasha. Frank is a Native and an/Irish-American 36-year-old male living in the Denver metro area. Frank is seeking counseling due to depression. He has recently experienced a breakup with his girlfriend and is also experiencing career dissatisfaction in his work as an attorney. Frank's presenting problem is depression and job dissatisfaction. Frank identifies as a Sioux Indian and lived on the reservation for some of the early years of his life. The remainder of his life has been spent off the reservation, but his identity resonates with both Indian and mainstream US cultures. Frank's overarching identity as he describes himself is that of a Sioux Indian, a son, a man, and an attorney. The client is experiencing a lack of motivation, and a clear direction in his life. He expressed an interest in working to resolve anger issues, work through feelings of isolation, and is also seeking closure for his recent breakup.

Frank has felt the effects of the oppression from the dominant cultural group. He still has family living on the Crow Creek Reservation, including his mother. Frank struggled with poverty in his childhood, and chose to pursue a career in law in order to help his people and himself. He continues to struggle mentally with the expectations of earning more money, and financially with the weight of student loan payments. Frank also seems to struggle with the topic of spirituality and living in a dual-culture.

Client Information

Name: Frank Wapasha (Red Leaf)
Age: *36*
Cultural Background: Dakota Sioux, Crow Creek Tribe

Presenting Problem

Frank came in due to his struggle with depression, due to a recent breakup with his girlfriend, and job dissatisfaction. Frank states he has had problems sleeping for the last month. He does not like to sleep in his bed because it reminds him that he is

A. Aron-Reno
University of Colorado Denver, Denver, CO, USA
e-mail: aareno@aimeearon.com

alone, and only sleeps for about 4-5 h per night. He has felt himself becoming more easily irritated with people and situations, and it affects his work. He said he feels sad and "transparent" most of the time. Frank stated, "I go to work where I am miserable, then I come home and watch television and I am sad and alone, and then get up and do it all over again. I feel like a robot… I can't focus on anything except being sad. I don't eat, and don't want to. I don't sleep, and don't want to. I just want it all to stop, but I don't know how to make it stop." When asked about weight loss Frank said, "Yeah, I think I've lost maybe 10 lb—my pants are a lot more loose."

Social/Educational Background

Frank is a Native American/Irish man who grew up mainly in South Dakota. He was born on the Crow Creek Reservation, but moved to Minneapolis with his father at the age of five. His parents were never married and have a strained relationship. His mother, Mary is full-blood Native American and his father, John is of Irish-American heritage. A Cherokee woman adopted his father, John, when he was a teenager, and he became attached to the Native American way of life. He moved to South Dakota in his late twenties and met Mary. They had a relationship for a few years, but due to Mary's alcoholism—John felt he needed to raise Frank on his own, and away from Mary.

John and Frank moved to Minneapolis, and continued to live there for 3 years. During this time, John realized how much he missed being connected to the Native culture in South Dakota. When Frank was 8 years-old, he and his father moved to Whitewood, South Dakota. Frank speaks fondly of the time he and his father spent in Minneapolis, but considers Whitewood his home.

After graduating from Whitewood High School, Frank attended Colorado State University. He studied political science and Native American studies. He said, "My grades were fair, but not exceptional." Upon graduating from college, Frank returned to Whitewood and worked on a few "meaningless jobs. For about a year he lived in Tucson, however, he returned home to Whitewood. Approximately 2 years later, Frank started applying to law schools and was accepted at the University of Montana. Upon completion of his law degree, he moved back to Fort Collins, Colorado and began applying for jobs and studying for the bar examination.

Frank met Susan, his girlfriend of two and one-half years while living in Fort Collins. She lived in Denver, and they met while skiing in Steamboat Springs, Colorado. In time, the two became closer and Frank ended up moving into Susan's apartment in Denver. They lived together for about 2 years until their breakup approximately 1 month ago. Frank is now living with a co-worker and friend. He said he feels like this was a "divorce." This was the second such relationship for Frank.

In the last year, Frank stated their relationship had become "tumultuous at best." They fought frequently, over things such as Susan's "flirtations with co-workers" and her "exploitive use of her body to get attention." Frank stated he knew his anger got out of control, but "she drove me to it." Frank mentioned punching a hole in the wall of their home. Also in the past year, Frank got his first job practicing law at a firm in downtown Denver. He liked it at first but said, "Once things started falling apart with Susan, everything seemed to fall apart." He has been at his current job for approximately 9 months and is feeling let down. "I expected to be making more money, and be doing more than answering phone calls and people's stupid questions all day," he noted. Frank shared that he hardly makes enough money to pay his bills.

Assessments

Cultural Identity Assessment

Frank seems to identify strongly with his Native American roots, but also seems to be in conflict about some of his values. During completion of the Cultural Identity Checklist-R© (CICL-R, Ibrahim, 2007, Appendix A), he stated the most significant part of his identity was as a Sioux. Frank seems to identify very strongly as a heterosexual male, and shows signs of power as a male (dominance over women—including his ex-girlfriend as well as his mother) and frustrations regarding respect for Native identified men.

The three main focal issues that were identified by Frank emerging from his cultural identity and their connection to the presenting problem were: (a) lack of balance between Frank's core beliefs and his current lifestyle; (b) lack of direction or motivation; and (c) feelings of alienation.

Worldview

Frank took the Scale to Assess Worldview© to clarify his core beliefs and values (SAWV; Ibrahim & Kahn, 1984). Frank's worldview seems to fit most in the optimistic and here-and-now categories of the SAWV (Ibrahim & Owen, 1994). Frank sees people as good, and acknowledges that some of his answers are "somewhat tainted by recent events." He believes strongly in harmony with nature, and attributes this to his Native American roots. These beliefs were also evident in his time orientation to favor the present. He says he "generally lives in the now—because you cannot change the past, and you never know what will happen in the future." He stated that his preferred time perspective has felt "somewhat off lately—maybe because I'm constantly reviewing what could've happened, or how I might have changed my current circumstances if I had done something differently in the past—with Susan, or my job."

Acculturation Level

Frank's level of acculturation was measured using the United States Acculturation Index© (Ibrahim, 2008, Appendix B). I chose to complete the assessment with Frank, to discuss his current situation, his upbringing, and his values more thoroughly. Results of the evaluation showed Frank's tendencies towards "Present Time Focus" a "Family-kinship Orientation" and "Mind/Body Connection." These resonate with Sioux traditions. On other topics on the Acculturation Index his responses were more individualistic, specifically some indefinite answers in the areas of "Individual or Community Focus," and "Authoritarian or Mutual Relationships". Reviewing the acculturation information, it is clear from a clinical point of view that these ambiguities may be related to the uncertainty Frank may be feeling about his life as a multiracial Native and Irish American living in, and identifying with two cultures.

Other Relevant Assessments

Gender identity: Frank identifies as a male, he is not struggling with any issues of gender identity no further assessment was pursued.

Spirituality: Frank stated he has "been thinking more lately about going home to The Hills where he feels more grounded." He notes, "it's hard to practice Native practices, when you are not surrounded by it—you get distracted." I asked Frank about how this was making him feel, since he had stated his spirituality was "innate" when we were completing the Cultural Identity Checklist-Revised© (Ibrahim, 2007). He seemed slightly surprised by this question and stated, "I had always identified my spirituality as Native, and it wasn't really a religion, it was a way of life. I went to church with Susan sometimes; she grew up Baptist… maybe that made me question some things. I guess I wasn't used to thinking of that element of my life as a choice, or optional." According to Genia (1990) and Hodge (2001), an individual can be in transition among the five stages of spiritual development. Using this tool, I assessed Frank to be in stage three or the Transitional Stage, in his spiritual journey. This is an area that may need follow-up to help resolve confusion for Frank.

DSM-5 Diagnosis

Initial assessment of Frank seems to conclude that he meets the criteria for Major Depressive Episode (American Psychiatric Association (APA), 2013). He exhibits six of the nine symptoms necessary for this diagnosis, and upon further examination I suspect he may possess more symptoms of Major Depressive Episode. He shared that he is generally in good health, and has not experienced these feelings in the past, therefore justifying a diagnosis of single episode.

Counselor Biases

An area of bias that I will need to evaluate is acculturation level. It would be easy to assume that Frank's acculturation level is very similar to White Anglo Saxon perspectives, because he currently lives in Denver, and has attended college, and law school at mostly White institutions. This presupposition would be unfair, and not based upon fact, or any cultural assessment. Another area of concern is transference. Native people are usually portrayed as having a past time orientation and stereotyped as lazy (Duran, 2006). These stereotypes can damage the therapeutic relationship that is usually difficult to establish with indigenous US citizens, and lead to a continuation of suffering caused by intergenerational trauma (Chavez Cameron & Turtle-Song, 2003). Due to ignorance of the experiences of Native Americans in the United States and their ancestors, their experiences may never be fully understood by a Euro-American therapist. As a culturally competent counselor, my goal will be to empathize and accept the client's views by researching the history and resulting social-cultural perspectives to understand him.

Another very important area of concern is the issue of "White racism." This topic is of concern not only because of the narrow-mindedness the concept exemplifies, but also because of the propensity for this phenomenon to occur among White counselors who work with a Native American client (Duran, Duran, & Brave Heart, 1998; Evans-Campbell, 2008). It will be critical for me to continuously remind myself and be aware of issue, and the need to take action not through denial or apathy, but to take action and responsibility for change. I will need to be respectful of our differences, and continuously check in with Frank to make sure he is comfortable with me, and our professional relationship.

Intervention Strategies

Overall Intervention Plan

Teaching resiliency in dealing with matters regarding living between two cultures, while honoring tradition, is a desired outcome in working with Frank (Gone & Alcantara, 2007; LaFromboise, Trimble, & Mohatt, 1990). In order to do this, I propose using a cultural perspective for understanding the client's story from his perspective (Castillo, 1997). I will use specific strategies such as narrative therapy (Denborough, 2014; Etchison & Kleist, 2000) to determine the core problems that Frank is experiencing, and where they are stemming from, in a manner that is respectful of indigenous culture (McAuliffe & Associates, 2012). I intend to recognize and reinforce strengths that Frank identifies with, both from the mainstream American culture, as well as Native American culture, and use these to help Frank to solidify and accept his strengths, and remind him of strategies he has used and were successful for him during previous challenging times (Ivey et al., 2008).

Specific Strategies

Since the first session could be challenging for a Euro-American counselor working with a Native American client it is important for me to be aware of basic issues that are important to Native Americans. For example, most indigenous people consider eye contact with an elder as a sign of disrespect (Chavez Cameron & Turtle-Song, 2003). If the client is younger, or very traditional, this could be a concern. Also, due to our cultural differences and our sociopolitical history, Frank may be hesitant about working with me as his counselor. I will pay special attention to nonverbal communication, since there is greater nonverbal, than verbal communication among Native Americans (Chavez Cameron & Turtle-Song, 2003; LaFromboise et al., 1990). I began the introductory session by asking Frank how comfortable he was in working with me, and to address any concerns he had about our cultural differences (Comstock et al., 2008; McAuliffe & Associates, 2012). I also encouraged him to discuss any concerns that emerge for him during counseling immediately, specially, given our sociopolitical history, and our cultural differences that misunderstandings may occur between us. This will reduce the chance of early termination (Ibrahim, personal communication, 2008). I reiterated that I appreciated him for coming to counseling, and trusting me. I told him I was honored by his trust, and reinforced to him for reaching out for assistance as an act of courage.

Asking Frank how comfortable he is with me, and acknowledging the differences between us was effective in helping him build trust. Frank took the opportunity to explore his concerns about my values, beliefs, socialization, and my approach to counseling and psychotherapy. I answered Frank's questions and concerns directly and openly. In cross-cultural encounters it is recommended that counselors focus on flexibility and have less rigid boundaries around sharing, especially about their beliefs, values, and assumptions as they pertain to faith, and spirituality as these may be of significant concern to clients, who may not be familiar with the culture of the counselor (Ibrahim, 2003). Frank was receptive and responded with appreciation to my "openness," and the therapeutic relationship began on a positive note.

Duran (2006) recommends that formal assessment with Native American clients should only be done after permission from the client is formally sought, and it is accepted. As a culturally competent counselor, I openly explained to Frank what each of the assessments were, and how I intended to use the information. I shared that it would help me to understand him, and to develop interventions that will be consistent with his values, beliefs, socialization, and his spirituality. I also asked Frank to provide his perspective on the assessment process and the results. Frank agreed to the proposed assessment tools and actively participated in the process. The following assessment tools were used: the Scale to Assess World View© (SAWV: Ibrahim & Kahn, 1984), Cultural Identity Check List-Revised© (CICL-R; Ibrahim, 2008) and the US Acculturation Index© (Ibrahim, 2007). He understood the reasoning for the use of the tools and said, "I guess if there are additional items to learn along the way we can figure those out as we go." These assessments are recommended with indigenous and nondominant cultural group members in counseling (Ibrahim, 2003).

My next step in working with Frank was to conduct my own research concerning family expectations, demographics of the Crow Creek Reservation, as well as tribal ceremonies and traditions. Understanding the context in which the client's life story takes place is an essential element of the multicultural counseling practice. As practitioners we must educate ourselves to a degree of knowledge about our client's culture. We must not solely rely on the client to educate us about that element of their personal experience (Chavez Cameron & Turtle-Song, 2003; LaFromboise et al., 1990; McAuliffe & Associates, 2012).

The Eight Questions posed by N.C. Ware and Arthur Kleinman (1992) proved to be an effective option and starting point for work with Frank. Using these questions in a culturally responsive manner would warrant revisions to traditional models of counseling would hope to bring a level of comfort for an indigenous client. I used the following questions, which are modeled after Kleinman:

1. What do you see and feel is the issue or problem?
2. What do you see and feel is unbalanced in your life?
3. Why do you think this unbalance is coming about?
4. What do you think causes this imbalance? What feeds it?
5. How severe is this imbalance?
6. What do you believe would help you to recover or heal? What do you hope for as a result of our work?
7. What do you think needs to heal? What are the main areas in your life affected by the imbalance?
8. What do you fear in regard to the imbalance?

To change the wording of these questions is important in order to respect the Native American belief that mental illness is an imbalance and especially given Frank's primary socialization (Chavez Cameron & Turtle-Song, 2003). Exploring the responses to the eight questions will assist me as the counselor in understanding what the central issues are for the client, and help the client assess the level of disequilibrium and its impact on his life, along with the solutions that he thinks would help (Castillo, 1997; Lonner & Ibrahim, 2008)

For Native Americans' the past, present, and future are fused together (Trimble & Gonzalez, 2008). This concept of time and it's relation to the depth of unresolved grief of loss of land, culture, languages, and foreign domination will more than likely be present for the majority of Native American clients throughout the counseling process (Duran, 2006). I will need to be mindful of this possibility and the resulting issues for Frank. In his 2006 work *Healing the Soul Wound*; Eduardo Duran reminds us that intergenerational trauma is called a "soul wound" by Native Americans. It is a concept that Duran believes may be the underlying variable in most American Indian mental health and social problems, since the trauma is unresolved for the Indian nation. The author goes on to explain that this unresolved trauma tends to increase over time and becomes more severe with each generation. Given this premise, within each session, this will need to be a ubiquitous concern for me to consider since it is a major issue in working with Native Americans. Specifically, Frank has not addressed this issue yet; however, I believe it will come up sometime during our work as he explores the plight of his people, and the challenges they have faced, and continue to face, and how exclusion and racism has affected his life.

If individual work towards building resiliency proved unsuccessful, group therapy may be another option for Frank. LaFromboise and Bigfoot (1988) found group work to be effective in working with Native American clients in order to relieve some of the burden of disclosure to an individual counselor; working in groups with culturally similar populations assists clients' to share because it provides a more comfortable setting, given the cultural commonality and validation from the other group members.

Evaluation of the Assessments and the Intervention

Overall Evaluation of the Assessments and the Interventions

Overall I consider the work with Frank a success. Frank did allow me into his life, and shared his struggles. He agreed to complete all of the assessments, and appreciated my willingness to honor and acknowledge our cultural differences. We continued our work through culturally consistent and sensitive methods of listening, empathy, and support, encouraging, active participation for both of us. All of which honored Frank's indigenous roots as well as his current occupational path, as an attorney in Denver.

Specific Strategies That Worked

Prior to beginning our work together, I had assessed that earning Frank's trust and his permission to enter into his life would be my first measure of success, since it would signify engagement (Chavez Cameron & Turtle-Song, 2003; McAuliffe & Associates, 2012). The initial step to enter into counseling may be the hardest step for the majority of Native American clients. As a counselor I helped Frank to feel comfortable with me, which then allowed me the space to earn his trust. Together we conquered the first and possibly most challenging hurdle (LaFromboise et al., 1990).

Another measure to evaluate the counseling process with Frank was to determine if questions 6, 7 and 8 (from Kleinman's list) were answered and/or addressed. Together, Frank and I were able to determine a few issues that would help him to heal, these included: (a) in order to heal, Frank suggested returning home to the Black Hills for a vacation. He had originally said a long weekend, but then determined he had enough vacation time to take a full week. We both agreed that if this helps him to feel grounded, this could be a positive step for him.

The desired outcome of this trip was my next concern. Is it purely relaxation and a getaway? This was certainly an acceptable and good motive for coping with the loss of his relationship (Bruce, Kim, Leaf, & Jacobs, 1990). Was this an opportunity to reconnect with friends and family? Was this a step towards returning to South Dakota permanently? I asked Frank to consider what he wanted out of the trip and how he wanted to feel when he returned to Denver. His answer was, "A little of all of it." He also shared that he wanted to return to Denver feeling refreshed, and to not dread returning to his home. I suggested that we begin our work with his second suggestion for healing—bringing closure to his relationship with Susan. We both agreed this might help in his recovery from loss, having addressed the closure of the relationship first; therefore allowing him to feel more relaxed during his trip home. The need for closure of his relationship with Susan arose when Frank said, "Things happened so fast, and we were both so angry—and I don't want to leave it like that." Our work included developing a plan to meet with Susan; when, where, and what outcome Frank wanted from this meeting. We role-played the interaction… giving Frank an opportunity to address best and worst case scenarios that may occur. I agreed with Frank's desire to heal. I believe a trip home would help him to reconnect with loved ones, as he feels fairly isolated right now. I also believe it may help Frank to bring closure to his relationship and breakup with Susan. Our continued work also brought out the depth and breadth of Frank's job dissatisfaction.

We will need to determine if he is truly unhappy with his current employer and wants to pursue employment elsewhere, or if he is unhappy with practicing law and may have other career interests. In summary, from our work together I hope to accomplish the following: (a) help Frank to gain closure on his relationship with Susan; (b) help Frank understand where his job dissatisfaction is coming from. This will help him in his current situation, and hopefully if he ever feels similar feelings in the future he will have the cognizance to handle that situation; (c) help Frank to determine where the imbalances are in his life, and how to recognize those feelings and work through them; (d) Frank and I both agreed that the current crisis in his life has made him not only sad, but also very angry; and this has led to acting inappropriately in certain situations. We planned to work together to determine what causes those feelings of intense anger, so we can try to determine what the unresolved issues are or him, either from the current situation, or from the past. We will also work to find alternative modes of coping for the intense anger he is experiencing. Frank said, "I don't like that feeling of anger—it is scary for me, so I'm sure it's scary to the person on the other end of it."

My fear for Frank is that the imbalance and anger that he is feeling could become deeper, therefore deepening his depression. I believe he may have been feeling this disparity for quite some time, but without recognition of the symptoms. I hope to help Frank find a meditative place, so he can stabilize the chaos he is experiencing in his life by discovering peace within himself. My hunch is that Frank is feeling quite torn between his two worlds and is unsure where he belongs. I hope that by working through these issues we will be able to resolve Frank's depression and anger and this should help him to see clearly the path he desires to follow.

Strategies That Failed

A strategy that failed was my hunch that Frank may want to participate in more of his tribe's spiritual practices, in order to try to reconnect, or to see if this was the missing element in his life. I asked Frank if when he returned home if there was a ceremony or some kind of spiritual practice in which he could participate. He looked surprised, and replied, "Why? This isn't about being an Indian—this is about me. I have to get some things figured out for myself before I can think about participating in anything else." He then followed up with, "Besides… if I was going to do something like that I would participate in my Mom's Sun Dance in August—and I'm not ready for that."

After this exchange, I realized that I might be pushing my agenda on Frank—rather than letting him lead. My imposition was making him defensive. I had assumed he may want to reconnect with his indigenous roots, but he had not necessarily communicated that to me. I apologized to Frank, and let him know that I realized I had made a mistake and would ask him what made the most sense to him in the future, rather than making a recommendation. From that point onwards, I was careful to ask Frank what *he* wanted rather than assuming he wanted to choose one path or another.

Summary

This case is a presentation of a Native American/Irish man living in a metro area. The client is seeking counseling due to the recent disintegration of his primary relationship, as well as job dissatisfaction. Upon evaluation, the client meets the criteria of a Major Depressive Episode.

The client presents with a worldview that was fairly consistent with indigenous beliefs, although, some elements of his worldview show evidence of acculturation to mainstream culture possibly derived from his Irish-American heritage. Other assessments used were the Cultural Identity Checklist-R© (Ibrahim, 2008), Scale to Assess Worldview© (Ibrahim & Kahn, 1984), and the Acculturation Index© (Ibrahim, 2007). Elements of a bicultural identity were evident from the results of each assessment.

Several strategies were used in order to work with the client in a culturally responsive and competent manner. These strategies were intended for use with bicultural clients, who primarily identifies as Native-American and secondarily as an Irish-American. All of the strategies were from a multicultural theoretical perspective. Specifics of each intervention were discussed, including the client's and the counselor's perspectives and the desired outcomes. Evaluation of the intervention was presented including successful and unsuccessful approaches and how the situation was resolved, when the intervention did not work.

Case 2: Counseling a Cross-Racial African American Adoptee

Kimberly Berkey

Introduction

Tara is an African American female enrolled in her second semester at a large university where approximately 30 % of students are from nondominant cultural groups. A German American family adopted her as an infant. She is the only child in her family. Tara grew up in an affluent community and was one of nine African Americans in her high school class of 300 students. The remainders of her classmates were from European origin. Tara is well adjusted, she relates well to others; she is outgoing, sociable, and makes friends easily. Tara was a model student and excelled in sports, and extracurricular activities. She was awarded an academic scholarship to a university that was her first choice, and she plans to pursue her undergraduate degree in Business. When asked how her friends would describe her, she answered that her friends would describe her as "a bit of a perfectionist."

Although Tara mentions that as a youth she was aware of her physical differences (in comparison to the majority of her nonadopted, European origin peers), she says that she was rarely confronted or emotionally affected by her difference from others within her immediate community. However, Tara later mentioned in the sessions that she has always felt a need to prove herself and be better than the "others." Tara defines this aspect of her personality as part of her "competitive spirit." Tara states that although she expressed some interest in finding out more about her biological parents when she was younger, she currently does not desire to meet her biological family. Tara explains that her adoptive parents are very loving and supportive of her academic, social, and athletic pursuits. Tara also states that while her adoptive parents were somewhat strict in her youth, she was the person who mainly pushed herself to achieve at the "highest level."

In the past year, Tara has made the adjustment from living with her family of European origin and attending high school in a community environment with limited cultural diversity to attending an out-of-state university with a significantly large diverse population. Tara is also noticing that with a new environment comes added privacy. Here, people do not automatically know she is adopted and assume her parents are of African American origin. However, Tara is also experiencing disconnect from her past interactions with others, i.e., how she viewed herself and how she believed others viewed her.

Though Tara has not had difficulty in making friends at college, she feels that it has been difficult to adjust and connect with her new circle of friends, which she perceives in a different light, than she sees herself. Tara states that she feels more

K. Berkey
BMGI International Consulting, Denver, CO, USA
e-mail: kimberlyberkey@gmail.com; kimberly.berkey@bmgi.com

comfortable with the circle of friends that are mainly White because they have similar upbringings and interests as the peers from her home community. However, she expresses that with this group, she is now very aware of her skin color, and how it separates her from becoming fully accepted as "one of them." Tara feels that this group views her differently than her friends from high school. Furthermore, though Tara expresses happiness at being invited and welcomed into another group that consists mainly of people who look more like her, and are from diverse backgrounds, she mentions her fear of being "found out" that her parents are not African American. Tara admits that she sometimes downplays the fact that she comes from an affluent family and does not mention that her nonbiological parents are White to fit in better with her new diverse friends. Tara expresses some feelings of guilt about what she has chosen not to share about herself with her new friends from both groups. Many of her diverse friends have come from lower social class, and are disadvantaged, and they have expressed disdain toward some of Tara's White friends. Sometimes Tara's White friends make negative comments about people from diverse backgrounds that cause Tara to become uncomfortable. Tara says that she thought she knew who she was, but is now beginning to feel lost, depressed, and caught in the middle of her two groups of friends and her two identities. She complains of feeling tired because she is constantly worrying about how she is perceived by the groups that she hangs out with. She states that she believes she acts differently with each group and is worried about being called fake. She is not sure how to go forward, and does not feel like she has control of her feelings and emotions related to her changing identities, and this issue, she feels has come to a head, and she needs resolution.

Tara decided to come to counseling after a faculty member noted the change in her. She had taken a class with this professor during her first semester in college, and now she was enrolled in another course in her class during her second semester. The professor discussed with Tara about her changed mood, she noted that Tara was distracted, and at times inappropriately emotional, this was significant, because she had noticed her upbeat personality in the first semester. She recommended that Tara speak with a counselor at the University Student Counseling Center to offer her assistance in adjusting to the new environment.

Client Information

Name: Tara B.
Age: 19
Cultural Background: African American female adopted by White (German American) family.
Presenting Problem: An adopted, female college student of African American origin, who was socialized in a White family from infancy onwards, is experiencing cultural identity issues.
Social/Educational Background: Affluent, upper-middle class family. Both parents have college degrees. Tara is currently in her second semester of school, and plans to pursue an undergraduate degree in Business.

Assessments

It is important for counselors to consider how the worldview of a clients' is shaped, i.e., beliefs, values, and assumptions that are important in understanding their cultural identity, race/ethnicity, gender, sexual orientation, acculturation, social class, environment, educational level, etc. (Ibrahim, 1999, 2003). Additionally, Ibrahim recommends that a cultural assessment needs to be conducted prior to setting goals, deciding on the counseling process, and implementing a counseling intervention. Tara grew up in an affluent, German American household. As a result, she currently holds many of the values and worldview of her adoptive White parents, such as family unity, support, loyalty, and a strong work ethic. However, though Tara is aware of the difference in skin color as it relates to her adoptive parents, neither she nor her parents may realize that racism in today's culture is subtle. Further, Tara seems to be in denial about emotions related to her identity. Tara is also not aware that she assumes the privilege that White Americans enjoy, now that she does not have her parents to shield her she is confused by the various viewpoints expressed by her friends at college.

In some ways Tara's upbringing separates her from her new African American and other diverse peers who grew up with different experiences, developed a cultural identity that recognized social hierarchies, oppressions, and had different socioeconomic status, which results in varying values, and worldviews. Furthermore, in her new, significantly larger and culturally diverse community setting, Tara is beginning to experience more overt oppressions and prejudice associated with being an African American woman, which she had not previously encountered on a consistent basis. Along with the process of trying to accept her adoption, Tara is presented with many conflicting cultural, socioeconomic, and sociopolitical conceptions of her identity, which she does not necessarily identify with.

Tara is confused, feels her identity is unraveling and she appears to be in a state of identity crisis; she identified several issues in her response to the questions on the CICL-R (Ibrahim, 2008), which indicated that she was not fully together. Since Tara does well academically and likes to explore material cognitively, I asked her to fill out several paper–pencil instruments in conducting the formal cultural assessments. I used the following instruments to help me understand how Tara sees herself, specifically The CICL-R (Ibrahim, 2008) to understand her cultural identity, USAI (Ibrahim, 2007) to find out about her acculturation to mainstream US values, and the Privilege/Oppression Continuum (Miami Family Therapy Institute, n.d.) to understand her privilege and oppressions. I reviewed the results of the cultural assessments and listened closely to Tara's narrative to identify her concerns, and the outcomes she was seeking; I used clinical judgment and conducted a review of the literature on counseling interventions specific to Tara's concerns, to develop a therapeutic intervention that was tailored to Tara's unique situation.

Cultural Identity Assessment

In reviewing her responses on the Cultural Identity Check List© (Ibrahim, 2008), it appears that Tara is caught between the cultural identity and traditions of her adoptive parents, and what she believes would be the cultural identity of her biological, African American parents. In her responses, she consistently wavers and often gives split answers because she is not certain of the "correct" answer. Three main issues are linked to the presenting problem from both Tara's and my perspective: (a) emerging inner conflicts related to cultural identity; (b) introduction to coping with racism and oppression as well as adoption; and (c) unrecognized & internalized self-hatred manifested in unhealthy perfectionism.

Worldview

After taking the "Scale to Assess Worldview" (Ibrahim & Kahn, 1984, 1987), Tara's primary Worldview is Optimistic, which indicates that she believes that human nature is basically good. She is balanced in her activity domain, as she values both inner (spiritual) and outer development (success as evaluated by external standards). She accepts the power of nature, desires to live in harmony with nature. When she cannot solve problems using her primary value system, she uses her secondary worldview, Here-and-Now (Spontaneous worldview), where Activity (Being-in Becoming, and Being) and time are valued, and more attention to present time than the past (Ibrahim & Owen, 1994).

Acculturation Level

After taking the *US Acculturation Index*© (USAI; Ibrahim, 2007), Tara discovered that her Acculturation Level is characterized by elements of both collectivism, and individualism. However, she takes the middle path, which is indicative of her generation (Marantz Henig, 2010). Since she was socialized in an affluent, White household, she shares many of the same values as her adoptive parents. She appears to be much more flexible, and is able to shift between interdependence and independence on many of the variables.

Other Relevant Assessments

Tara reviewed her response to the Privilege-Oppression continuum, she noted that she has been socialized in a privileged life style and she expects more from life, than the average person. Upon reflection, she expressed guilt that her life was more privileged, than many of her other diverse friends.

Counselor Biases

I am motivated to work with those of dissimilar backgrounds from me, partly because I am aware of the privilege I have enjoyed, and in a way, I want to help others access opportunities that may have been denied to them. However, I recognized that my privilege and pride/shame issues might at times negatively affect my counseling; both in how I counsel others, and how my clients may view me, since I do not fit within their cultural framework. Understanding my biases as well as researching my own cultural history, identity, worldview, and acculturation are imperative to my success as a counselor, and my client's experience. I realize that individual clients' beliefs, worldviews, etc., will vary from mine. However, confronting and recognizing all aspects of my cultural identity help me to hear the client accurately, without imposing my own perspectives on the client. It is important to acknowledge my strengths and my challenges, to help me in identifying my personal issues and pursue counseling to make an effort to close this gap as much as possible, to grow in my ability to be culturally competent and responsive, and to enhance my abilities to recognize issues of social oppression.

Intervention

Overall Intervention Plan

Tara is emotionally stable, although she is dealing with a transition, because she is having trouble accepting the identity that is being imposed upon her, to match her physical appearance. She has moments when she is confused, and upset, however, she is able to bring the issues to counseling. Considering her conflict and desire to come to terms with how she sees herself and how others define her, I decided to use Feminist Counseling and the Multicultural Identity Development Model (Harper & McFadden, 2003). Our therapy session is a partnership between equals, and our counseling relationship is egalitarian. Together we focus on education, with an emphasis on critical thinking because given Tara's socialization, this is the most productive, and efficient way to help her bring congruence to her identity (Corey, 2009, pp. 340–369). I use an approach to Feminist Therapy, with a relational-cultural emphasis (Miller & Stiver, 1997; Rosenberger, 2014) that recognizes the diversity among women, and the effect of the various contexts of women's lives. We work together to consider the social, cultural, and political context as contributing factors to her new emerging feelings, and try to understand the impact of society and culture in the environment where she lives. We additionally discussed understanding multiple oppressions, multicultural awareness, multicultural competence, and working towards acceptance of her multiple identities related to race, ethnicity, gender and socioeconomic class (Corey, 2009). I also chose Feminist Therapy because it focuses on the importance of intersectionality of identity and relationships. Additionally, we focused on strengths and reformulated her definition of psychological distress. In therapy, all types of oppression are recognized and Tara learned to understand that in the context of her sociocultural environments, social and political inequities have a negative effect on all people, including her. Other goals Tara worked on: (a) become aware of her gender-role socialization; (b) identification of negative internalized messages, and replace them with self-enhancing beliefs; (c) understand sexism and oppressive beliefs; (d) acquire social activism skills; (e) recognize the power of relationships and interconnectedness; and (f) trust in her own experiences and intuition.

Specific Strategies

Specific strategies I used with Tara included empowerment, and gender-role intervention. I provided insight on how social issues affect her, power analysis of how unequal access to power and resources influence personal realities, and assertiveness training. This was designed to help Tara become aware of interpersonal rights, transcend stereotypes, change negative beliefs, and implement change, as well as reframing and relabeling by shifting "blaming the victim" to an analysis of social/political factors. I also recommended group counseling as the next step in this work.

I believe bibliotherapy (with nonfiction books, autobiographies, self-help books, educational videos, films and novels), related to her biological parents and adoptive parents, cultural identity, adoption, racism and oppression, and other books with themes, messages related to her experience. Bibliotherapy helped encourage critical thinking and self-reflection and proved helpful for Tara's continued growth and personal development.

I also recommended that since Tara is such an excellent student, she might want to consider taking courses towards a minor related to diversity and social change, where she could have the opportunity to further research many of the newly developing questions about her identity. Additionally, membership in specific clubs or groups may help Tara's discovery and acceptance of her unique identity.

Evaluation of the Assessments and the Intervention

Tara responded very well to Feminist Therapy and bibliotherapy. Since her professor noticed the change in Tara's behavior at the beginning of the semester, related to her emotional stress, and referred her to counseling. Therapy served as a positive intervention, and helped her obtain more information about her questions. Her time in therapy mainly focused on discovery of new feelings, and emotions related to her current experience in college. Some time was spent discussing how to respond, and cope with both the positive, and negative experiences of her diverse identity in her new environment. We took time to explore her experiences with racism and how people treat her differently due to her skin color. We additionally explored how she both consciously and unconsciously internalized factors about her identity. At times, we borrowed from other theories and practiced the "empty chair" where she had conversations with the friends from each of the cultural groups (White and African American) to discuss how what they said affected her, and what she needed from them to feel accepted in the relationship.

Specific Strategies That Worked

Tara enjoyed bibliotherapy and actually was the most responsive to this form of therapy, specifically, in relation to critical thinking, reflection, and growth. However, with the mounting homework and assignments in school, she started to become stressed with taking time for therapy. We decided to slow down on some of the readings designated for her therapy homework, and focused more on short stories and articles. I additionally provided Tara with a list of books that ranged in topics related to various aspects of her developing identity that she could select and read at her leisure. This change alleviated some of her anxieties related to time management. The shorter readings allowed for reflection without consuming a majority her time outside her therapy sessions.

Strategies That Failed

Tara was not as receptive to opening up about her adoption and the emotions associated with her adoptive and biological parents. Discovering and feeling comfortable with discussing one's identity is a continuous process, and while Tara felt comfortable discussing certain issues, she was still very closed about others. Feminist Therapy was a positive starting point to help Tara build understanding and self-confidence, other strategies from different theories might be beneficial to further explore her emotions as it relates to adoption when she is ready to address this issue.

Summary

Tara was able to come to terms with her identity as a transracial adoptee with the help of bibliotherapy and a strong therapeutic relationship. Building a strong therapeutic relationship was facilitated due to an accurate identification of her cultural identity, as a visibly African American young woman, it would have been difficult to recognize that since she was socialized by her White adoptive parents, she would share a cultural identity, similar to theirs. Bibliotherapy was helpful, because she is bright college student who prefers to figure things out on her own, and it was not intrusive. Feminist therapy, especially at this stage of her life was empowering for her and helped her in finding her voice, and not being intimidated by her peers. As noted above, identity resolution and integration is a process that takes time, and over time, Tara, given her strengths will be able to accept all parts of her identity, and voice her perspectives, without fear of being judged.

Case 3: Counseling a Bicultural Native American Client

Jennifer Anne Blair

Client Information

Name: John A. Silversmith
Age: 20
Cultural background: American Indian (Navajo)

Presenting Problem

John presents with symptoms of depression, anxiety, and possible alcohol abuse. He states, "I have not been sleeping well, my future seems hopeless, I have no appetite, nothing seems fun anymore, I experience difficulty concentrating, and I feel really tense most of the time." John adds that he "feels gloomy" and no longer enjoys his work. Additionally, John states that he has lost interest in his usual pastimes. "I seem to have very little energy and sometimes people tell me that I am speaking somewhat slowly." John states, "I had started to notice that something was missing from my life about 9 months ago. When my brother got promoted to senior partner at his architectural firm; I started to wonder what I was doing with my life." Shortly after his brother's promotion, he indicated that he began experiencing difficulty falling asleep and staying asleep. "I often wake up 2–3 times during the night." John reports that he has little appetite and has lost almost 15 lb in the previous 6-week period. He adds that he finds his work boring and feels somewhat isolated at his place of work, because he is the only employee of American Indian heritage. He goes on to state that he feels trapped in his job, and his future seems hopeless, all of this leads to irritability and feelings of worthlessness. John indicates that these issues have created difficulties in functioning both socially and professionally. John states "I used to get off of work and go to the gym, or play some basketball with my friends. Now when I get home I sit in front of the television, and have a few beers. I dread going into work each day, and my manager tells me that my productivity has dropped noticeably in recent months. Sometimes just thinking about going to work makes me feel very tense. When I am at work I have a hard time concentrating." John adds, "When I have trouble sleeping I will start to think about my future and my heart will begin to beat rapidly, I become short of breath, and feel sick to my stomach. Sometimes it gets so bad that I get chest pains, and feel like I might be having a heart attack." On a 1–10 scale, John rates the difficulties he experiences are at an 8.

J.A. Blair
Jennifer Blair Counseling, Denver, CO, USA

University of Colorado Denver, Denver, CO, USA
e-mail: Jennifer.blair.counseling@msn.com; estrojenn@msn.com

Social/Educational Background

Childhood and Adolescence

John A. Silversmith was born and raised in Lakewood Colorado by his birth parents, Robert Silversmith (age 49), and Dana Silversmith (age 44). John's father, Robert, is employed by the city of Lakewood as the Assistant Director of Social Services. John's mother, Dana, is a teacher at a local elementary school. John's father is of the Azee'tsoh Dine'é clan, which translated into English means, Big Medicine People. His mother is of the Ats'osi Dine'é clan, which translated into English means, The Feather People (Lapahie, 2001). Consistent with Navajo tradition, John is considered a member of his mother's clan, the Ats'osi Dine'é (Lapahie, 2001). John has two siblings, one sister and one brother. His brother, Thomas Silversmith (age 24) is married, and lives in Albuquerque, New Mexico, he is employed with a large architectural firm. John's sister, Mary Lomack (age 26), is married, and employed as the director of a day care center, and resides in Casper, Wyoming. John, along with all members of his family, was schooled in both Catholicism and traditional Navajo spiritualities.

While growing up John would typically spend much of the summer on the reservation in northeast New Mexico with his grandparents, cousins, and numerous aunts and uncles. Although raised predominantly in a White suburb, he speaks fluent Athapaskan, the native language of the Navajo Nation (Winson, 2002). Additionally, by virtue of spending every summer on the reservation for the past 20 years, he is well versed in the beliefs, traditions, values, and spirituality of the Navajo people (as are his parents and siblings). Throughout his life he has successfully retained the culture of the Navajo people while thriving in the world of the dominant White culture of the suburbs.

John graduated from Lakewood Central High School in 2005. He performed well academically graduating with a 3.85 grade point average. John graduated with honors and was in the 90th percentile amongst his classmates. While in high school, he was active in numerous campus activities and sports. Additionally, he maintained several meaningful interpersonal relationships.

Psychosocial History, Life as an Adult

Subsequent to graduating from high school, John spent the summer on the reservation with his relatives, while struggling with what he should do with his life. Upon returning to Lakewood that fall, he was still undecided about going to college, or start work. He chose to find a job until he was able to make a definitive decision regarding his future. Lacking a college education, the only job he could find was as a telemarketer. Although John had an excellent academic record he was unable to get a better paying job. He continues to live with his parents and pays them rent, as well as contributing to household chores. Although he enjoys numerous sports, and goes dancing with his friends on weekends, in the previous 1-year period he has lost interest in most of those activities. John spends most of his leisure time in seclusion now, playing video games, watching television, and "having a few beers." He infrequently socializes with a few close friends. John indicates that he is dissatisfied with his current employment and is exploring alternative opportunities including going back to school. He notes that he enjoyed being in school as a teenager, but has serious doubts about his ability to succeed in college.

Assessments

As recommended by several culturally responsive experts, prior to a counseling intervention, cultural assessment must be conducted to evaluate the client's cultural orientation (APA, 2013; Lonner & Ibrahim, 2008). Given that this case would be a cross-cultural encounter, the client was encouraged to participate in the assessment process to assist the counselor in understanding his acculturation level, cultural identity, worldview (beliefs, values, and assumptions). The client agreed to participate in the cultural assessments.

Worldview

Although cognizant of the ongoing atrocities perpetrated upon American Indians John also acknowledges the strength and resilience engendered in his people by virtue of surviving (Chavez Cameron & Turtle-Song, 2003.) In contrast to the symptoms he is currently experiencing, his overall worldview is predominantly "Optimistic" (Ibrahim & Owen, 1994; Ibrahim, Roysircar-Sodowsky, & Ohnishi, 2001).

> This worldview is characterized by values in three areas: Human Nature, Activity Orientation, and Relationship with Nature. There is a belief that human nature is essentially good, that human activity must focus on inner and outer development (i.e., spiritual and material), and that there is a need to be in harmony with nature with an acceptance of the power of nature. (Ibrahim et al., 2001, p. 430)

Cultural Identity Assessment

The second instrument administered was the Cultural Identity Check List-Revised© (CICL-R, Ibrahim, 1990, 2008). This is an 18 item, self-report, qualitative questionnaire, designed to understand the client's psychosocial identity within the context of his or her cultural and historical background. The following salient data were gleaned from this instrument. John, his immediate family, and extended family, are all 100 % Navajo. Although brought up in a typical American suburb, he was also brought up in a Native cultural context and identifies most strongly with his tribal roots. John is fluent in both Athapaskan (Native Navajo language (Winson, 2002)), and English. He can speak, write, and read in both languages. His summers are spent on the reservation with members of his extended family. This has further served to solidify his bonds with his native culture, traditions, beliefs, and values. It was through these extended stays that he was able to learn of his cultural history. Through stories, song, dance, and rituals, he learned of the struggles, the genocides, traditional Navajo spiritualities, and healing ceremonies (Boxer, 2009; Chavez Cameron & Turtle-Song, 2003). He understands the significance of the resiliency of his native culture. John has successfully integrated the beliefs of these two disparate cultures without compromising his connection with either.

His dual spiritual beliefs, with a primary emphasis on traditional Navajo spirituality should prove to be a therapeutic strength, as he has two sources of support (Catholicism and Navajo spirituality); both are positive influences on his worldview. John's social class is also an asset since it provided access to most of the resources afforded to the dominant culture. Although he self-identifies as heterosexual male he is open-minded regarding sexual and gender identity as embraced by Navajo values and beliefs (Sutton & Broken Nose, 2005). John's openness is conducive to his neutrality regarding gender roles. He is accepting of both the traditional patriarchal hierarchy of the White dominant culture and of the "matriarchal structure seen among the Navajo, where women govern the family…" (Sue & Sue, 2003, p. 313).

Information gleaned from this questionnaire, along with other data, proved to be invaluable in structuring the framework of a treatment plan for John. As recommended in the literature the therapist began to conceptualize a treatment plan which would "integrate Western and indigenous healing techniques in order to address the multidimensional mental health needs of Native American peoples" and to be responsive to his bicultural identity (Chavez Cameron & Turtle-Song, 2003, p. 75).

Acculturation Index

As a precursor to starting a counseling intervention, the therapist wanted to first "have an authentic understanding" of her own acculturation level (Chavez Cameron & Turtle-Song, 2003, p. 76). Thus, she evaluated her own level of acculturation and administered the United States Acculturation Index© to herself (Ibrahim, 2007). The following day she met with the client for the first time and administered the same instrument to the client. The therapist then compared her results with the client's results to establish a baseline of their similarities and differences. This comparison revealed that although similar in most areas there were important differences. John's score was very high in the area of "Community Focus" whereas the therapist's score was midway between "Community Focus" and "Individual Focus." The client highly endorsed being "Interdependent" vs. the therapist who endorsed "Independence." John strongly endorsed being "Highly family and kin oriented" whereas the therapist endorsed "Taking care of self." Lastly, the client scored very high on "Age is revered" vs. the therapist endorsed "Youth is revered." This comparison provided a valuable template highlighting both cultural differences, and similarities. This in turn served as a basis for establishing a relationship by using the similarities as strengths that will help build a positive therapeutic relationship while remaining vigilant regarding areas of dissimilarity, as these can lead to disengagement and ultimately termination of counseling (Ibrahim, 1991, 2003).

Trauma History

John denies any history of physical trauma, direct psychological trauma, or sexual abuse, either as a child or as an adult. It is noteworthy however, that he may suffer effects of intergenerational trauma, as an artifact of the historical genocides, and ongoing atrocities, and abuse perpetrated upon the Navajo Nation by the dominant culture (Ibrahim & Ohnishi, 2001; Keoke & Porterfield, 2003; Navajo World, n.d.; Boxer, 2009).

Center for Epidemiological Studies—Depression Assessment

Data gathered from the intake, in addition to all of the abovementioned assessments, strongly supported a diagnosis of a mood disorder. Thus, the Center for Epidemiological Studies—Depression (CES-D; Radloff, 1977) was administered. The client scored 36 out of a possible 60 points. Scoring protocols for this instrument suggest the diagnosis of Major Depressive Disorder (MDD) (APA, 2013, pp. 160–168). It should be noted that this instrument has strong reliability, and validity, and is available on the internet.

Clinical Interview

Data collected during the clinical interview served to interweave and support hypotheses developed from information gathered to this point. During the assessment, and consistent with the recommendations in the psychological literature, the therapist was vigilant in employing active listening skills (McGoldrick, Giordano, & Garcia Preto, 2005). Current areas of emotional distress were identified and explored using free association. Case conceptualization was based on data gathered during the interview, and was validated with empirical data. Additionally, self-report of symptoms justified the use of a mood chart (www.TherapistAid.com© (2012–2014)), to confirm or deny the presence of depression. It is noteworthy that the clinical interview served to firmly establish the trust, and collaboration endemic to a strong therapeutic alliance, while constructing a contextual framework by which to diagnose and treat John's presenting problem.

Behavioral Observations

John presented for the interview comfortably and appropriately attired in blue jeans, sport shirt, and athletic shoes. He is of medium build and height. His voice inflection was normal with appropriate timing, tone, volume, and pressure. His posture suggests that he was both attentive yet comfortable. John presents as being lucid, cognizant, and well oriented to person, place, time, and date. A full mental status exam was deemed unnecessary at this time.

Risk Assessment

John was screened for symptoms of suicidality. John admits to having occasional thoughts of suicide, with the last episode occurring approximately 4 months ago. Further investigation revealed mild suicide ideation, with no specific suicide plan, no actual intent, and no chosen method(s). When asked if I, "should have any concerns regarding his personal safety and well-being at this time" he responded "no." His response was made with good eye contact, and conviction in his voice. John was very clear in stating that he has no intention of committing suicide, or possible self-harm, as it would be against his spiritual beliefs and would bring shame to his family. John provided insufficient reasons to believe he is at imminent risk of self-harm or harm to another at this time.

DSM-5 Diagnosis

It is my clinical impression that John suffers from MDD, and generalized anxiety disorder (GAD) (APA, 2013). Regarding MDD, the information gathered suggests that John meets, and exceeds the criteria for this disorder. Of the possible nine symptoms five are required for this diagnosis. Information provided by the client indicates that he endorses seven items out of the nine thereby meeting and exceeding the criteria for this diagnosis. Regarding the diagnosis of GAD, there are six possible symptoms three of which are required for diagnosis. John endorses five of the necessary criteria, and thus meets the criteria for this diagnosis (APA, 2013): Major Depressive Disorder, Recurrent, Moderate (296.22). Generalized Anxiety Disorder (300.22).

Rule Outs (Differential Diagnoses): It is posited, by virtue of psychological and physical trauma experienced by his extended family, and other members of the Navajo Nation, that John may experience subclinical symptoms of intergenerational Posttraumatic Stress Disorder, i.e., 309.81 (Ibrahim & Ohnishi, 2001). Additionally, many of the symptoms that he experiences mimic the criteria for Adjustment Disorder, With Mixed Anxiety and Depressed mood (309.28). Lastly, although John admits to using alcohol 4 days a week (on average), and consuming 2–3 beverages per episode, he fails to meet the necessary criteria for a diagnosis of an Alcohol Use Disorder.

Counselor Biases

Positive biases: In working with John, I learned that there are more similarities between the American Indian population, and myself than I had previously envisioned. Additionally, I have learned that my spiritual beliefs (which are highly eclectic) are, generally speaking, compatible with those of American Indians. In sum, I have come to recognize that I have a great affinity for the American Indian people and their culture. In the future, should I have the privilege of working with persons from this population, I will approach my work with a new appreciation of soul wounds (Duran, 2006).

Negative biases: First, prior to studying multicultural counseling, the sum total of my knowledge of the American Indian Population was limited to stereotypes perpetrated by the media. I was oblivious to the systematic ongoing genocide, and marginalization that the dominant White culture had perpetrated upon the American Indian population. I am now embarrassed to state that my vision of American Indian people was that they had little ambition, were content to panhandle, and consume copious quantities of alcohol. Had it not been for my thorough investigations of this population, and my coursework in multicultural counseling, these biases may have remained; possibly would have had a negative influence upon my clinical work.

Client Goals

John has entered therapy at this time in hopes of ameliorating his symptoms of depression and anxiety. Additionally, he seeks to have a better understanding of himself, while exploring the prospects for a line of work that might be more satisfying, and rewarding to him. Lastly, he indicates that it is important for him to achieve these goals without compromising the beliefs, and traditions of his cultural heritage; given the cultural assessment he is bicultural. Therapeutically, John's bicultural identity is culturally consistent with the literature which acknowledges that, "It would be unrealistic for Native Americans to relinquish the positive aspects of western culture, just as it would be ridiculous to expect a total return to traditional/indigenous healing" (Chavez Cameron & Turtle-Song, 2003, p. 75).

Intervention

Overall Intervention Plan

Examination of the client's psychosocial background, cultural contexts, qualitative assessments, and quantitative assessments, suggest two primary areas of clinical focus, and two secondary areas. The two primary areas are the client's MDD and GAD. It is noteworthy that the literature suggests that Mood Disorders, including MDD are often comorbid with Anxiety Disorders (APA, 2013). Secondary areas of clinical focus include an action plan to address John's ambiguity regarding his future, addressing intergenerational trauma, and his subclinical, but potentially harmful use of alcohol. It is hypothesized that all of these areas of clinical concern are inextricably intertwined and therapeutic success in any given area may have a significant and positive effect on the remaining issues. It is further hypothesized that the dissonance John is experiencing, because of his indecisiveness regarding his future, may be at the epicenter of the remainder of his presenting problems. Lastly, it is hypothesized that the primary areas of clinical focus should be addressed first as they may be impinging on his ability to successfully address the secondary issues. All interventions were designed to reflect therapeutic strengths found within his cultural heritage (Chavez Cameron & Turtle-Song, 2003).

Theoretical frameworks to be utilized in addressing John's presenting problems will include Cognitive Therapy (Beck, 1995), Behavioral Therapy, and Problem Solving Skills (Goldfried & Davison, 1994), Liberation Therapy (Duran, Firehammer, & Gonzalez, 2008), and Motivational Interviewing (Miller & Rollnick, 2002). Thus, the overall treatment plan is both cognitive and behavioral in nature. As the literature suggests, it is of paramount importance that the clinician is able to make minor modifications in the process, and application, of these interventions within the scope of the client's racial, cultural, and ethnic background (Goldfried & Davison, 1994). Lastly, it is recommended that traditional Navajo interventions, administered by a Navajo healer, be incorporated into the treatment plan (Chavez Cameron & Turtle-Song, 2003).

Specific Strategies

Major Depressive Disorder

The primary intervention strategy chosen for MDD was Cognitive Therapy. Cognitive therapy (also known as cognitive behavioral therapy [CBT]), works on the assumption that depression may be the result of irrational or dysfunctional cognitive processes (Beck, 1995). John's belief that "he doubts as to whether or not he could succeed at college" is inconsistent with his academic performance in high school. It is hypothesized that the source of John's depression may be a result of dysfunctional thoughts. The therapist chose this theoretical orientation based on a variety of criteria. First, it qualifies as an evidence-based intervention strategy. In her seminal book, *Cognitive Behavioral Therapy and Beyond*, Judith Beck notes that cognitive therapy is "one of the very few systems of psychotherapy that have been empirically validated" (Beck, Preface, xi). Mood charting, which is an integral part of CBT provides support for the efficacy of the intervention while directly involving the client as an active participant in her/his/zir own healing process. Second, the intervention obviates the need for psychopharmacological interventions and their associated side effects. Although, Seligman, Walker, and Rosenham (2001) state, "meta-analysis shows no difference [in outcome] between CBT and antidepressant medication" (pp. 282–283). Perhaps most importantly, the literature suggests that CBT is consistent with the values, beliefs, traditions, and therapeutic preferences of the American Indian population (Renfrey, 1992).

Generalized Anxiety Disorder

The primary intervention in addressing John's symptoms in this area is based on a theoretical orientation grounded in Behavioral Therapy, more specifically Relaxation Training (Goldfried & Davison, 1994). Much of the distress John is experiencing is manifested as physiological symptoms. Relaxation training provides the client with concrete skills which, when employed, often have immediate effect in relieving the symptoms of distress. The primary intervention involves training the client in the use of diaphragmatic breathing techniques (deep breathing), and progressive muscle relaxation. As with CBT, the data strongly supports this intervention is evidence-based. "Data are plentiful demonstrating that relaxing one's muscles does markedly reduce anxiety" (Goldfried & Davison, 1994, p. 82).

Career Change

Although, as a stated therapeutic goal, John indicates that he would like to explore the possibilities of a better career, he is also considering ongoing education in the form of college. John seems torn between these two disparate options. Unable to arrive at a favorable conclusion he became *stuck*. A two-stage approach was initiated in resolving this dilemma. The first intervention, Problem Solving (Goldfried & Davison, 1994), is designed to facilitate the decision making process. The second intervention, Motivational Interviewing (Miller & Rollnick, 2002), is designed to evoke proactive behavior in initiating the desired change. Problems Solving as an intervention is defined by Goldfried and Davison (p. 187) as "a behavioral process, whether overt or cognitive, which (1) provides a variety of potentially effective responses to the problem situation, and (2) increases the likelihood of selecting the most effective response from among these various alternatives." Although there are numerous variations on the protocols of problem solving as a theoretical orientation meta-analysis reveals a set of recurring themes. "The following five stages represent a consensus view: (1) general orientation, (2) problem definition and formulation, (3) generation of alternatives, (4) decision making, and (5) verification" (Goldfried & Davison, 1994, p. 187). Motivational Interviewing, which is used to initiate change, may be employed in addressing John's alcohol use. Ultimately, there may be merit in referring John to a professional career counselor to assist in his quest for a more fulfilling source of employment.

Trauma

Liberation Psychology (Duran et al., 2008) provides a cultural template for therapeutic work with oppressed and colonized people (Tate, Rivera, Brown, & Skaistis, 2013). It can be integrated with a variety of psychological and indigenous interventions. According to Duran et al. (2008), clinicians who utilize traditional western interventions, in a culturally insensitive manner, are inflicting "soul wounds"

(p. 289) on a cultural being, given that Native Americans have already suffered generations of genocide, and concomitant psychological trauma. It is suggested that by re-conceptualizing psychopathologies as soul wounds, and treatment as soul healing, therapists are able to reframe their work as one of healing the spirit, often using metaphors from Native culture. Using interventions viewed through this lens a therapist is more favorably positioned to work with persons with indigenous beliefs, and oppressed culture more successfully. In this instance, the authors specifically suggest this modality as appropriate for the American Indian population (Duran et al., 2008). Thus, Liberation Psychology is incorporated into the present treatment plan as an underlying guiding principle. All interventions were conducted within the framework of Liberation Psychology.

Alcohol Use

Motivational Interviewing is a systematic method of initiating change in which the therapist indirectly elicits motivation for change through a series of both open-ended and closed-ended questions (Miller & Rollnick, 2002). Although no specific data were available regarding the application of this intervention across cultures, Miller and Rollnick suggest that if administered within the context of the client's primary culture, the intervention is applicable to persons from a wide variety of racial, cultural, and ethnic backgrounds. Since John is bicultural, and well acculturated to both the dominant White culture, and his own Navajo culture, there is little reason to doubt the efficacy of this intervention considering John's cultural background.

Adjunct Interventions

The therapist, although well versed in multicultural counseling, wisely choose to seek consultation regarding her proposed treatment plan. Specifically she sought feedback from her colleagues regarding the possibility of recruiting the services of a traditional Navajo healer as part of John's treatment plan. Her colleagues confirmed the merits of this plan. With John's permission a Navajo Medicine Person, from John's family reservation, was contacted and he agreed to see John professionally during the upcoming Christmas Holiday. John had already planned on spending the holiday with his immediate, and extended family on the reservation.

Evaluation of the Assessments and Interventions

The battery of cultural and psychological assessments that were administered proved to be invaluable to the clinician. Cultural differences and similarities were identified and ultimately served to inform the entire treatment plan. The CICL-R©

(Ibrahim, 2008) in particular was beneficial in that it provided a conceptualization of the client's sociocultural, and historical context, and background. Facts gleaned from this tool were the cornerstone of the therapeutic intervention. The time spent on clarifying the client's cultural identity also solidified the therapeutic relationship. Quantitative instruments such, as the CES-D (Radloff, 1977) served to solidify hypotheses into concrete diagnoses.

Prior to Christmas break the therapist was able to initiate CBT intervention strategies (Beck, 1995), and Behavioral interventions in the form of Relaxation Skill Training (Goldfried & Davison, 1994). As was evidenced by John's Mood Chart, his symptoms of depression showed a steady and significant improvement. Assessment of his progress was confirmed by re-administration of the CES-D (Radloff, 1977), which yielded a score of eight. This score places John in the "depression free" category. It was concluded that this intervention was successful.

The behavioral intervention, using relaxation, was also successful as John reports using the skills daily, with documented results and improvement in functioning. The efficacy of the intervention was confirmed using the Mood Chart. John's scores on the anxiety section of the Mood Chart went from a range of 2–3 to a consistent 1 (the lowest possible score) over a period of 5–6 weeks.

Although the therapist had begun to integrate problem solving and Motivational Interviewing into her work with John, little progress was being made. John remained *stuck* in his decision making regarding a career change and/or college. It was at this time that John visited his reservation over Christmas, and had several meetings with his tribe's healer, Sam Yazzie. It was during one of those visits that Mr. Yazzie told John the metaphorical story of the Coyote and the Giant (Navajo World, n.d.). When John asked the meaning of the story, Mr. Yazzie declined to explain and instructed John to "listen to his heart" to find the meaning. Upon returning to Lakewood, John shared the story and his interpretation with his therapist. John believed the story spoke to him of the futility of his internal struggles. He stated that he "now knew that his soul wound was merely a result of not listening to his heart." In listening to his heart, his soul had called him to embark on a journey. Intrigued, the therapist inquired as to what his journey was to be. John replied,

> Ms. Doe, both you and Mr. Yazzie have done me a great service and healed my soul wound. My heart has told me to follow in the footsteps of those who healed me. I have decided to go back to college to study to be a therapist. After that I will study traditional healing methods of the Navajo people. It is my goal to then move back to the reservation and help others as I have been helped.

Having successfully resolved the ambivalence regarding his future, John stopped using alcohol, and had no additional episodes of either depression, or anxiety. John had reconnected with his cultural background in a way that he could have never anticipated. No additional services were required.

Summary

Initially six interventions were proposed in the treatment plan. In conclusion, CBT, Relaxation Skills, and involving an indigenous healer had been successful. Regarding Problem Solving and Motivational Interviewing little progress was made. This was attributed to these interventions being misapplied from a cultural contextual perspective. Ultimately, these and the remaining interventions became obviated, subsequent to referring John to Mr. Yazzie.

Case 4: Counseling a Colombian Immigrant Client

Carlo A. Caballero

Client Information

Name: Juan Hernandez
Age: 26

Cultural Background

Juan was born in Colombia but moved to the United States when he was 13, with his father, and brother. He identifies as Colombian since he was born there and both his parents are Colombian.

Presenting Problem

Juan presented to counseling after being involved in a car accident that killed two people. Juan felt responsible for this accident, and became extremely depressed because of his feelings of guilt and eventually he had to be admitted to a hospital for a 72 h-hold. During the 72 h-hold, Juan was seen by a therapist to get a better understanding of his situation. The therapist was able to obtain a lot of information about Juan's current life situation, and history. Juan informed the therapist that he moved to New Jersey from Colombia when he was 13 years old with his father and brother.

C.A. Caballero
University of Colorado Denver, Denver, CO, USA
e-mail: carlo.caballero@ucdenver.edu

He also noted that he has not seen his mother since he left Colombia. Also, Juan mentioned that his father was an alcoholic, and would physically abuse him, and his brother when he was drunk. This went on until Juan turned 18 and he moved to Florida, with his brother and close friend.

Juan currently lives in Florida with his brother and friend, but he has no other significant relationships. Juan also is currently unemployed because he used to be a truck driver, but since the accident he has been laid off, and is currently living on disability, since he was injured in the accident, which occurred while he was on the job.

Juan stated that he feels he has no valuable skills that will help him find a good job again, and it has stressed him out, because he does not know how he will pay rent. Juan reported that most of the time when he is at home he lies in bed, and cries quite often because he stated "I do not feel happy with my life." Even though he lies in bed all day, he has a trouble sleeping because he stated that all he thinks about is "those people I killed." Juan reported that he finds no pleasure in most of the things that used to give him pleasure, and he has no energy most of the time. After he found out that two people died in the accident, he felt a lot of guilt and he realized that he did not want to live anymore because he felt like a murderer. His brother advised him to go to counseling, and he finally decided to pursue counseling and came to see me. During the initial visit he spoke about his "wish to be die" so I decided to conduct a suicide risk assessment. After discussing with other colleagues and further evaluation I decided it would be best to hospitalize him and put him on a 72 h-hold. After he was stable, he was referred back to me to continue counseling.

Social/Educational Background

Juan completed high school when he was in New Jersey but did not continue his education after he graduated from high school. He shows some desire to go to college to obtain more knowledge and skills to acquire a meaningful career. Juan stated besides his brother, and friend, he has no other social network. He seems to be lacking a strong support network and doesn't seem to have many friends or family that can support him through this process. He has lost contact with his immediate and extended family, and has not established any romantic relationships, and he identifies as a single heterosexual male.

Assessments

Cultural Identity Assessment

The results from Ibrahim's (2008) *Cultural Identity Check List-Revised*© showed that Juan's culture derives mostly from his country of origin, i.e., Colombia. Even though he arrived to the United States when he was 13, his values and beliefs still derive from his Colombian background. In the checklist there were many questions that focused on Juan's culture, and how it relates to his identity. Juan described one of his most salient features of his identity was the fact that he is a Colombian male, and I think that it describes his cultural orientation, because in Latin cultures being male comes with a lot of privilege, and authority (Rojano & Duncan-Rojano, 2005). It seems that Juan knows the privilege that come with being male in US society, and that is why he considers it to be an important aspect of his identity. Also, he mentioned how his family was received with prejudice and exclusion, because of their Colombian background, and it shows that he has resilience to deal with oppression, which is one of his strengths. This checklist helped better understand Juan's cultural identity, which is important for me in working with him as a client.

Worldview

Juan's worldview reflects his Colombian culture, and his acculturation to the US. Juan's beliefs, values and assumptions make up a big part of his identity, and it affects how he views the world especially in this society. I used Ibrahim & Kahn's *Scale to Assess Worldview*© (SAWV, 1984) to assess Juan's worldview. After scoring Juan's responses, it is obvious that a significant part of his worldview derives from his Colombian culture. It also reflects some traumatic events that occurred during his childhood. Living in the United States also influenced Juan's worldview, mostly because of his minority status here in this country.

According to the results of the SAWV, Juan's primary worldview is best characterized by worldview IV, i.e., the Pessimistic or realistic worldview. This worldview has values from three cultural orientation domains, i.e., Human Nature, Social Relationships and Nature" (Ibrahim & Owen, 1994). People who hold this worldview usually see human nature as primarily bad, and allow that there may be some good qualities mixed with the bad (Ibrahim & Owen). People who adopt this worldview know that they are living in an unjust world, and if they were treated as equals, then they would be able to accomplish their goals. Most people from nondominant cultures hold this worldview, usually as a secondary worldview, because they are dealing with oppression on a daily basis, and they know they will not be treated as equals (Ibrahim et al., 2001). Since Juan's cultural identity mostly derives from his Colombian culture, and most of his beliefs come from his culture of origin, he appears to perceive a significant amount of the injustice.

Juan's secondary worldview is Traditional World View, or World View II. This worldview focuses on Social relationships, Time, and Nature. Social relationships are considered primarily lineal-hierarchical here (top down), with some expectations for collateral-mutual relationships (if you give me respect, then I will give you respect). Time is mostly future oriented, with some emphasis on the past. Regarding Nature, there is a belief that it can be controlled.

This is a Calvinistic point of view; it comes from patriarchal power relationships, and is focused on social control, and a very strong future time orientation (McKim, 2001). The perspective is found in highly traditional societies, where for the good of the social order controlling everyone in the social system is valued. There is also a belief that nature can be controlled (Ibrahim, personal communication, 2014).

Juan's primary and secondary worldviews definitely coincides with Juan's cultural values, beliefs, and assumptions. Further, due to the fact that he has experiences of oppression as an immigrant, as well as trauma and physical abuse form his alcoholic father, it has made him more of a pessimist.

Other Assessments

I implemented the "Cultural Formulation Interview" (CFI; APA, 2013) with Juan because the "CFI follows a person-centered approach to cultural assessment by eliciting information from the individual about his or her own views" (APA, p. 751). Also, the CFI is "designed to avoid stereotyping, in that each individual's cultural knowledge reflects how he, or she interprets the illness experience, and guides how he or she seeks help" (APA, p. 751). The CFI allowed me to view Juan's mental illness from his own cultural perspective, and to see how he interpreted his own problems, and what he believes will improve his situation.

During the assessment Juan explained that he knows that is dealing with a lot of stress and guilt, and he was also quite lonely. He stated that he missed his family from Colombia, and it was difficult for him to not be around his mother, and other family members. Also, he feels it is very difficult for him to get a job, especially because he does not want to be a truck driver anymore, because it reminds him of the accident. He reports that he has no other skills besides truck driving, so it is difficult for him to find something worthwhile, especially because he is an immigrant and a person of color, and people judge him negatively. He also stated that his guilt at "killing" those people has been overwhelming for him, and has made him unable to function, and all he wants to do is sleep, and forget what happened. We then moved the focus on strengths and support, and he told me that he was very spiritual, but he lost that along the way, but would like to regain it. He told me he had no supports except for his brother, and friend, but since he was able to overcome past problems by himself, he doesn't like to depend on others. He stated that he wants to build stronger relationships with others, and also reconnect with his family. Also, he noted that he must to focus on getting better and moving past his guilt so he can function again, and then maybe he will apply to a community college, and move toward getting higher education to get a better job in the future.

It seems that Juan has a good understanding of what his issues are, and also how he can fix them. Juan seems to have plenty of strengths such as, desire to regain his spirituality, resilience, and ability to adapt. These strengths will be useful for Juan to overcome some of his issues with guilt, which seemed to be causing the depression. Helping Juan regain his sense of spirituality will be helpful for him, especially, to move past the guilt, and move towards healing. Also, he knows how important it is for him to obtain a meaningful career path, to help him in accomplishing his goals, which would eventually help in improving his mood. It is positive that Juan knows how he is going to be able to overcome his problems because counseling can help facilitate, and guide him to overcome this current situation. This cultural formulation helped me in understanding Juan's problems, from his perspective, and what we can do together to get him to the place he needs to be in his life.

DSM-5 Diagnosis

296.22 MDD, Single episode, Moderate with melancholic features (APA, 2013)

This is the diagnosis that Juan and I agreed on. I think this diagnosis best fits Juan's condition. He has probably dealt with mild depression because of his loneliness, due to his family not being around, but I think it became a major depressive episode due to the accident (Bhugra & Becker, 2005). At this point I would not consider it recurrent, because there is not enough evidence for it. If his guilt is resolved, and he still shows signs of major depression, migration and loss of family may be the contributors (Bhugra & Becker, 2005; Lin, Dean, & Ensel, 1986). Caplan et al. (2012) note the influence of culture, and how it was a factor in depression among Latino immigrants. The results showed that there were several factors that contributed to depression, especially in the Latino/a immigrant community, these included: trauma and loss of loved ones, lack of faith in God, and the migration experience, the stress of negotiating a new cultural environment. The participants also discussed the difficulty of being away from their home country, their family and friends. Some of the participants discussed the difficulty in adapting to this new culture, especially when they did not have the education, and resources needed to succeed, and having to take care of their family on a low income. It was difficult to provide for their family, and it contributed to their depression because they realized that they were oppressed, which made it difficult to succeed in this country.

Overall Intervention Plan

Psychiatric evaluation: First, I think it would be important to obtain a psychiatric evaluation for Juan to check on the severity depression, and if medication, or hospitalization is required. After the evaluation is done I would have him come in and develop a safety plan/no self-harm contract. This will help Juan establish a successful plan to prevent suicidal behavior.

Specific strategies: In individual therapy I implemented culturally adapted cognitive behavioral techniques (Interian, Allen, Gara, & Escobar, 2008) to help Juan diminish suicidal ideation, and boost his self-worth. These techniques helped Juan diminish irrational thinking about his life, and increased positive thinking, which helped him cope with his depression. Also, I worked with Juan to identify maladaptive, negative thoughts, and replace them with positive thoughts. I taught him techniques to identify these thoughts, and when he is not in session, I assigned homework assignments to provide a check that Juan is continuing to use these coping strategies between sessions. This therapeutic modality helped Juan identify the thoughts that made him suicidal and depressed. Further these techniques helped erase the guilt from the accident. I helped him understand that the accident was not his fault, and that even though it was a tragedy, he needs to deal with his grief over the death, and loss of his job, and try and move forward in his life.

Group therapy: After Juan had worked through some of the issues, and dealt with depression, grief, and loss issues, I recommended he join a group to help him further explore any lingering issues caused by the accident. I helped provide resources to help him select a group, specifically I ensured that the group is culturally diverse and deals with issues pertaining to grief and loss. I explored any concerns that he might have about joining a group, and make sure that he is ready to talk about his issues pertaining to grief and loss. I think group counseling will be very helpful for Juan, he will be able to talk about his feelings, and just get support from other members who may have had similar experiences. Also, he will be able to gain a strong support network that will be helpful for Juan, since he is quite isolated.

Relationship building: I think for Juan it is important to help him build a strong support system and reconnect with his family. In therapy I implemented some brief psychodynamic therapy to help Juan become aware of his thoughts and feelings regarding his family members. Especially since his dad physically abused him and he felt abandoned by his mother, it was beneficial to explore these feelings with Juan to evaluate how it would be to reconnect with his family in Colombia. I also helped Juan to join a relationship/communication skill-building group, to help him in developing relationships in his life, and a strong support system. I think it is important for Juan to work on his relationship-building skills, and to reconnect with his family in Colombia, because culturally he comes from a collectivist society and he needs to be able to bond with his family to feel happy. Also, he needs these relationships because he has not been able to maintain them and has become susceptible to depression as a result of it.

Vocational counseling: After we deal with Juan's depression and guilt, I wanted to focus on his vocational goals. It is important for Juan to have a job, to help him be self-sufficient again. I would refer him to a career counselor, who can conduct a vocational/career assessment and help identify his strengths within his current skill set. Further, a career counselor can help him find a job through the resources that are available to him or her. I think helping Juan find a job will be very beneficial to him and will help get his life back on track, enhance his self-concept, and steer his focus away from the accident.

Summary

The interventions were helpful in addressing the depression and the grief. The culturally adapted CBT not only helped him work on his irrational thinking, but also helped with the depression. The focus on his cultural identity and context really helped me, because he felt truly understood and supported. Being involved in group counseling helped Juan in establishing some relationships, and reduced his sense of isolation. The goal of reconnecting with his family was a very positive motivator and it helped him get engaged with group counseling, and relationship-building skills. As Juan symptoms of depression and guilt dissipated, he was motivated to work on his vocational goals. In essence, Juan was able to overcome several obstacles in his life, he has resilience and once he gets a job he will be able to have a fuller, and more meaningful life.

Case 5: Counseling a Lesbian Latina Client

Bryce Carithers

Client Information

Client: Salina Knox
Ethnicity: Mexican-American
Age: 32

Background Information

Salina's maternal grandparents emigrated to the United States from Mexico, making Salina a second-generation US citizen. While Salina's grandparents were fluent in Spanish, her mother speaks and understands only some Spanish, and Salina is monolingual in English. She identifies as a lesbian, and is healthy, and able, with no physical or cognitive disabilities. Salina lives in an area of town with a high population of Latino/as' with her ex-brother-in-law, who is a source of support for her. Salina currently has a stable and secure job working in cellular technology, with high potential to advance within her company.

History of Presenting Problem

The presenting problem that brought Salina to counseling is chronic depression and anxiety that stems from an intense fear of being viewed negatively by others in numerous areas of her life. Salina states that she has battled with these concerns for

B. Carithers
University of Colorado Denver, Denver, CO, USA
e-mail: Bryce.carithers@ucdenver.edu

years, that her anxiety has gotten to the point of being debilitating when it comes to her social, and personal life, and that this fear of being seen in a negative light influences or determines many of her decisions. For example, Salina actively avoids situations or places that are not within a close distance to medical care, new or unfamiliar situations, and a situation in which she doubts her ability to perform well. Salina has experienced these feelings on some level since adolescence, and several times throughout the years has entertained suicide ideation, and once attempted suicide at age 14. Additionally, Salina recently went through the breakup of a 3-year marriage, which has accentuated her feelings of depression and anxiety, and ultimately pushed her to seek counseling.

Family Structure

Salina's immediate family consists of her mother, two older sisters, her 3-year-old nephew, and her older brother. Salina is very close to her mother and sisters, because she grew up with them, and especially now, since the breakup of her relationship, she feels closest to them. Salina's mother presently lives with her oldest sister, and both her mother and sisters have spent significant amounts of time living with Salina in the past. Both of Salina's sisters and her brother have a history of drug abuse that extends through Salina's childhood, and into the present, and her sisters and mother have all been treated for depression, at least once. Salina has minimal contact with her brother, and even less with her father, who has spent most of his life in prison.

Although close to her mother and sisters, Salina has identified these relationships as contributing to her presenting problems in several ways. During her childhood, Salina was witness to her siblings abusing drugs, going to jail, and the unhealthy relationship that her mother was in with her stepfather (now deceased). Throughout her adulthood, Salina has been the primary source of emotional and financial support for her family, including opening her home to her mother and sisters, and helping them out in many logistical ways (lending her car, giving rides, doing home repairs, etc.). Salina also recognizes the role that these family dynamics played in the breakup of her 3-year marriage, stating that her partner became drained by the constant issues, needs, and arguments that arose with Salina's mother, sisters, and cousin, who were all living with the couple at the time. This left little time or energy for the couple to focus on their own needs and their relationship, and also it became financially draining. Since the breakup of her marriage, Salina has slowly been working toward creating emotional and financial boundaries with her family members.

Client Strengths

Salina has many strengths that will be beneficial in the counseling process. One of her greatest strengths throughout her life has been her ability to learn not only from her own mistakes, but also from observing others' mistakes. Due to witnessing her family's struggles with drug use, finances, and incarceration, Salina realized at a young age that she possessed a strong desire to follow a different path that included being financially stable, and free of drug abuse. She has been successful in following that path, she prides herself on this, and her strong work ethic has assisted her in achieving her GED at 21 years-old, completing some college coursework, and securing a job that allows her to meet her financial needs and wants. At present, Salina is the first and only member in her immediate family who owns a home, which she was able to buy at age 21. One of Salina's biggest sources of pride is how far she has been able to advance in her jobs, and her present career despite not having the required education, an accomplishment that she attributes to her own determination to be a responsible, and a "good" person.

Salina shows a level of emotional resilience that has allowed her to survive and thrive despite her struggles with family, relationships, mental health concerns, and belonging to more than one vulnerable population in the United States. Salina is observant, thoughtful, and describes herself (even as a child) as always analyzing, and thinking about why people do the things they do. Salina is self-reflective and has a level of self-awareness that has given her insight into what constitutes healthy functioning for her. She is motivated to grow, is highly intelligent, and possesses an emotional vocabulary that aids in her keen awareness of her internal experience. When faced with adversity (such as the breakup of her marriage), Salina is able to seek out ways to help her cope and adjust, e.g., seeking counseling.

Assessments

Cultural Identity Exploration

Salina identifies as a Mexican-American, lesbian female, with an orientation towards spirituality. Salina's responses on CICL-R© (Ibrahim, 2008) reveals a general lack of understanding of the history of her cultural group, or her family's migration experience. The progression of English replacing Spanish as the primary language in Salina's family is an example of her family's experiences with acculturation and assimilation into US culture.

Worldview

Salina's results on the Scale to Assess World View© (SAWV: Ibrahim & Kahn, 1984, 1987) indicate her primary worldview to be Optimistic (4.33), followed by Pessimistic (or Realistic, 3.29), Here-and-Now (2.6), and Traditional (1.7). Having a primarily Optimistic worldview is common among people born and raised in the United States, as this worldview holds a belief that people are essentially good, and activity or work focuses on personal (including spiritual), and material development. It is also common for women, and people belonging to nondominant populations to score high on the Pessimistic worldview (Ibrahim et al., 2001), and this is true for Salina as well. As a female, a lesbian, and a person of color, it is likely that Salina has experienced oppression in numerous areas of her life, although she reports that she has very rarely felt oppressed. Ultimately, she has a sense of realism about her place in the system.

Acculturation

Salina's responses on this USAI (Ibrahim, 2007) continuum reflects a blend of collectivistic values, endorsed by Mexican culture, and values that she and her family have adopted from mainstream US culture, Salina's possible experiences of oppression due to her ethnicity, sexual orientation, and gender, and her own unique personality and belief system. Salina displays high acculturation and assimilation in that she identifies as future-time-oriented, independent, valuing mutual relationships, attributing success to personal effort, and valuing youth, over age. She shows less acculturation and assimilation in that she views mind and body to be connected, she is more oriented toward family; she has permeable boundaries, and recognizes her lack of control over life events. On all other variables, Salina scored near, or exactly in, the middle of the spectrum, likely reflecting her bicultural acculturation.

Resilience Scale

The Connor–Davidson Resilience Scale was used to assess Salina's resilience. On a scale of 1–100, Salina scored a raw score of 56 on this resiliency scale. This score indicates that in spite of her success in life, her resilience is not very high. A higher score (closer to 100), indicates high resilience. Examination of individual item responses on this scale reveals some discrepancies in self-perception. For example, Salina responded with "True nearly all the time" to the item, "When things look hopeless, I don't give up," and "Often true" to the item "I can handle anything that comes," indicating that she has a sense of determination and perseverance within herself. However, Salina's responses to the items "I see myself as a strong person" and "I am not easily discouraged by failure" were "Rarely true," indicating self-doubt about her strengths. Salina explains this discrepancy by stating that even though she doesn't see herself as strong, and at times does feel discouraged by failure, she keeps pushing through difficult situations anyway, which in itself is a sign of resilience.

The Privilege-Oppressed Continuum

Salina's self-ratings on the Privileged-Oppression Continuum (Miami Family Therapy Institute, n.d.) reveal that she identifies as having privilege in the area of her health and ability, but on all other variables she scored between 3 and 5 on the continuum (range 1 [oppressed] to 7 [privileged]). Salina explains that a score of 4 means that she doesn't feel that she experiences oppression, or privilege in that area of her life. Salina identifies as experiencing the same, or similar, amounts of oppression in the areas of ecology, and environment, sexual orientation, culture, and gender, and the similarly in the areas of religion, or spirituality, ethnicity, class or SES, and race.

DSM-5 Diagnosis

296.32	Major Depressive Disorder, Recurrent, Moderate
300.23	Social Anxiety Disorder

Intervention

Overall Intervention Plan

As Salina's counselor, it will be necessary to broach the differences that exist between us, and establish an open, and honest dialogue around these issues. Similarly, I will also want to pay attention throughout assessment to identify areas of common ground between us that will help facilitate rapport, and trust. I will need to be aware of the internal biases that I hold regarding people of color, Latina/o people, lesbians, and women in general, so as to make sure that I am being as open-minded and unbiased as possible. I will also need to be very aware of my own feelings towards my client since I have a propensity for physical attraction to Latinas, and this would certainly influence the counseling process, unless I am aware and monitor my behavior. Self-disclosure with Salina would likely be beneficial when talking about our differences, as it might be helpful for her to know that I've spent significant amounts of time in Central, and South America, that I have some basic knowledge about the Latino/a culture, or that I also identify as primarily lesbian. While it will be necessary for me to familiarize myself further with Mexican culture, Salina will be the one to educate me on her unique experience of living in, and between two cultures in the United States.

I will also need to be aware of the power dynamics that exist within our relationship to make sure I am not abusing this power, or intentionally using it to sway my client in any way. First, a power differential will exist due to my being in the position of "the expert," so I will want to make sure that Salina understands how the counseling process generally works, that she will be the expert on her own life and experiences, and will educate me and that we will work collaboratively. Secondly, I am in a power position because of the privilege I have due to being a White female. When working with a person of color, I will need to be very aware of this difference so as not to unintentionally use my privilege in unproductive or harmful ways, commit microaggressions, or invalidate my client's experience. Additionally, there is a significant difference in education levels between us, this will be another difference for me to be actively aware of to not let it negatively affect the therapeutic process.

In practice, I will put these concepts into action and work towards building a therapeutic relationship with Salina by empathically listening to her, accepting and validating her experience without challenging the truth behind it, and by being aware of my vocabulary and the underlying message behind my words. Should I slip up with a microaggression, I will directly acknowledge it, and apologize, and I will encourage my client to confront me on any of my words or actions that are overtly or covertly offensive. Empowering Salina to address these concerns as a mutual other will be important. Further, therapy from cognitive behavior therapy and strengths-based perspective will help battle the stigma, stereotypes, and negative self-perception that often come with depression, and anxiety, especially in having a vulnerable identity (LGBT), being a person of color, and female. This client is a great candidate for this approach, as she clearly possesses many strengths, and internal resources, as evidenced by her past struggles and successes.

Goal 1

Salina will experience reduced levels and severity of anxiety and depressive symptoms, as evidenced by:

Prior to initiating work on goal 1, Salina was asked to complete a full medical psychiatric evaluation to rule out physical problems, or if medication would be helpful in reducing her symptoms. She went through with the evaluations and was given a clean bill of health. No medication was needed for her psychological problems at this time.

Goal 1a. When compared with initial results prior to therapy, Salina will show lowered scores on measures assessing anxiety and depressive symptoms during and following treatment.

Goal 1b. Salina will be able to identify the triggers for her anxiety, and know how to prepare for, and cope with these situations.

Counseling strategies for goal 1a and 1b: "Practicing Mindfulness" involved a compassionate or nonjudgmental awareness of one's internal, and external experience in the present moment (Roemer & Orsillo, 2009). This can be practiced by intentionally focusing on one's experience during either a formal mindfulness activity (yoga, meditation, etc.,) or during an informal mindfulness activity (eating, walking, washing dishes, etc.). With practice, this skill becomes more habitual, increases the client's self-awareness, and brings them more fully into their life overall.

Goal 1c. Salina will be able to attend new situations, or go to new places that are far from medical facilities, without experiencing panic attacks or debilitating anxiety.

Counseling strategy for goal 1c. "Stress Inoculation Training" will be used with Salina to help her learn how to initially cope with mild stressors, and eventually with more stressful experiences in her life, e.g., venturing far from medical facilities. This technique boosts clients' coping skills, and enhances their belief in their ability to cope, by examining: the nature of the stressor, its conceptualization, its purpose, and the role it plays in maintaining the anxiety, and how to break down stressful situations into more specific and manageable goals (Erford, Eaves, Bryant, & Young, 2010).

Goal 2

Salina will work toward and strengthen an integrated cultural identity, as evidenced by:

Goal 2a. Salina will be able to identify the values, beliefs, and customs from each of the cultures she identifies with, and wants to maintain in her life.

Goal 2b. Salina will gain a more thorough understanding of her family's heritage, and how this has shaped her values, beliefs, and customs today.

Counseling strategy for goal 2a and 2b. During counseling sessions, Salina and I will work on several genograms to explore different parts of her family's history, and heritage such as ethnicity, family history with mental illness, and substance abuse, family occupational history, beliefs and customs, etc.

Goal 2c. Salina will be able to recognize the interplay of variables (both personal and social) that contribute to her present struggles, as opposed to taking full responsibility for all the events and experiences she had in her life.

Counseling strategies for goal 2c. (a) "Cultivating Self-Compassion" is a technique that comes from mindfulness and acceptance-based therapies. It encourages the client to recognize the ways in which socialization plays a role in becoming self-critical. The goal is to learn to be more forgiving and loving to oneself (Roemer & Orsillo, 2009). Cultivating self-compassion will be a theme throughout therapy with Salina. Compassion is initially communicated to the client by the therapist by consistently responding to the client in a empathic, and nonjudgmental manner, without trying to eliminate the client's negative experience, thereby communicating that the client's struggles are neither good nor bad, but simply part of the human experience. Specific mindfulness and breathing exercises will be used to focus on self-compassion, and how to foster it.

(b) Bibliotherapy will be used to help Salina understand privilege and oppression in the United States, and to better understand the sociopolitical environment she lives in, and how this influences her experiences as an individual, and at the social level. Because this client identifies as having minor struggles with maintaining focus while reading, alternative forms of media and information will likely be used such as videos, documentaries, art exhibits, etc. Salina and I will follow up on her reading by discussing these readings, and in helping her identify the ways in which she sees these privileges and oppression play out in her life.

Goal 3

Salina will improve her familial relationships and support network, as evidenced by establishing boundaries:

Goal 3a. Establishing emotional, and financial boundaries with her mother and sisters, as identified by Salina, which she considers as necessary for her own healthy functioning.

Counseling strategy for goal 3a. "Role Play" exercises will be used to practice conversations, and will focus on helping Salina "no" to family members to establish or reinforce a boundary.

Goal 3b. Salina will become involved in at least one social activity that she is interested in.

Goal 3b. Salina will develop and strengthen her social network by engaging in a social activity with a family member/friend(s) at least once a week.

Counseling strategy for goal 3a and 3b. Salina will keep a log of her social activities during the week and discuss her experiences, positive and negative each week with me. This will help her in empowering herself to select activities and interactions that empowering and will help her in expanding her world to develop new interests and relationships.

Summary

Salina possesses the necessary strengths and resources to be able to reach her treatment goals if therapy is conducted in an empowering, culturally sensitive, and empathic manner. As Salina's counselor, it is my goal to support, encourage, and advocate for my client while providing guidance, skills, and psychoeducation on the topics related to Salina's overall mental health. Through collaboration, empowerment, and a strong therapeutic relationship, I feel absolutely confident that Salina will successfully reach her treatment goals.

Case 6: Counseling a Transgender Client

Jianna R. Heuer

Client Information

Client: Cindy Gates
Race/Ethnicity: Argentinean/Italian
Age: 41
Clinician: Jianna Heuer, LMSW

J.R. Heuer
La Guardia Community College, New York, NY, USA

New York University, New York, NY, USA
e-mail: Jiannaheuer@gmail.com; http://www.jiannaheuer.com

Informed Consent was obtained using the following:

State of New York Disclosure

- Fee Structure Business and Emergency Protocols
- Statement of Confidentiality

Presenting Problem

Cindy presents with sexual performance issues. She has been in treatment for the last 2 years for addiction issues related to Heroin and Crack-Cocaine. Cindy reports being sober consistently for the 2 years, she was in in-patient treatment. She has been living on her own for 3 months, and she fears she is in danger of relapse. Also, she reports since leaving treatment she has not been able to ejaculate with a partner but masturbates up to 5× a day and she feels this is an unhealthy way to live. Cindy currently works for a nonprofit organization, facilitating support groups for transgender women, and also works as a hairdresser. She is trying to figure out what to do with her future. She feels she has never really made a decision about what she wanted to do with her life, and her career ambitions; she notes she "just rolled with what was presented to her." Cindy reports that besides the sexual issues, she is happy with her life.

Psychosocial History, Childhood and Adolescence

Cindy was born and raised to her birth parents in a countryside town in Argentina. Her mother worked as a cook and cleaned homes, and her father was a business owner. Both of her parents were originally from Italy. She was born a boy but reports always feeling like a girl. Her parents were extremely unsupportive and embarrassed by her behavior; because she acted very feminine as a child. Her father dismissed her when he realized she was "weird," and her mother was always striving to change her. Cindy reports her family was middle class but her peers were all very wealthy so she always felt she needed to pretend to be wealthy as well. Her father died when she was in her mid-30s. Her mother died recently. Cindy has one older brother and he is unemployed and still lives in Argentina.

Cindy was sexually abused by a neighbor, a male, from the age of 6 until she was in her late teens. She thinks her parents were "willfully ignorant" about what was going on. Her abuser was the only person who accepted her as a girl. Cindy always felt she acted different from the other kids, more "queer" but did not come out until she left Argentina.

Cindy graduated from high school in Argentina and has almost completed a Bachelor's degree in Music from a University in Argentina. She lived as a boy until she left Argentina when she was 21 years old and moved to Miami. In Miami she was a drag queen in the club scene, and she initiated a series of surgeries to begin her transition from male to female gender.

Psychosocial History, Life as an Adult

In Miami, Cindy reports being a famous drag queen. She also started working as an escort, and this became her main source of income until she was 38 years old, and arrested for possession of Heroin and prostitution in New York City. She lived in Miami and did well for herself for 10 years, but in those 10 years her drug use amplified from just social use to addiction. While living in Miami, she got involved with a man who stalked her. At the age of 32, she moved to New York City to get away from him. After the move Cindy continued working as an escort, but the drug use got out of control, and she went from being a high-priced call girl to doing whatever she could to get to the next bag of heroin. This led to her arrest, and she was offered treatment instead of incarceration, which she accepted. She stayed in treatment for 2 years and is now a hairdresser living in Queens, NY.

Assessments

This case presents a cross-cultural encounter between therapist and client on several levels, i.e. gender identity, culture of origin, migration status, and drug addition. In order to provide the best possible service, the therapist offered a few cultural assessments that may help with the therapeutic process. The client agreed that the following assessments would be helpful in our work.

Cultural Identity Assessment

The first instrument administered was the Cultural Identity Index© (CICL, Ibrahim, 1990, 2008). This 18 item self-report, qualitative questionnaire is designed to shed light on client's psychosocial identity within the context of her/his/zir cultural and historical background. The following data was obtained from this instrument. Cindy grew up in Argentina; her parents had emigrated from Italy before her birth. As a child she related strongly to her Italian heritage. In adolescence she started to identify as Latina, and has since felt a closer kinship to Latin American culture. She is the only one in her family to migrate to the United States, and she feels this transition has been positive, and she has been well received. She has exceeded her parents in education; they both finished primary school while she went on to finish her bachelor's degree. While she says her family accepts her gender identity she has also indicated, they are very uncomfortable with her transgender status, and how she has chosen to live her life. Cindy identifies as a transperson first and foremost. Her secondary identity characteristics are as a Latina, and as an immigrant.

Worldview

In congruence with how Cindy has described her past and current situation her worldview is skewed significantly towards Pessimistic (Realistic). This perspective reflects the values of Human Nature, Social Relationships, and Nature that the client deems important and significant. Due to Cindy's migration, struggle with her gender identity, and sexual orientation, lack of support from her family of origin, and her social class, this worldview of seeing the community she lives in as a place that is not cooperating with her, based on who she is, and what she believes in, seems more a realistic stance then pessimistic in terms of her cultural identity. Her secondary worldview is a combination of Here-and-Now (Spontaneous) and Optimistic. She prefers to live in the moment, and does feel that things will work out. She has gone through several challenges in her life, and has managed to make it. These assumptions seem to reflect how Cindy's life has evolved.

Acculturation Index

The therapist assessed her own level of acculturation using the United States Acculturation Index (Ibrahim, 2007) prior to meeting with Cindy and found her acculturation level to be significantly distant from mainstream US cultural assumptions. In assessing Cindy's acculturation level she found her to be closer to mainstream US cultural assumptions on many levels. However, there was a significant similarity in values between the client and the therapist, in regard to expressing emotion, present time focus, and having a highly individual orientation and beliefs.

Trauma History

Cindy has a significant trauma history. Her father was psychologically abusive from a very early age. He would put her down, call her names, and often ignored her. There also is a sense of abandonment from her mother, who was always trying to change her to meet her father's expectations. Further, a middle-aged male neighbor, sexually abused her from age 6 to 19 years-old. Although, she does not consider her history with drugs or prostitution as traumatic experiences, it is possible because drugs helped her cope with the reality of her childhood experiences. She also does not consider her gender transition as a traumatic event. However, being a transgendered woman has led to some traumatic experiences such as verbal, emotional, and physical assault/abuse from strangers, as well as being forced to seek asylum in the United States in order to gain legal status, a common path transgender individuals have to take due to the threat of violence against them in their own country (Cerezo, Morales, Quintero, & Rothman, 2014).

Clinical Interview

The case conceptualization was based on tying together aspects of the information gathered, assessments used, and the clinical interview. Using motivational interviewing and active listening the therapist completed an assessment of the current distressing factors affecting the client's life (Ivey, Ivey, & Zalaquett, 2009; Miller & Rollnick, 2002; Miller & Rose, 2009). The diagnosis and treatment plan were formulated mutually with the client and information collected. By creating a therapeutic alliance with Cindy, and understanding the acculturation differences between client and therapist, this provided a framework, for how best to intervene with Cindy's current emotional distress (Horvath & Luborsky, 1993).

Behavioral Observations

Cindy presented as calm, collected, and sure of herself. She was well dressed, and her attire was appropriate for the weather. Cindy was aware of the time, date, and place. She did not require a mental status exam.

Risk Assessment

A brief risk assessment was conducted with Cindy. She showed no signs of engaging in risky behavior. She is currently in Narcotics Anonymous (NA) and has a sponsor she speaks to quite often. She seemed secure in her recovery. She has a strong support system, and does not suffer from depression. She is currently experiencing no suicidal ideation. She does not pose a threat to herself or anyone else at the moment.

DSM-5 Diagnosis

It is my clinical assessment that Cindy is working with a diagnosis of Gender Dysphoria: Post-Transition 302.85 (F64.1) as well as Post Traumatic Stress Disorder (PTSD) 309.81 (F43.10), (APA, 2013). In terms of the Gender Dysphoria, Cindy meets five out of the six criteria to qualify for this diagnosis. The diagnosis of Posttraumatic Stress Disorder is more complicated. I think the original trauma included being born as a male, and being sexually abused from age 6 until her teen years, but Cindy also describes traumatic experiences in adulthood (prostitution and violence), that could have contributed to symptoms of PTSD. She meets most of the criteria but most significant are her experiences of the traumatic events, recurring dreams of events, physiological reactions to the trauma, avoidance of stimuli associated with the trauma, and the long-term distress and stress this has caused throughout Cindy's life (Resnick, Nisith, Weaver, Astin, & Feuer, 2002; Rowan & Foy, 1993; Rowan, Foy, Rodriguez, & Ryan, 1994).

Counselor Biases

Negative biases: I fancy myself as a culturally competent clinician. However, I admittedly knew very little about transgendered people. I did not have a particularly coherent grasp on Argentina, and its political, and social climate, during the time Cindy was growing up. I also had never encountered anyone in my life, or in my work that had been a prostitute. I did have concerns that I would not be able to connect with Cindy, because I could be judgmental about her past drug use, and the prostitution. After learning more about Cindy, her worldview, the experiences she has had, and her views on sex work, and transgendered individuals, I came to not only understand, but also empathize with Cindy's view on these issues. I believe my ability to be open, and truly be with her, and hear what Cindy was saying, allowed me to overcome any negative biases I may have had, when we began our work.

Positive biases: I consider myself a feminist, a person who accepts people for who they are, and one who is open to many different ways of being. This ability to understand and welcome difference really contributed to Cindy and I creating a successful therapeutic relationship. Also, as a woman I felt a kinship with Cindy who expressed similar beliefs about love, and relationships, to my own. Our worldviews were very similar which allowed me to have more insight than one would think considering our obvious differences.

Client Goals

Cindy entered therapy in order to continue her recovery, as well as work on her sexual dysfunction issues. She has indicated her most important goal is staying sober. She believes being able to have a healthy sexual relationship with someone would help her to maintain sobriety, at this point in her recovery. She indicated that she would also like to work on exploring her past issues, including her family dynamics, and the sexual abuse she endured as a child.

Intervention

Overall Intervention Plan

Based on the clinical interviews, as well as the assessments completed by Cindy there are four major areas to focus on in therapy; Gender Dysphoria Disorder, PTSD, Sexual Dysfunction, and Substance Use Disorder. Cindy is interested in long term treatment therefore the main orientation used will be psychodynamic. We will also utilize mindfulness, Motivational interviewing, CBT techniques, and Narrative Therapy to aid in our work.

The main goal Cindy has is exploring why she is encountering sexual issues and how to mitigate them. It is the clinician's belief that her childhood sexual abuse, lack of acceptance of her gender identity by significant others, and the effects of PTSD have contributed to Cindy's current sexual issues (Browne & Finkelhor, 1986). We utilized psychodynamic therapy to create a true therapeutic alliance it is the therapist's belief that working through some of these historically significant issues will help to resolve the sexual dysfunction, and also aid in Cindy remaining sober (Horvath & Luborsky, 1993).

Specific Strategies

Gender dysphoria disorder: In Cindy's case she seems to have fully accepted her gender identity. Unfortunately the society she grew up in, i.e., Argentina did not accept her, her family did not accept her, and even though she is comfortable in the United States, she finds an abundant lack of acceptance here, which makes her question her choices, surgeries, and identity. She has shown interest in writing her story, and enjoys journaling, so narrative therapy, along with hormone treatment seemed to be the best intervention to mitigate these issues.

Posttraumatic stress disorder: Using psychodynamic psychotherapy, mindfulness training, and CBT to help Cindy work through the traumas she has experienced should help to eventually lessen the issues of sexual dysfunction Cindy describes (Fletcher & Hayes, 2005; McCabe et al., 2010; Resnick et al., 2002). Cindy explained that in her rehab program, one of the most useful techniques she utilized was meditation and yoga. Engaging in mindfulness, meditation, deep breathing, and practicing these skills in a therapeutic setting will allow Cindy to be able to discuss her traumas in a safe environment, where she will have the tools to deescalate, if memories become too intense in therapy (Deatherage, 1975; Fletcher & Hayes, 2005). Cognitive behavioral techniques including keeping a record of her thoughts, identifying patterns of behaviors that are not healthy, and replacing those behaviors with more healthy mindful activities, will help Cindy to move forward in her therapeutic work (Resnick et al., 2002).

Sexual dysfunction: Engaging in a psychodynamic, therapeutic relationship where Cindy feels she can explore her childhood sexual abuse, history of prostitution, and how her past may relate to her current sexual issues will result in her being able to have a better understanding of what she wants from a sexual relationship, and how she can get it in a healthy manner (Manetta, Gentile, & Gillig, 2011).

Substance use: Cindy is utilizing her sponsor and Narcotics Anonymous as her main source of support for her recovery. The clinician will use motivational interviewing to help Cindy to explore any issues that may arise in terms of her substance use and issues of relapse.

Evaluation of the Assessments and Interventions

Using the Scale to Asses Worldview and the Acculturation Checklist were instrumental in Cindy's treatment. These instruments gave me a very clear understanding of where Cindy has been, what she has had to overcome, and who she is as a person. I gleaned a better understanding of the sociopolitical environment she emerged from, and how different it was for her in the United States, this understanding helped me to develop a culturally responsive treatment plan that could best serve Cindy in alleviating the various symptoms she presented in her initial interview.

Intervention Evaluation

Psychodynamic treatment is ongoing and seemingly productive for Cindy. She has explored issues surrounding her childhood sexual abuse, her family, relationship with her mother, history of drug use, and prostitution, and her future plans. She continues to be motivated and reflective in sessions and has made many important life changes since beginning treatment. She now works for a nonprofit organization with transgender clients, and feels a great sense of fulfillment from this work, and envisions a successful future working in this field. She lives on her own, a goal she has had since leaving her drug rehabilitation program. She is staying sober and using meditation, fitness, and relaxation methods, to remain in control of her sobriety, as well as work on her sexual dysfunction issues. Motivational interviewing and mindfulness have proved to be incredibly helpful tools in treatment with Cindy. We have not yet utilized any CBT methods in treatment. She reports deriving more pleasure from sexual experiences currently, than she did when she started treatment, and believes working through her history of sexual abuse in therapy has helped in this area of her life.

Summary

Overall Cindy has made vast improvement since beginning therapy. She is willing and capable of exploring deeper meaning in her revelations about the past and present. She is excited about being in treatment and rarely misses appointments. Cindy has shown great growth, and continues to discuss difficult topics with much insight. The therapeutic alliance shared between clinician and client is strong and transference reactions are usefully utilized in therapy. Cindy does exhibit some resistance in accepting good things, into her life and believing they will sustain.

Case 7: Counseling an Iranian Immigrant Client

Lisa Taggart

Client Information

Name: Saeed
Age: *25*

Cultural Background

The client, Saeed, is a 25-year-old, able-bodied, heterosexual male who identifies as Persian-American. He reports no religious or spiritual orientation. When the client was 11, his family emigrated from Iran to the United States, and they settled in Utah, when he was 14, they moved to Denver, CO. The client reports that the socioeconomic status of his family was upper class in Iran; he describes the family as middle class in the United States. He is fluent in both English and Farsi.

Presenting Problem

The client came to counseling to discuss his primary concerns about feelings of alienation from his parents. He also noted that he feels isolated in his job as a software developer; he spends the day writing computer code in a tiny cubicle at work. He is concerned about his physical health, because he has difficulty sleeping at night, which he attributes to having to go to the toilet, several times during the night. Further, he is concerned about his social skills, and how people perceive him, this makes him nervous in social situations. Lastly, he mentioned that once he starts thinking about how he acts, or what he says around other people, he cannot make himself stop.

Social/Educational Background

The client states that he refers to himself as Persian, so people will not associate him with the "bad" parts of Iran (Mirkin & Kamya, 2008). In addition, he does not identify with any particular religion, although he experiences some internal and external

L. Taggart
Four Directions Counseling LLC, Denver, CO, USA

University of Colorado Denver, Denver, CO, USA
e-mail: lisa@lisataggart.com

conflict about the traditional beliefs of his family, such as the unquestioned authority of his father (Frank, Plunkett, & Otten, 2010). His family identifies as Shiite Muslim, which is the majority religion in Iran, but he states he has distanced himself from his family's religious beliefs.

Currently, the client is alienated from his family because of conflicts over his Western beliefs, such as his personal independence, and his love of music. He is financially independent. He lives by himself and identifies two friends as part of his social support system; one of his friends is counseling him, informally. The client is currently also working on completing his undergraduate degree. However, he is struggling with his coursework, and he is fearful he will fail some of his courses. This worry also contributes to his difficulty in sleeping; and he states that his anxiety is beginning to affect many parts of his life, especially his relationships with people at work.

According to Jalali and Boyce (1980), Iranian families adapt to US culture in several different ways: (a) Iranian families may denigrate the old culture by denying their cultural origins, and adopting the cultural norms of the United States (b) Iranian families may reject the new culture, by reproducing the familiar culture of their homeland; and (c) Iranian immigrant families may choose to integrate the cultures of both countries (Jalali, 2005). In addition, there may be several other characteristics of Iranian culture that may be important to note in this case. It is important to be aware that there is no collective profile of Iranian immigrants, and regional roots are highly influential in shaping the culture of Iranians (Jalali). In addition, Frank et al. (2010) suggest that the pride of the individual may lead to difficulty in interpersonal relationships due to an inability to admit mistakes. Jalali & Boyce points out that friendships in the Iranian culture are close knit, and often of long duration and evoke strong emotions. The father is the traditional head of the Iranian family, and other family members hesitate to question his authority (Jalali, 2005). Lastly, Jalali maintains that higher education can be a source of pride for Iranian immigrants. Awareness of each of these cultural considerations will be important in counseling Saeed (Bushfield & Fitzpatrick, 2010).

The client demonstrates a number of strengths that will be useful in overcoming the difficulties he has identified. Saeed exhibits awareness and insight about himself, as well as the difficulties with his family. In addition, he is resilient as evidenced by his desire and ability to be independent, as well as surviving his journey of immigration. He also demonstrates a willingness to form relationships and is interested in improving his social skills to create new friendships. He is able to ask for help when he needs it, as evidenced by coming to counseling. Furthermore, he is bilingual. His interpersonal strengths include his close friendships and his video game community. His environmental strengths include a love of music and the university community (Hays, 2008).

The client's current adjustment level may be described as somewhat compromised. Over the last year, the client has felt alienated from his family of origin and forced to rely on his own financial and interpersonal resources. For instance, he lives alone and works to support himself financially. The client considers his alienation is contributing to his difficulty in getting adequate sleep and his heightened anxiety. He also notes having difficulty in social interactions, and he wants to increase his social skills. While he has been able to maintain employment, he expresses concern that his performance will continue to deteriorate, if he does not learn new ways of relating to his peers.

Assessments

Cultural Identity Assessment

The Cultural Identity Checklist has revealed the need for further exploration of Saeed's immigration experience (Ibrahim, 2008). It is possible there is some underlying trauma that occurred either prior to, or during the migration from Iran, or there may be intergenerational historical trauma. Further exploration of the reason and means by which Saeed's family left Iran may help identify a connection to his feelings of alienation and isolation. In addition, Saeed has revealed some internalized oppression with regard to his hesitancy to identify himself as being from Iran, as evidenced by his desire to be called Persian American. The cultural assessments reveal three significant issues to consider in working with Saeed and these are his ethnicity, his national origin and his gender.

Worldview

An assessment using the Scale to Assess Worldview (Ibrahim & Kahn, 1984) exhibits several noteworthy attributes that will be helpful in developing treatment goals. For instance, while Saeed's score, 3.11, on World View I (Optimistic worldview) indicates a degree of optimism. He also exhibits realism, as evidenced by his score of 3.71 on the World View IV (Pessimistic or Realistic worldview). In addition, Saeed has a score of 2.8 on World View II (Traditional worldview), indicating nontraditional cultural beliefs and perspectives. These perspectives will be important to explore further, especially as they relate to his relationship and frustration with his family. Lastly, Saeed demonstrates an orientation toward spontaneity and being in the moment, evidenced by his score of 3.4 on the World View III (Here-and-Now or Spontaneous worldview). This orientation will be important to incorporate into the assessment of his feelings of anxiety, because a here-and-now focus, it may indicate the consideration of meditation, as a possible intervention.

Acculturation Level

Saeed demonstrates a high level of acculturation in the United States. He has moved out and independent from his immediate family, and is self-supporting. In addition, he is very optimistic about his future, especially the opportunities that exist in the world of software development. At times, his present financial success makes him question the need to further his education. Saeed demonstrates what Hoffman (1991) describes as a division of self that allows Iranian immigrants to reveal the inner self to close friends, as evidenced by the informal counseling he is receiving from a friend who is a student pursuing a Master's in Social Work. In addition, he feels that "while he looks put together on the outside, on the inside he is a mess." The United States Acculturation Index shows Saeed's movement away from his culture of origin, and this may be an important consideration in assessing his disconnection and alienation from his family of origin (Ibrahim, 2007).

DSM-5 Diagnosis

It appears that given the information shared by the client, Saeed is suffering from GAD, possibly due to acculturation issues, which have created a rift between him and his family (Baumeister, 1986). The isolation, and the anxiety about grades, along with not feeling close to his primary support system, has left him adrift (Cokley, McClain, Enciso, & Martinez, 2013).

Counselor Biases

There are several areas of bias that may affect my therapeutic relationship with Saeed. As a woman, I want to be aware of Iranian cultural assumptions about the place of women, and I need be aware of not imposing my beliefs on the counseling relationship. In addition, I must also be open to Iranian attitudes regarding same-sex relationships within Muslim communities, and not let my values around this part of my identity as a lesbian, get in the way. It will be important to be respectful of Iranian beliefs, such as the existence of patriarchy among Iranian families, and support Saeed's role within his family. Even though anxiety may not involve somatic expression within my culture, it is possible that in Saeed's primary culture experiencing somatic symptoms, like frequent urination, as a result of his anxiety is socially conditioned (Castillo, 1997). In addition, I want to be aware of my unconscious racism that I may exhibit, especially in monitoring my nonverbal communications with the client. I also want to be aware of any biases that I may hold regarding 9/11, and how that may come across to Saeed. In addition, I share a nonreligious perspective with Saeed and this may be a strength that will help create some common ground between us. However, the three significant characteristics of my identity are female, lesbian and White, which will require a high level of awareness and education about Iranian American culture, as well as the Shiite Muslim culture. I may need to be prepared to refer this client to a more competent therapist or obtain supervision to manage the differences, if Saeed expresses concern about working with me.

Intervention

Client Insights and Strengths

In addressing the presenting concerns that Saeed brings to counseling, it is critical to give consideration to his level of acculturation, as opposed to the level of acculturation found within his family of origin. Saeed is aware of his feelings of alienation and isolation, and, while he has not directly attributed it to his evolving acculturation, it may be a result of it. In addition, he identifies lacking social skills, and attributes this to his work as a software developer, living inside his head on a regular basis. Furthermore, Saeed is interested in understanding his acculturative immersion in the United States. His adopted cultural norms have strained his relationship with his family, as well as challenging the beliefs that his family holds around collectivism and patriarchy. Lastly, the insight Saeed exhibits about his anxiety is a strength, which makes him aware of how it manifests itself in social situations.

Specific Strategies

CBT will be used as the theoretical orientation in working with Saeed. According to Hays (2008), CBT helps create realistic and helpful thinking that assists clients in changing irrational thoughts and self-defeating behaviors. In addition, CBT may help eliminate distressing physical symptoms (Hays). Hays maintains that CBT can help build specific skills while focusing on the cultural identity, and strengths of the client. In addition, Hays makes the case for emphasizing the role of the environment in shaping behaviors, while articulating and assessing a cross-cultural perspective. Since Saeed believes some of his isolation may be indirectly related to racism, it will be important to evaluate the role of his social, familial, and work environment to identify how behavioral changes can take place.

Saeed has identified three goals that he would like to accomplish over the course of his treatment. First of all, he wants to increase his social skills, and use them to improve his interpersonal relationships. Secondly, he wants to improve his quality of life by managing his anxiety. Lastly, he wants to improve the quality of interactions he experiences with his family of origin.

There are several strategies, such as assigning homework, that have been identified to attain the goals that Saeed has set out for himself. In my opinion, it is important to acknowledge that any distorted thoughts may be responses to cultural oppression, and more externally based. In an effort to reduce the acute symptoms of stress, such as sleeplessness, Saeed will utilize the technique of progressive muscle relaxation (Erford et al., 2010). In my opinion, Saeed can use this skill in conjunction with other assigned homework. De-catastrophizing is one strategy that may be effective for Saeed as he engages with his family (Truscott, 2010). For instance, if Saeed experiences worry about what will happen when he meets with his family, it will be important to offer some problem-solving techniques, such as setting boundaries around the amount of time he will spend with his family. Appropriate boundaries need to be influenced by cultural factors and I want to listen to Saeed for direction as to what those may be.

Identifying and testing automatic thoughts (Truscott, 2010) is another strategy to assist Saeed in reaching his goal of improving social skills. For instance, Saeed has verbalized that no one at work likes him and to test this assumption, he will need to record how often his co-workers treat him nicely (Truscott, 2010). By testing his thoughts, he may discover the people who do like him at work. De-centering is another technique offered by Truscott (2010) as a way to mitigate anxiety. This technique may be useful in dealing with anxious feelings that accompany much of Saeed's life. For instance, Saeed thinks people are talking about him, and that he is at the center of their lives, particularly at work. Again, if Saeed will agree to test his belief, by recording positive and negative interactions, he may discover that he is not at the center of anyone's lives (Truscott, 2010).

Another technique that will be employed during this intervention is the use of thought stopping (Truscott, 2010). When Saeed makes arrangements to visit his parents and he experiences the cognitive distortion that his family does not value him, or want to spend time with him, it will be important to identify a positive thought, such as how attached he was to his parents as a child. This thought will replace the thought, which is causing him distress (Truscott, 2010). All of these strategies will require adaptation to Saeed's cultural orientation (Hays, 2008). For instance, collaborating with Saeed may require referring to his thoughts with regard to the helpfulness he feels in dealing with his family and coworkers, instead of calling them cognitive distortions (Hays, 2008). In addition, the intervention will utilize his cultural and personal strengths, and the social and environmental supports as identified by him (Hays, 2008).

Evaluation of Assessments and Intervention

Implementation of the intervention and assessments required a slight shift in perspective. For instance, my hunch that his frequent urination may have been a result of his anxiety was incorrect. It turned out to be the result of a urological problem that Saeed investigated with his physician. In addition, Saeed revealed that he had been bullied as a teenager about his weight and his nationality. This information clarified why he is anxious about his cultural heritage.

Saeed was uncomfortable setting boundaries with his parents as a problem solving method, because he thought it would be disrespectful, and would dishonor his family. However, he was able to successfully use the thought stopping measure as a way to control his anxiety, and he is very invested in continuing the practice. Overall, Saeed considered the de-centering technique to be successful, because it helped him feel more comfortable in social settings. This new level of comfort enabled him to improve his interpersonal relationships and make new friends. Saeed still had difficulty relating to his parents and appreciated his new skill of identifying his thoughts, especially as it related to his parents' desire to keep both feet planted in Iranian culture.

Specific Strategies That Worked

Saeed especially appreciated the progressive muscle relaxation technique and he was able to determine other situations in which to use this strategy. For instance, he reported using it at work when he felt anxiety creeping into his interactions with coworkers. In addition, he was able to use it as a way to wind down at the end of the day, and used this method as a way to replace video games, as a coping skill.

Strategies That Failed

Saeed found the thought stopping exercise difficult to implement because it was difficult for him to devise positive thoughts, to replace his negative thinking. In an effort to become more aware of his thoughts, Saeed chose to use his journal to track his thoughts, and relate the onset of those thoughts to particular negative incidents in his life (Truscott, 2010). One strategy I reworked was the boundary setting approach by encouraging Saeed to write in a journal instead, and keep track of the types of interactions he had with his family, tracking the number of positive interactions, as well as the number of the negative interactions. This strategy allowed Saeed to have a record of the quality of interactions with his family, especially when negative thoughts flooded his cognitions. Furthermore, the journal allowed Saeed to see the quality of his relationship with his family in a very concrete way.

The collaborative goal setting increased Saeed's investment in obtaining his goals. By the end of our sessions, he had developed new friendships, and was visiting his family once every other month, as well as feeling more comfortable with his co-workers. Both of these outcomes were a result of our work together. The cultural assessments yielded useful information with regard to the Saeed's bicultural and multiple identities. For instance, it was helpful to know that Saeed has a high level of acculturation, and the impact of this on his relationships with his family. Although the assessment for posttraumatic stress disorder did not result in a diagnosis, it remained important to be aware of any trauma related behaviors or feelings.

Summary

Saeed presented with problems of anxiety, low self-concept, internalized oppression, and interpersonal and relational difficulties with family and coworkers. Cultural assessments, such as the Cultural Identity Checklist and the United States

Acculturation Index, accurately revealed a high level of acculturation, as well as other concerns associated with his identity. The diagnosis of GAD is based on western constructs of the DSM-5, and attention to his cultural context proved helpful (Castillo, 1997). In addition, the use of CBT, as a theoretical orientation, was adapted for a cross-cultural intervention, by establishing collaborative goals and modifying strategies. Saeed lives at the intersection of many identities, which include his ethnicity, his gender, his level of acculturation, and his national origin. Our work together helped Saeed to weave together his strengths, allowing him to control, and modify his negative thoughts, and led to lowering and managing anxiety.

References

American Psychiatric Association. (2013). *Diagnostic and statistical manual of mental disorders* (5th ed.). Washington, DC: Author.

Arnold, K. M. (2010). *A qualitative examination of African American counselors' experiences of addressing issues of race, ethnicity, and culture with clients of color*. Doctoral dissertation, Virginia Polytechnic Institute and State University.

Baker Miller, J. (2012). *Five good things*. Wellesley, MA: Jean Baker Miller Training Institute at the Wellesley Centers for Women.

Baumeister, R. F. (1986). *Identity: Cultural change and the struggle for self* (p. 153). New York: Oxford University Press.

Beck, J. S. (1995). *Cognitive therapy: Basics and beyond*. New York: The Guilford Press.

Bhugra, D., & Becker, M. A. (2005). Migration cultural bereavement and cultural identity. *World Psychiatry, 4*, 18–24.

Boxer, A. (2009). *History today: Native Americans and The federal government*. Retrieved from http://www.historytoday.com/andrew-boxer/native-americans-and-federal-government.

Boysen, G. A., & Vogel, D. L. (2008). The relationship between level of training, implicit bias, and multicultural competency among counselor trainees. *Training and Education in Professional Psychology, 2*(2), 103–110.

Browne, A., & Finkelhor, D. (1986). Impact of child sexual abuse: A review of the research. *Psychological Bulletin, 99*(1), 66–77.

Bruce, M. L., Kim, K., Leaf, P. J., & Jacobs, S. (1990). Depressive episodes and dysphoria resulting from conjugal bereavement in a prospective community sample. *American Journal of Psychiatry, 147*, 608–611.

Bushfield, S., & Fitzpatrick, T. R. (2010). Therapeutic interventions with immigrant Muslim families in the United States. *Journal of Religion & Spirituality in Social Work: Social Thought, 29*(2), 165–179.

Caplan, S., Escobar, J., Paris, M., Alvidrez, J., Dixon, J., Desai, M., et al. (2012). Cultural influences on causal beliefs about depression among Latino immigrants. *Journal of Transcultural Nursing, 24*(68), 68–76. doi:10.117/1043659612453745.

Cardemil, E. V., & Battle, C. L. (2003). Guess who is coming to therapy? Getting comfortable with conversations about race and ethnicity in psychotherapy. *Professional Psychology: Research and Practice, 34*(3), 278–286. doi:10.1037/0735-7028.34.3.278.

Castillo, R. J. (1997). *Culture & mental illness*. Pacific Grove, CA: Brooks/Cole Publishing Company.

Cerezo, A., Morales, A., Quintero, D., & Rothman, S. (2014). Trans migrations: Exploring life at the intersection of transgender identity and immigration. *Psychology of Sexual Orientation and Gender Diversity, 1*(2), 170–180.

Chang, D. F., & Yoon, P. (2011). Ethnic minority clients' perceptions of the significance of race in cross-racial therapy relationships. *Psychotherapy Research, 21*(5), 567–582. doi:10.1080/10503307.2011.592549.

Chavez Cameron, S. C., & Turtle-Song, I. (2003). Native American mental health: An examination of resiliency in the face of overwhelming odds. In F. D. Harper & J. McFadden (Eds.), *Culture and counseling: New approaches* (pp. 66–80). Boston: Allyn & Bacon.

Cokley, K., McClain, S., Enciso, A., & Martinez, M. (2013). An examination of the impact of minority status stress, and impostor feelings on the mental health of diverse ethnic minority college students. *Journal of Multicultural Counseling and Development, 41*(2), 82–95.

Comstock, D. L., Hammer, T. R., Strentzsch, J., Cannon, K., Parsons, J., & Salazar, G., II. (2008). Relational-cultural theory: A framework for bridging relational, multicultural, and social justice competencies. *Journal of Counseling and Development, 86*(2), 279–287.

Connor, K. M., & Davidson, J. R. T. (2003). Development of a new resilience scale: The Connor-Davidson Resilience Scale (CD-RISC). *Depression and Anxiety, 18*, 76–82.

Corey, G. (2009). *Theory and practice of counseling and psychotherapy* (8th ed.). Belmont, CA: Brooks/Cole.

Cornish, J. A. E., Schreier, B. A., Nadkarni, L. I., Metzger, L. H., & Rodolfa, E. R. (Eds.). (2010). *Handbook of multicultural competencies*. New York: Wiley.

Cunningham-Warburton, P. A. (1988). *A study of the relationship between cross-cultural training, the Scale to Assess World Views© and the quality of care given by nurses in a psychiatric setting*. Unpublished doctoral dissertation, University of Connecticut, Storrs.

Dana, R. H. (2008). National and international professional resources. In R. H. Dana & J. Allen (Eds.), *Cultural competency in a global society* (pp. 43–66). New York: Springer.

Day-Vines, N. L., Wood, S. M., Grothaus, T., Craigen, L., Holman, A., Dotson-Blake, K., et al. (2007). Broaching the subjects of race, ethnicity, and culture during the counseling process. *Journal of Counseling & Development, 85*(4), 401–409.

Deatherage, G. (1975). The clinical use of "mindfulness" meditation techniques in short-term psychotherapy. *Journal of Transpersonal Psychology, 7*(2), 133–143.

Denborough, D. (2014). *Retelling the stories of our lives: Everyday narrative therapy to draw inspiration and transform experience*. New York: W. W. Norton.

Duran, E. (2006). *Healing the soul wound: Counseling with American Indians and other native peoples*. New York: Teachers College Press.

Duran, B., Duran, E., & Brave Heart, M. Y. H. (1998). Native Americans and the trauma of history. In R. Thornton (Ed.), *Studying Native America: Problems and Prospects in Native American Studies* (pp. 244–278). Madison, WI: University of Wisconsin Press.

Duran, E., Firehammer, J., & Gonzalez, J. (2008). Liberation psychology as the path toward healing cultural soul wounds. *Journal of Counseling and Development, 86*, 288–295.

Erford, B. T., Eaves, S. H., Bryant, E. M., & Young, K. A. (2010). *35 techniques every counselor should know*. Upper Saddle River, NJ: Pearson Education.

Etchison, M., & Kleist, D. M. (2000). Review of narrative therapy: Research and utility. *The Family Journal, 8*(1), 61–66.

Evans-Campbell, T. (2008). Historical trauma in American Indian/Native Alaska communities: A multilevel framework for exploring impacts on individuals, families, and communities. *Journal of Interpersonal Violence, 23*, 316–338.

Fletcher, L., & Hayes, S. C. (2005). Relational frame theory, acceptance and commitment therapy, and a functional analytic definition of mindfulness. *Journal of Rational-Emotive & Cognitive Behavior Therapy, 23*, 315–336.

Frank, G., Plunkett, S. W., & Otten, M. P. (2010). Perceived parenting, self-esteem and general self-efficacy of Iranian American adolescents. *Journal of Child and Family Studies, 19*, 738–746.

Gaztambide, D. J. (2012). Addressing cultural impasses in rupture resolution strategies: A proposal and recommendation. *Professional Psychology: Research and Practice, 43*(3), 183–189. doi:10.1037/a0026911.

Genia, V. (1990). Religious development: A synthesis and a reformulation. *Journal of Religion and Health, 29*(2), 85–99.
Goldfried, M. R., & Davison, G. C. (1994). Rational-emotive & cognitive behavior therapy. In M. R. Goldfried & G. C. Davison (Eds.), *Clinical behavior therapy: Expanded edition* (pp. 315–336). New York: Wiley.
Gone, J. P., & Alcantara, C. (2007). Identifying effective mental health interventions for American Indians and Alaska Natives: A review of the literature. *Cultural Diversity and Ethnic Minority Psychology, 13*, 356–363.
Greenwald, A. G., Nosek, B. A., & Banaji, M. R. (2003). Understanding and using the implicit association test: I. An improved scoring algorithm. *Journal of Personality and Social Psychology, 85*, 197–216.
Harper, F. D., & McFadden, J. (Eds.). (2003). *Culture and counseling: New approaches*. New York: Pearson Eduction.
Hays, P. A. (2008). *Addressing cultural complexities in practice*. Washington, DC: American Psychological Association.
Hodge, D. R. (2001). Spiritual assessment: A review of major qualitative methods, and a new framework for assessing spirituality. *Social Work, 46*(3), 203–214.
Hoffman, D. M. (1991). Beyond conflict: Culture, self, and intercultural learning among Iranians in the U.S. *International Journal of Intercultural Relations, 14*(3), 275–299.
Horvath, A. O., & Luborsky, L. (1993). The role of therapeutic alliance in psychotherapy. *Journal of Consulting and Clinical Psychology, 61*(4), 561–573.
Howard, K. I., Krasner, R., & Saunders, S. (1999). The evaluation of psychotherapy. In B. J. Sadock, V. A. Sadock, & P. Ruiz (Eds.), *Kaplan and Sadock's comprehensive textbook of psychiatry* (7th ed., pp. 2217–2224). Philadelphia, PA: Lippincott Williams & Wilkins.
Howard, K. I., Moras, K., Brill, P. L., Martinovich, Z., & Lutz, W. (1996). Evaluation of psychotherapy: Efficacy, effectiveness, and patient progress. *American Psychologist, 51*(10), 1059–1064.
Ibrahim, F. A. (1990). *Cultural Identity Check List©*. Unpublished document, Storrs, CT.
Ibrahim, F. A. (1991). Contribution of cultural worldview to generic counseling and development. *Journal of Counseling and Development, 70*, 13–19.
Ibrahim, F. A. (1999). Transcultural counseling: Existential world view theory and cultural identity: Transcultural applications. In J. McFadden (Ed.), *Transcultural counseling* (2nd ed., pp. 23–57). Alexandria, VA: ACA Press.
Ibrahim, F. A. (2003). Existential worldview counseling theory: Inception to applications. In F. D. Harper & J. McFadden (Eds.), *Culture and counseling: New approaches* (pp. 196–208). Boston: Allyn & Bacon.
Ibrahim, F. A. (2007). *United States Acculturation Index©*. Unpublished document, Denver, CO.
Ibrahim, F. A. (2008). *Cultural Identity Check List-Revised©*. Unpublished document, Denver, CO.
Ibrahim, F. A. (2010). Innovative teaching strategies for group work: Addressing cultural responsiveness and social justice. *The Journal for Specialists in Group Work, 35*, 271–280.
Ibrahim, F. A., & Heuer, J. R. (2013, August). *Social justice and cultural responsiveness: Using cultural assessments*. Poster presentation at the American Psychological Association, Honolulu, HI.
Ibrahim, F. A., & Kahn, H. (1984). *Scale to Assess World View©*. Unpublished document, Storrs, CT.
Ibrahim, F. A., & Kahn, H. (1987). Assessment of world views. *Psychological Reports, 60*, 163–176.
Ibrahim, F. A., & Ohnishi, H. (2001). Posttraumatic stress disorder and the minority experience. In D. R. Pope-Davis & H. L. K. Coleman (Eds.), *The intersection of race, class, and gender in multicultural counseling* (pp. 89–119). Thousand Oaks, CA: Sage.
Ibrahim, F. A., Ohnishi, H., & Wilson, R. (1994). Career counseling in a pluralistic society. *Journal of Career Assessment, 2*, 276–288.
Ibrahim, F. A., & Owen, S. V. (1994). Factor analytic structure of the Scale to Assess World View©. *Current Psychology, 13*, 201–209.
Ibrahim, F. A., Roysircar-Sodowsky, G., & Ohnishi, H. (2001). Worldview: Recent developments and needed directions. In J. G. Ponterotto, M. J. Casas, L. A. Suzuki, & C. M. Alexander (Eds.), *Handbook of multicultural counseling* (2nd ed., p. 430). Thousand Oaks, CA: Sage.

Interian, A., Allen, L., Gara, M., & Escobar, J. (2008). A pilot study of culturally adapted cognitive behavior therapy for Hispanics with major depression. *Cognitive and Behavioral Practice, 15*(1), 67–75. doi:10.1016/j.cbpra.2006.12.002.

Ivey, A. E., Ivey, M. B., & Zalaquett, C. (2009). *Intentional interviewing and counseling*. Belmont, CA: Wadsworth/Cengage.

Ivey, A. E., Pedersen, P. B., & Ivey, M. B. (2008). *Intentional group counseling: A microskills approach*. Belmont, CA: Cengage.

Jalali, B. (2005). Iranian families. In M. McGoldrick, J. Giordano, & N. Garcia-Preto (Eds.), *Ethnicity and family therapy* (3rd ed., pp. 451–467). New York: Guilford.

Jalali, B., & Boyce, E. (1980). Multicultural families in treatment. *International Journal of Family Psychiatry, 4*, 475–484.

Kazdin, A. E. (2006). Childhood depression. *Journal of Child Psychology and Psychiatry, 31*(1), 121–160. doi:10.1111/j.1469-7610.1990.tb02276.x.

Keoke, E. D., & Porterfield, K. M. (2003). *Brainwashing and boarding schools: Undoing the shameful legacy* (n.d.). Retrieved November 26, 2008, from http://www.kporterfield.com/aicttw/articles/boardingschool.html

LaFromboise, T. D., & Bigfoot, D. S. (1988). Cultural and cognitive considerations in the prevention of American Indian adolescent suicide. *Journal of Adolescence, 11*, 139–153.

LaFromboise, T. D., & Foster, S. L. (1992). Cross-cultural training: Scientist-practitioner model and methods. *Counseling Psychologist, 20*(3), 472–489.

LaFromboise, T. D., Trimble, J. E., & Mohatt, G. E. (1990). Counseling intervention and American Indian tradition: An integrative approach. *Counseling Psychologist, 18*(4), 628–654.

Lapahie, H., Jr. (2001). *Dine' clans*. Retrieved November 24, 2008, from http://www.lapahie.com/Dine_Clans.cfm

Leong, F. T. L., Leach, M. M., & Malikiosos-Loizos, M. (2012). Internationalizing the field of counseling psychology. In F. T. L. Leong, W. E. Pickren, M. M. Leach, & A. J. Marsella (Eds.), *Internationalizing the psychology curriculum in the United States* (pp. 201–224). New York: Springer.

Lin, N., Dean, A. R. C., & Ensel, N. (Eds.). (1986). *Social support life events and depression*. New York: Academic.

Lonner, W. J., & Ibrahim, F. A. (2008). Appraisal and assessment in cross cultural counseling. In P. B. Pedersen, J. G. Draguns, W. J. Lonner, & J. E. Trimble (Eds.), *Counseling across cultures* (6th ed., pp. 37–55). Thousand Oaks, CA: Sage.

Lopez, E. C., & Rogers, M. R. (2007). Multicultural competencies and training in school psychology issues, approaches, and future directions. In G. B. Esquivel, E. C. Lopez, & S. G. Nahari (Eds.), *Multicultural handbook of school psychology: An interdisciplinary perspective* (pp. 47–67). Mahwah, NJ: Lawrence Erlbaum.

Manetta, C. T., Gentile, J. P., & Gillig, P. M. (2011). Examining the therapeutic relationship and confronting resistances in psychodynamic psychotherapy: A certified public accountant case. *Innovations in Clinical Neuroscience, 85*(5), 35–40.

Marantz Henig, R. (2010, August 18). What is it about 20-somethings? *The New York Times*.

Marsella, A. J., & Pedersen, P. (2004). Internationalizing the counseling psychology curriculum: Toward new values, competencies, and directions. *Counselling Psychology Quarterly, 17*(4), 413–423.

Maslow, A. H. (1987). *Motivation and personality* (3rd ed.). New York: Harper & Row.

McAuliffe, G., & Associates. (2012). *Culturally alert counseling: A comprehensive introduction*. Newbury Park, CA: Sage.

McCabe, M., Althof, S. E., Assalian, P., Chevret-Measson, M., Leiblum, S. R., Simonelli, C., et al. (2010). Psychological and interpersonal dimensions of sexual function and dysfunction. *The Journal of Sexual Medicine, 7*(1–2), 327–336.

McGoldrick, M., Giordano, J., & Garcia Preto, N. (Eds.). (2005). *Ethnicity and family therapy* (3rd ed.). New York: Guilford Press.

McKim, D. K. (2001). *Introducing the reformed faith*. Louisville, KY: Westminster.

Miami Family Therapy Institute. (n.d.). *Privilege-oppression continuum*. Unpublished document, Miami, FL.

Miller, S. D., Hubble, M. A., Chow, D. L., & Seidal, J. A. (2013). The outcome of psychotherapy: Yesterday, today, and tomorrow. *Psychotherapy, 50*(1), 88–97. doi:10.1037/a0031097.

Miller, W. R., & Rollnick, S. (2002). *Motivational interviewing: Preparing people for change* (2nd ed.). New York: Guilford Press.

Miller, W. R., & Rose, G. S. (2009). Toward a theory of motivational interviewing. *American Psychologist, 64*(6), 527–537.

Miller, J. B., & Stiver, I. P. (1997). *The healing connection: How women form relationships in therapy and in life*. Boston: Beacon.

Mirkin, M. P., & Kamya, H. (2008). Working with immigrant and refugee families. In M. McGoldrick & K. V. Hardy (Eds.), *Re-visioning family therapy* (2nd ed., pp. 311–326). New York: Guilford Press.

Mollen, D., Ridley, C. R., & Hill, C. L. (2003). Models of multicultural counseling competence. In D. B. Pope-Davis, H. L. K. Coleman, W. M. Liu, & R. L. Toporek (Eds.), *Handbook of multicultural counseling competencies in counseling and psychology* (pp. 21–37). Thousand Oaks, CA: Sage.

Navajo World. (n.d.). *Alcohol and poverty: Daily life on the rez* (p. 3). Retrieved November 25, 2008, from http://www.navajoworld.com/newsletter/earth3.htm

Navajo World. (n.d.). *The Navajo people: A brief history* (p. 2). Retrieved November 26, 2008, from http://www.navajoworld.com/newsletter/earth2.htm

Ponterotto, J. G. (1996). Multicultural counseling in the twenty-first century. *The Counseling Psychologist, 24*(2), 259–268.

Project Implicit. (2011). Retrieved from https://implicit.harvard.edu/implicit/

Radloff, L. S. (1977). The CES-D scale: A self-report depression scale for research in the general population. In *Counseling resource*. Retrieved November 27, 2008, from http://counsellingresource.com/quizzes/cesd/index.html

Renfrey, G. S. (1992). Cognitive-behavioral therapy and the Native American client. *Behavior Therapy, 23*, 321–340.

Resnick, P. A., Nisith, P., Weaver, T. L., Astin, M. C., & Feuer, C. A. (2002). A comparison of cognitive-processing therapy with prolonged exposure and a waiting condition for the treatment of chronic posttraumatic stress disorder in female rape victims. *Journal of Consulting and Clinical Psychology, 70*(4), 867–879.

Reynolds, S., Stiles, W. B., Barkham, M., Shapiro, D. A., Hardy, G. E., & Rees, A. (1996). Acceleration of changes in session impact during contrasting time-limited psychotherapies. *Journal of Consulting and Clinical Psychology, 64*, 577–586.

Roemer, L., & Orsillo, S. M. (2009). *Mindfulness and acceptance-based behavioral therapies in practice*. New York: Guilford Press.

Rojano, R., & Duncan-Rojano, J. (2005). Colombian families. In M. McGoldrick, J. Giordano, & N. Garcia-Preto (Eds.), *Ethnicity and family therapy* (3rd ed., pp. 311–346). New York: Guilford Press.

Rosenberger, J. B. (Ed.). (2014). *Introduction. Relational social work practice with diverse clients* (pp. 3–12). New York: Springer.

Rowan, A. B., & Foy, D. W. (1993). Post-traumatic stress disorder in child sexual abuse survivors: A literature review. *Journal of Traumatic Stress, 6*(1), 3–20.

Rowan, A. B., Foy, D. W., Rodriguez, N., & Ryan, S. (1994). Posttraumatic stress disorder in a clinical sample of adults sexually abused as children. *Child Abuse and Neglect, 18*, 51–61.

Sadlak, M. J. (1986). *A study of the impact of training in cross-cultural counseling on counselor effectiveness and sensitivity*. Doctoral dissertation, University of Connecticut, Storrs.

Seligman, M. E., Steen, T. A., Park, N., & Peterson, C. (2005). Positive psychology progress: Empirical validation of interventions. *American Psychologist, 60*(5), 410–421. doi:10.1037/003-066X.60.5.410.

Seligman, M. E. P., Walker, E. F., & Rosenham, D. L. (Eds.). (2001). *Abnormal psychology* (4th ed.). New York: W. W. Norton.

Stiles, W. B. (1980). Measurement of the impact of psychotherapy sessions. *Journal of Consulting and Clinical Psychology, 48*, 176–185.

Stiles, W. B., Gordon, L. E., & Lani, J. A. (2002). Session evaluation and the Session Evaluation Questionnaire. In G. S. Tryon (Ed.), *Counseling based on process research: Applying what we know* (pp. 325–343). Boston: Allyn & Bacon.

Stiles, W. B., Reynolds, S., Hardy, G. E., Rees, A., Barkham, M., & Shapiro, D. A. (1994). Evaluation and description of psychotherapy sessions by clients using the Session Evaluation Questionnaire and the Session Impacts Scale. *Journal of Counseling Psychology, 41*, 175–185.

Stiles, W. B., & Snow, J. S. (1984). Dimensions of psychotherapy session impact across sessions and across clients. *British Journal of Clinical Psychology, 23*, 59–63.

Stiles, W. B., Tupler, L. A., & Carpenter, J. C. (1982). Participants' perceptions of self-analytic group sessions. *Small Group Behavior, 13*, 237–254.

Suarez-Balcazar, Y., Durlak, J. A., & Smith, C. (1994). Multicultural training practices in community psychology programs. *American Journal of Community Psychology, 22*, 785–798.

Sue, D. W., & Sue, D. (2003). *Counseling the culturally diverse: Theory and practice* (4th ed.). New York: Wiley.

Sue, S., Zane, N., Hall, G. C. N., & Berger, L. K. (2009). The case for cultural competency in psychotherapeutic interventions. *Annual Review of Psychology, 60*, 525–548.

Sutton, C. E., & Broken Nose, M. A. (2005). American Indian families: An overview. In M. McGoldrick, J. Giordano, & N. Garcia-Preto (Eds.), *Ethnicity & family therapy* (3rd ed., pp. 43–54). New York: Guilford Press.

Tate, K. A., Rivera, E. T., Brown, E., & Skaistis, L. (2013). Foundations for liberation: Social justice, liberation, and counseling psychology. *Interamerican Journal of Psychology, 47*(3), 373–382.

Therapist Aid. (2012–2014). *Daily mood chart.* Retrieved December 17, 2014, from http://www.therapistaid.com/therapy-worksheet/daily-mood-chart/none/none

Tosone, C. (2004). Relational social work: Honoring the tradition. *Smith College Studies in Social Work, 74*(3), 475–487.

Trimble, J., & Gonzalez, J. (2008). Cultural considerations and perspectives for providing psychological counseling for Native American Indians. In P. B. Pedersen, J. Draguns, W. J. Lonner, & J. Trimble (Eds.), *Counseling across cultures* (6th ed., p. 96). Thousand Oaks, CA: Sage.

Truscott, D. (2010). *Becoming an effective psychotherapist: Adopting a theory of psychotherapy that's right for you and your client.* Washington, DC: American Psychological Association.

Ware, N. C., & Kleinman, A. (1992). Culture and somatic experience: The social course of illness in neurasthenia and chronic fatigue syndrome. *Psychosomatic Medicine, 54*(5), 546–560.

Winson, T. (2002). *The Navajo.* Retrieved November 25, 2008, from http://www.anthro4n6.net/navajo/

Zegley, L. A. (2007). *An investigation of the relationship between self-reported multicultural counseling competence and middle school counselors' efforts to broach racial, ethnic, and cultural factors with students.* Doctoral dissertation, Virginia Polytechnic Institute ad State University.

Zhang, N., & Burkard, A. (2008). Discussions of racial difference and the effect on client ratings of the working alliance and counselor. *Journal of Multicultural Counseling and Development, 36*(2), 77–87. doi:10.1002/j.2161-1912.2008.tb00072.x.

Appendix A
Cultural Identity Check-List-Revised©

Cultural Identity Checklist-Revised© (CICL-R)

Farah A. Ibrahim (2007)

Name: ______________________ Age: _________ Gender:__________

Cultural Background:_____________ Religion:____________________

Please respond to the following questions in the most direct manner, as you see yourself, rather than how others define you.

1. What is your ethnic background? Please list ethnicities of both parents and their parents.
2. (a) Which ethnic group has influenced your values and beliefs the most?
   (b) Which ethnic group do you identify with personally?
3. Is your cultural group indigenous to the USA? YES NO.
4. If your answer is no, when did your family or ancestors migrate to the USA?
   (a) Was migration a free choice or was it forced?
   (b) How was your ethnic group received?
5. How did your primary group establish itself in the USA?
6. What do you know about the sociopolitical history?
   (a) How do you feel about the sociopolitical history of your primary group?
7. What was the socioeconomic status of your family of origin?
8. What is your socioeconomic level?
9. What was the educational level of your parents?
10. What is your educational level?
11. Is your family monolingual? If your family is bilingual or trilingual, please list the languages they speak?
12. Are you monolingual? If you are bilingual or trilingual, please list the languages you speak, read, and write.

F.A. Ibrahim, J.R. Heuer, *Cultural and Social Justice Counseling*,
International and Cultural Psychology, DOI 10.1007/978-3-319-18057-1

13. Do you have a religious faith/affiliation?
    (a) Do you actively practice your faith and believe in it?
14. What is your birth order in your family of origin? Oldest? Middle? Or Youngest? Or are you an only child ? (please circle)
15. What is your sexual preference? Heterosexual? Homosexual? Bisexual?
    (a) How does your family relate to your sexual preference?
16. Do you have any disabilities? YES NO (please circle)
    (a) If yes, how does your family relate to your disability? Accept Y N (please circle)
17. How do you relate to your own gender identity? Do you accept it? Y N (please circle)
18. Does your family accept your gender? Y N (please circle)

Identify the three most salient features of your identity for you:

1.
2.
3.

The Cultural Identity Check List is not a test per se; it is a checklist to gather data that is usually overlooked in mental health settings; it has significance in a pluralistic society because it taps into all aspects of a person's identity, i.e., the concept of multiple identities. It can be used to gather demographic data on aspects that have relevance to culture, ethnicity, migration status, and provides a contextual analysis. Primarily, it helps in identifying the meaning of the various aspects of identity in terms of privilege and oppression. It also helps identify assets and challenges that a person possesses and how these facilitate or obstruct her or his life. Further, it helps in identifying significant areas of common ground that the therapist may share with the client. It can facilitate not only the counseling process, and development of goals, but also help in creating a shared worldview.

Some important issues to think about for helping professionals: (a) what are your cultural differences? What are your similarities? (b) When clients list the three significant areas of their identity, it can help in understanding the presenting problem, and what professionals need to be aware of in working with a specific client; and (c) exploring the CICL-R with the client will help in understanding the client's core values or worldview. The client's worldview is at the core of her/his/zir cultural identity.

Appendix B
Scale to Assess World View©

Scale to Assess World Views-II©

Farah A. Ibrahim & Steve V. Owen (1994)

Demographic Data:

ID#: Last four digits of ID (any ID including Driver's License):________

Age: ___________

Gender: Female____ Male___ Transgender___ Intersex____

Ethnicity: Asian (specific ethic group_________)

_____Black (African American) ______Black (International)

_____Latino/a _____Multiracial ______Native-American (Indian)

_____Pacific Islander (Specific group______)

_____White (Non-Hispanic) _______White (Hispanic)

_____Other (List:)

Religion_____________________ Spiritual not religious_________________

Region(s) of the country where you grew up_____________________________

Are you an immigrant? Y N

If yes, at what age did you migrate? ___________________________________

F.A. Ibrahim, J.R. Heuer, *Cultural and Social Justice Counseling*,
International and Cultural Psychology, DOI 10.1007/978-3-319-18057-1

Political affiliation: ____

Parents Economic Status: ____Upper class ____Middle class ____Lower class

Your Economic Status: Status: ____Upper class ____Middle class ____Lower class

Parents' educational level: Mom________ Dad_________________

Your educational level: ____________

Do you live in: ____Urban environment ____Suburban environment ____Rural environment

Scale to Assess World View© (SAWV)

This is a survey to assess some of your attitudes toward the world and people. Of course, there is no right or wrong answer. The best answer is what you feel is true of yourself.

Please respond to each of the questions according to the following scheme:

1	2	3	4	5
Strongly Disagree	Disagree	Undecided	Agree	Strongly Agree

CIRCLE THE ANSWER THAT BEST DESCRIBES YOUR ATTITUDE.

1. No weakness or difficulty can hold us back if we have enough will power.

   1 2 3 4 5

2. Human nature being what it is there will always be war and conflict.

   1 2 3 4 5

3. Women who want to remove the word obey from the marriage service do not understand what it means to be a wife.

   1 2 3 4 5

4. The past is no more, the future may never be, the present is all we can be certain of.

   1 2 3 4 5

5. Beneath the polite and smiling surface of human nature is a bottomless pit of evil.

   1 2 3 4 5

6. I believe life is easier in the cities where one has access to all modern amenities.

   1 2 3 4 5

7. When you come right down to it, it is human nature never to do anything without an eye to one's own profit.

   1 2 3 4 5

8. The reason you should not criticize others is that they will turn around and criticize you.

   1 2 3 4 5

9. The forces of nature are powerful enough to destroy everything that people can build.

   1 2 3 4 5

10. If I spend 14 years pursuing my education, I will have a good job in the future.

    1 2 3 4 5

11. Basically, all human beings have a great potential for good.

    1 2 3 4 5

12. The relationship between people and nature is one of mutual coexistence.

    1 2 3 4 5

13. It is important that people be involved in the present rather than concerned with the past or the future.

    1 2 3 4 5

14. The fact that I am in existence is enough for me, I do not necessarily also have to have major accomplishments in life.

    1 2 3 4 5

15. Although people are intrinsically good, they have developed institutions which force them to act in opposition to their basic nature.

    1 2 3 4 5

16. I plan for tomorrow, today is of no consequence, and the past is over with.

    1 2 3 4 5

17. I prefer to relax and enjoy life as it comes.

    1 2 3 4 5

18. The father is the head of the household; every person in the family should follow his lead.

1 2 3 4 5

19. We are healthier when we live in harmony with our natural world.

1 2 3 4 5

20. We can find happiness within ourselves.

1 2 3 4 5

21. Every person has the potential to do good.

1 2 3 4 5

22. When natural catastrophes occur, we have to accept them.

1 2 3 4 5

23. Planning for the future allows one to accomplish all of one's goals.

1 2 3 4 5

24. I believe that feelings and human relationships are the most important things in life.

1 2 3 4 5

25. Some people will help you and others will try to hurt you.

1 2 3 4 5

26. Top management should make all the decisions: everyone in the company should follow these directives.

1 2 3 4 5

27. I feel quite powerless when faced with the forces of nature.

1 2 3 4 5

28. We need to model our lives after our parents and ancestors and focus on our glorious past.

1 2 3 4 5

29. I believe it is more important to be a good person rather than a successful person.

1 2 3 4 5

30. Nowadays, a person has to live pretty much for today and let tomorrow take care of itself.

1 2 3 4 5

Scoring Instructions

Please add your scores on the following items and divide by the number given:

- WV I: Item# 1, 11, 12, 19, 20, 21, 22, 24, 29 divide by 9
- WV II: Item# 3, 6, 7, 8, 10, 16, 18, 23, 26, 28 divide by 10
- WV III: Item# 4, 13, 14, 17, 28, 30 divide by 6
- WV IV: Item# 2, 5, 7, 9, 15, 25, 27 divide by 7

The Four Worldviews

Optimistic Worldview (OWV I)

This perspective is characterized by values in three areas: Human nature, activity orientation, and Nature. There is a belief that human nature is essentially good. Activity must focus on inner and outer development (i.e., spiritual and material). There is a need to be in harmony with nature, with an acceptance of the power of nature.

This is a very common worldview among US born and raised individuals. The way you responded to the SAWV, in this case may reflect your ideal values as propagated by the culture. You need to reflect on this as it may simply be the way you are conditioned to respond, rather than what you actually do in terms of living by these assumptions. We all have an ideal set of values and analysis of our behavior in the past, and the present will help us see if this is really how we live and interact with others in our world.

Traditional Worldview (TWV II)

The emphasis in this perspective is on Social Relations, Time, and Nature. Social relationships are primarily lineal-hierarchical in this worldview (top down), with some expectations for collateral-mutual relationships (if you give me respect, then I will give you respect). Time is both mostly future oriented, with some emphasis on the past. Regarding Nature, there is a belief that it can be controlled.

This Calvinistic point of view represents patriarchal power relationships, social control, and a very strong future time orientation. This perspective is found in highly traditional societies, where controlling everyone in the social system is valued for the good of the social order. There is also a belief nature can be controlled, along with the environment, and the world we live in. For example, deciding to drive out in the midst of a blizzard with no regard to danger.

Spontaneous Worldview (SWV III)

This worldview reflects core values from two dimensions, Activity and Time. The Activity focus is primarily on spontaneity. Time emphasis is mainly on present time, with some attention to the past. This WV has emerged mostly after the end of the Vietnam War and is a reflection of the social movements of the 1960s and 1970s that challenged the TWV II, Calvinistic assumptions, and ideals of high social control.

There is also an influence of the Gestaltist worldview with the "here and now" focus of living in the moment. In addition, there is the influence of Eastern philosophy with a focus on meditation, focusing on the self to monitor emotions and manage oneself, and being spontaneous, instead of a rigid being that only lives for the future.

Pessimistic Worldview (PWV IV)

This perspective reflects core values from three dimensions: Human Nature, Social Relations, and Nature. Human nature is considered primarily bad, with some allowance for it being a combination of good and bad qualities. There is an acceptance of the power of nature. The relationship orientation is collateral-mutual. This worldview usually emerges as the secondary worldview for individuals who have the same ideals as people with the OWV I, but their place in the "system" is not one where they can achieve all that they value. There is also a feeling that if only "I lived in a fair world with compassionate beings" I could achieve all my goals and be happy.

Originally, this was named Pessimistic, but after reviewing the results of several research studies using the SAWV, it was learned that women and cultural nondominant groups in the USA generally come up with this as their secondary worldview. It was concluded that this actually represents a realistic perspective based on the realities of a person's life, and the limits that their gender, sexual orientation, SES, religion, or some other socially constructed vulnerability in their cultural identity brings this WV to the forefront.

The following readings can provide the philosophical and research background information on the scale.

Ibrahim, F. A. (1999). Transcultural counseling: Existential world view theory and cultural identity: Transcultural applications. In J. McFadden (Ed.), *Transcultural counseling* (2nd ed., pp. 23–57). Alexandria, VA: ACA Press.

Ibrahim, F. A., Roysircar-Sodowsky, G. R., & Ohnishi, H. (2001). World view: Recent developments and future trends. In J. G. Ponterrotto, M. Casas, L. Suzuki, & C. Alexander (Eds.), *Handbook of multicultural counseling* (2nd ed., pp. 425–456). Thousand Oaks, CA: Sage.

Ibrahim, F. A. (2003). Existential worldview theory: From inception to applications. In F. D. Harper, & J. McFadden (Eds.), *Culture and counseling: New approaches* (pp. 196–208). Boston: Allyn & Bacon.

Lonner, J., & Ibrahim, F. A. (2008). Assessment in cross-cultural counseling. In P. B. Pedersen, J. Draguns, W. J. Lonner, & J. Trimble (Eds.), *Counseling across cultures* (6th ed., pp. 37–57). Thousand Oaks, CA: Sage.

Appendix C
United States Acculturation Index©

United States Acculturation Index

Farah A. Ibrahim (2008)

Assessing Acculturation: A Rough Guide©

Acculturation has become a significant variable in understanding clients' worlds and the meaning they ascribe to various events. It is significant because you may underestimate the meaning of an event or situation based on your own level of acculturation to mainstream US society. It is important to not assume that everyone has the same level of acculturation; simply because they were born and raised here, or have so many degrees, or speak English without an accent, etc.

Acculturation in general refers to how close or distant one is from the host culture in terms of cultural knowledge, beliefs, values, assumptions, etc. In counseling, it has become essential to understand the acculturation level of all clients, to understand how this compares to mainstream cultural knowledge, beliefs, values, and assumptions. When I refer to "mainstream," I am really talking about White Anglo Saxon male heterosexual assumptions as these undergird the values of the majority of the population (Takaki, 1979). "Majority" here refers to the people who hold the power in the USA, i.e., the government, the legislature, the judiciary, multinational conglomerates, and the banks. Although, now women exceed men in the workforce (64 %), they are still a nondominant group, in terms of power and privilege.

So when you try to understand your acculturation level to "mainstream" assumptions, rate yourself on the following variables, depending on how close you are to the right side of the continuum will give you a fairly good index of your level of acculturation to mainstream assumptions. Similarly, when you sit with your clients, you can use this gauge to determine where they are on this variable and also how distant or close to you is the client's acculturation level.

F.A. Ibrahim, J.R. Heuer, *Cultural and Social Justice Counseling*,
International and Cultural Psychology, DOI 10.1007/978-3-319-18057-1

United States Acculturation Index©
Farah A. Ibrahim (2008)

Community focus	Individual focus
Show feelings	Stoic
Pessimistic	Optimistic
Social	Personal space valued
Relaxed	Rigid
Permeable boundaries	Strict boundaries
Interdependent	Independent
Present time focus	Future time focus
Recognizing lack of control	Can control life/situations
Highly family and kin oriented	Self-oriented
Success tied to all who helped made it happen	Success due to personal effort
Authoritarian relationships	Mutual relationships
Age is revered	Youth is revered
Mind/body connected	Mind/body separate

Reference

Takaki, R. (1979). *Iron cages: Race and culture in 19th-century America.* New York: Oxford University Press.

Scoring the USAI

The USAI has items on a continuum, it reflects information that represent two opposing perspectives. There are no right or wrong answers, it helps you determine how close or distant your perspectives are from the "official" mainstream assumptions.

Divide the continuum into three thirds: ………/………/……….

The first third represents that the left quadrant has been chosen reflecting collectivism.

The middle third represents a position that indicates the person accepts both ends of the spectrum as meaningful

The last third represents commitment to the items at this end of the continuum reflecting individualism.

Look at the scores and identify where the you/client stands, write a summary of acculturation or privilege and oppression.

Index

A

Acculturation
- and adaptation, 6, 149
- assessment, 86–89
- assumptions, 84–85
- attitudinal and behavioral adherence, 81
- categorization, 81
- client's adaptation, 7
- cognitive/behavioral, 81
- counseling implications, 90–91
- cultural competency, 78
- cultural differences, 77–78
- cultural hierarchies, 7
- culture shock, 82–83
- definition, 79–80
- depression and mental illness, 83
- ethnic identity, 80, 83–84
- human diversity, 77
- identity resolution, 154
- marginalization, 80–81
- migration, 78–79
- multidimensional and multidirectional, 82
- nondominant cultural groups, 155
- personal identity, 84
- positive/negative experiences, 7
- privilege and oppression status, 170
- and psychological well-being, 85–86
- social identity theory, 83
- stress, 82, 83
- U-curve, 82
- US residents, 78

Acculturative stress
- cultural contexts, 79–80
- marginalization, 85
- and mental health data, 83

Advocacy. *See also* Social justice
- ACAs, 104
- in counseling and psychotherapy, 104
- counseling theory and practice, 104–105
- counter-discourses, 21, 22
- cultural competence principles, 135
- knowledge and skills, 91
- mental health professions, 105
- social institutions, 138
- social justice principles
  - ACA and APA, 106
  - counseling psychology, 107–108
  - CSWE, 105
  - human development, 106
  - modern societies, 107
  - NASW, 105
  - operationalization, 108–109
  - recommendations, 106–107

Age
- and developmental stage, 19–20
- global knowledge bases, 29
- life stages, 1, 3, 15
- retirement, 139

American Counseling Association (ACA), 67
- advocacy competencies, 107
- and APA, 106
- mental health professional organizations, 1
- multicultural competencies, 55

American Psychological Association (APA), 1, 3, 9, 16, 20, 23, 24, 30, 78, 106
- and ACA (*see* American Counseling Association (ACA))
- DSM-IV, 3
- "gender non-conformity", 20

F.A. Ibrahim, J.R. Heuer, *Cultural and Social Justice Counseling*, International and Cultural Psychology, DOI 10.1007/978-3-319-18057-1

Assimilation
and acculturation, 213
acculturative stress, 85
classical assimilation theory, 130
mental health problems, 89
stages, process, 131
US cultural assumptions, 89
Association for Multicultural Counseling and Development (AMCD), 55, 67, 135
Assumptions
Catholics, 30
pathology, 22
socioeconomic levels, 35
superficial knowledge/understanding, 26–27
worldview (*see* Worldview)
Attitudes, 5–6, 19, 20, 31, 82, 88, 115

B
Behavior
CBT, 200
dialectical behavior therapy, 8
gender, 20–22
oppression, 24
Bicultural effectiveness training (BET), 90
Bicultural native American client (case study)
acculturation index, 196
adjunct interventions, 202
alcohol use, 202
anxiety disorder, 201
assessment process, 195
assessments and interventions evaluation, 202–203
behavioral observations, 197
CES-D, 197
childhood and adolescence, 194
clinical interview, 197
counselor biases, 198–199
cultural identity assessment, 195–196
depression, anxiety and alcohol abuse, 193
DSM-5, 195
intervention plan, 199–200
liberation psychology, 201–202
MDD, 200
motivational interviewing, 201
psychosocial history, 194–195
risk assessment, 198
trauma history, 197
worldview, 195
Birth order
behavioral characteristics, 32
educational level, 32
in family, 16
female children, 32
parental and marital stability, 32
Broaching, 169

C
Center for Epidemiological Studies—Depression (CES-D), 197
Center for Substance Abuse Treatment (CSAT), 161
Chronic stressors, 83
Cognitive
affective, and behavioral aspects, 62
and cultural schemas, 58
disabilities, 30
functioning, 90
Cognitive behavioral therapy (CBT), 200, 201, 203, 204, 209, 224, 229
Colombian Immigrant Client (case study)
CFI, 207
cultural identity assessment, 205–206
DSM-5, 208
group therapy, 209
problem presention, 204–205
psychiatric evaluation, 208
relationship building, 209
social/educational background, 205
vocational counseling, 209
worldview, 206–207
Competency statements, 1, 106
Connor–Davidson Resilience Scale, 213
Council on Social Work Education (CSWE), 105
Counseling. *See also* Refugees
AMCD, 135
BET, 90
biculturalism, 90
CICL-R, 54
contextual-structural barriers, 133
CSAT, 161
cultural identity, 54
cultural malpractice, 54
cultural trauma, 160
ecological systems, 134
evidence-based treatments, 133
five-level intervention program, 135–136
implications, 90–91
interventions
client cultural information, 60
cultural identity, 59
diagnosis and treatment, 59
ethnic groups, 59
OWV (*see* Optimistic Worldview (OWV))

process and goals, 60
SAWV, 60
TWV (*see* Traditional worldview (TWV))
macrosystem, 134
MAIP Model, 160
mental health problems, 132
mesosystem, 134
MLM, 135
multicultural competencies, 55
personal identity, 91
psychohistorical paradigm, 134
psychological assessments, 132–133
psychological well-being, 90
SAWV, 55
skills, 161–162
social–cultural barriers, 133
therapeutic relationship, 54
trauma awareness, 161
treatment modalities, 162–163
worldview assessment
hypothesis, 56
information, 57
SAWV, 56
Counseling interventions
cultural assessments (*see* Cultural assessment)
cultural identity, 16
evaluation, 170
multicultural/social justice, 137
SAWV, 60
worldview information, 59–60
Counseling modalities
group level, 110
individual level, 109–110
societal and global contexts, 111–112
theoretical frameworks, 19
therapist characteristics, 112–114
Counselor biases
bicultural native American client (case study), 198–199
cross-racial African American adoptee (case study), 190
Iranian immigrant client (case study), 228
native American client (case study), 180
transgender client (case study), 222
Cross-racial African American adoptee (case study)
acculturation level, 189
assessments, 188
counselor biases, 190
cultural identity assessment, 189
description, 186–187
empowerment, 191
feminist therapy and bibliotherapy, 191–192
gender-role intervention, 191
intervention plan, 190–191
worldview, 189
Cultural acculturation. *See* Acculturation
Cultural assessment
APA, 3
broaching cultural issues, 169
CFI, 3
CICL-R, 170
client's identity, 171
counseling process, 169–170
depression
healing systems, 7–9
identity (*See* Cultural identity)
mental health service providers, 1
paper–pencil assessments, 170
privilege and oppression, 5–6
psychological interventions, 171–175
psychotherapy and counseling, 1
Cultural background, 4, 16, 25, 58, 204, 204, 225
Cultural Formulation Interview (CFI), 36, 207
Cultural identity. *See also* Cultural assessment; Gender
AAMFT, 16
ability/disability status, 30–31
age and developmental stage, 19–20
assessment, 219
Cultural Identity Check List-Revisedc, 16
developmental counseling theory, 19
DSM-5 CFI, 36
ethnicity, 16–18
exploration, 212
helpers and client, 169
human suffering, 35
intersectionality, 15–16
mental health professionals, 36, 138
multicultural identity development model, 155
multidimensionality, 156
positive/negative experiences, 15
psychological literature, 36
psychological theories, 2
refugee, 157
SAWV, 4
social construction, 15
social–cultural identity, 154–155
SPH, 157
tribes/ethnic groups, 15
variables, 4, 112, 170
and worldview, 2, 156
Cultural Identity Check List-Revised© (CICL-R), 2, 4, 35, 170, 181, 189
Cultural malpractice, 22, 54, 57, 59

Cultural responsiveness. *See also* Cultural assessment
- client assumptions, 55
- social justice
  - counseling, 109
  - interventions, 1
- therapeutic process, 89

D

Demographics
- Crow Creek Reservation, 182
- cultural psychology, 4
- ethnicity, 68
- SAWV, 4
- and social factors, 127
- US, 103–104

Diagnostic and statistical manual-V (DSM 5)
- bicultural native American client (case study), 198
- CFI, 36
- Colombian immigrant client (case study), 208
- DSM-IV-TR categorization, 23
- Iranian immigrant client (case study), 228
- lesbian Latina client (case study), 214
- native American client (case study), 179
- transgender client (case study), 221–222

Disability
- and ability, 3, 59
- mental health professionals, 5
- multicultural counseling, 30
- multicultural movement, 31
- sensitivity, 30
- therapy models, 31
- worldview, 69

E

Ethnic identity (EI)
- acculturation
  - hyphenated American, 80
  - individuals, 83–84
  - intercultural contact, 80
  - process, 80
  - psychosocial changes, 80
  - social identity theory, 83
- counseling and psychotherapy, 78
- development and maintenance, 18, 124
- government agencies, 17
- immigrants/sojourners, 18
- interaction, 18
- and worldview, 80

Ethnicity
- cultural identity assessment, 16
- and gender, 3
- monocultural societies, 16–17
- negative feelings, 125
- political community, 17
- and sexuality, 34
- social relationships, 17

Eurobarometer, 27

Exclusion
- acculturative stress, 83
- and discrimination, 86
- hyphenated American, 80
- and isolation, 24
- and prejudice, 9
- and racism, 26
- stressors, 24

F

Family
- AAMFT, 16, 78
- composition, 31–32
- and friends, 132
- living arrangement, 3
- nonbiological parents, 187
- values and assumptions, 55

G

Gender
- anthropology, 21
- biological sex, 20
- cultural conceptualizations, 22
- cultural identity, 15
- and ethnicity, 3
- "gender non-conformity", 20
- identity, 2, 22–23, 219
- linguistic anthropology, 21
- men and women, 21
- multicultural counseling, 21
- psychological research, 20
- social–cultural contexts, 21
- transgender identity, 23–24
- transsexual concerns, 8

Gender dysphoria disorder, 222–223

Geographical environment, 3, 33–34

Global context, 11–112, 109

H

The Harvard Program in Refugee Trauma (HPRT), 163

Healing
- Client's Cultural World, 7–9
- Far East Asian healing method, 137

Navajo people, 203
traditional healing practices, 135–136
traditional Navajo spiritualities, 196
Here-and-now/spontaneous worldview (SWV)
collectivistic cultures, 65
process and goals, 65–66
time and activity, 65
Homophobia, 112
Host culture
acculturation, 3, 126–128
adaptation, 80, 127
assimilation, 127
BET, 90
bicultural identity, 125, 128
cultural awareness, 79
ethnicity, 125–126
hypothesis, 127
immigrant identity development, 126
immigrants, 84
marginalization, 127–128
personal/ethnic identity, 128
psychological adaptation, 126
religion/spirituality, 30

I
Identity development. *See also* Phases, identity development; Refugees
acculturation process, 124
adolescence, 154
commitment-making and identification, 155
cultural identity, 156
ethnic/personal identity, 124–125
homosexual, 24
host culture and adaptation, 123–124
"ideal" family, 32
individual, 154
integrated identity, 155
integration, host culture (*see* Host culture)
LGBT, 25
multidimensional identity, 156
psychological acculturation, 124
psychological interventions, 154
psychosocial and relational identity, 157
refugee, 157
social identity development models, 155
SPH, 157
Western context, 155
Immigrants. *See also* Identity development
acculturation (*see* Acculturation)
challenges, 136–137
in host culture, 123
identity (*see* Identity development)
indigenous people, 25
positive immigrant identity development, 138–140
social–cultural conditions, 123
sojourners, 18
Western European immigrants, 25–26
Implicit bias, 175
Individual level, 20, 83, 109–110
Integration. *See also* Host culture
acculturation, 82, 85, 88
bicultural identity, 82
ethnic group, 18
monocultural societies, 16–17
US society, 26
Internalized oppression, 107, 227, 231
Intersex and transgendered (IT) refugees, 148
Interventions. *See also* Cultural assessment
BET, 90
personal identity, 91
Iranian immigrant client (case study)
assessments and intervention evaluation, 230–231
CBT, 229
client insights and strengths, 229
collaborative goal setting, 231
counselor biases, 228
cultural identity checklist, 227
DSM-5, 228
level of acculturation, 227–228
muscle relaxation technique, 231
posttraumatic stress disorder, 231
problem presention, 225
social/educational background, 225–227
socioeconomic status, 225
worldview, 227

L
Language
emotional expression, 27
Eurobarometer, 27
globalization, 27
knowledge and skills, 27
non-English speaking client, 28
Lesbian gay bisexual and transgendered (LGBT), 24
Lesbian Latina client (case study)
acculturation, 213
CFI, 207
client strengths, 211–212
Connor–Davidson Resilience Scale, 213
cultural identity assessment, 205–206
cultural identity exploration, 212
depression and anxiety, 211
DSM-5, 214

Lesbian Latina client (case study) (*cont.*)
family structure, 211
goals, 215–217
intervention plan, 214–215
privileged-oppression continuum, 213–214
social/educational background, 205
worldview, 206–207, 212–213
Liberation psychology, 201–202
Lifespan, 23, 25, 31, 154, 161

M
Major depressive disorder (MDD), 197–200, 208
Microaggressions
ethnic/racial nondominant populations, 9
social justice variables, 99
Migration status
acculturation, 78–79
immigrant generation, 26–27
mental health professionals, 26
orthodox religions, 26
shame and anxiety, 26
sociopolitical changes, 26
Western European immigrants, 25–26
Multicultural assessment intervention process (MAIP) model, 160
Multidimensionality of identity, 36, 37, 156
The multilevel model (MLM), 135, 136
Multiple identities, 16, 231
acculturation, 80
sexual orientation, 24

N
National Association of Social Work (NASW)
and APA, 16
cultural competency, 78
health disparities, 105
professional standards, 105
Native American client (case study)
assessments and intervention evaluation, 183–185
counselor biases, 180
cultural identity assessment, 178
description, 176
DSM-5 diagnosis, 179
gender identity, 179
intervention, 180
level of acculturation, 179
sleeping, 176
social/educational background, 177–178
spirituality, 179
worldview, 178

O
Oppression. *See also* Privilege
and emotional abuse, 23
individual and group counseling, 109
and privilege, 3, 5–6
psychological adjustment, 24
social construct, 100
social justice variables, 99
societal attitudes, 30
and victimization, 23
Optimistic worldview (OWV)
activity, 61
human nature, 61
nature dimension, 61
process and goals, 62

P
Personal identity, 84, 86, 124–126, 128
Pessimistic worldview (PWV), 66–67
Phases, identity development
acculturation, 129
assimilation model, 131
classical assimilation theory, 130–131
communication, 129
cross-cultural identity, 130
developmental and positivist models, 130
ethnic group membership, 132
immigrant children, 130
multicultural model, 131
multivariate model, 129
psychological adaptation, 129
second–culture acquisition, 131–132
Posttraumatic stress disorder, 223
Prejudice
discrimination, 80
and exclusion, 206
hyphenated Americans, 80–81
Presenting problem
bicultural native American client, 193
Colombian immigrant client (case study), 204–205
identity, domains, 35–36
Iranian immigrant client, 225
native American client, 176–177
stress, 170
transgender client, 218
Privilege. *See also* Oppression
advocacy and activism, 109
anger/defensiveness, 101
APA, 106
Client's perception, 5
description, 101
non justice-related, 102

and oppression analysis (*see* Oppression)
and oppression function, 24
social justice and equity issues, 5
social justice variables, 99
"spared injustice", 102
training programs, 5–6
"valued" gender, 6
Psychological acculturation
attitudes, approaches, 88
"black box", 87
definition, 79
imposter phenomenon, 89
individualism and collectivism, 88
mental illness, 89
methodological issues, 86
proxy variables, 87
qualitative approaches, clients, 87
social desirability, 87
in USA, 89
Psychological interventions
authenticity, 171–172
client, empathy, 172
client strengths, 173
cross-cultural counseling relationships, 173
cultural responsiveness, 175
effectiveness, evaluation, 174
mutual relationship and co-construction, 172–173
"not knowing" perspective, 171
Psychological well-being, acculturation, 85–86
Psychotherapy. *See* Counseling

Q
Quick Discrimination Index (QDI), 114, 115

R
Racism, 81
African Americans, 83
exclusion, 6
and oppression, 188
and sexism, 5
Refugees. *See also* Identity development
classification, immigrants, 149
counseling (*see* Counseling)
ethnic studies and psychology, 149
identity development, 154–157
IT, 148
language and culture, 154
mental health professionals, 148–149
politics and perceptions, 149–154
"social group", 148
trauma, 158–160
UNHCR, 147–148
Religion
Bedouin culture, 30
counseling, 29
invaders and colonizers, 29
mental health assessment, 28
mental health practitioners, 29
parents' faith/spiritual beliefs, 29
worldview, 29

S
Scale to Assess World View© (SAWV), 4, 37, 51, 67, 69, 181, 212
Sexism, 5, 9, 112, 114, 115, 191
Sexual orientation
homosexual identity, 24
LGBT, 24
stage models, 25
Shared worldview, 57, 173
Social class
bidirectional interaction, 34
cultural identity, 34
culture and class boundaries, 34
culture stratification, 34
interpersonal and internalized classism, 35
therapist assumptions, 35
Social Class Worldview Model (SCWM), 34
Social construction, 2, 15, 17, 22, 100, 101
Social contexts, 6, 34, 99, 105, 128, 131, 134
Social identity
acculturation, 83
definition, 17
group, 100
and personal, 91
Socialization
beliefs and values, 29
client's culture, 3
collectivistic system, 4
discrimination and prejudice, 80–81
in geographical region, 33
graduate schools culture, 5
and life experiences, 9
social–cultural contexts, 21
Social justice. *See also* Counseling modalities
acculturation (*see* Acculturation)
and advocacy in counseling (*see* Advocacy)
assessment, 114–115
capitalism, 100
categories and hierarchies, 100–101
cultural differences, 99
democratic society, 103
equality, 100

Social justice. *See also* Counseling modalities (*cont.*)
humanity, 99
human rights, 101
issues, 104, 108, 109, 112, 114, 140
male *vs.* female, 101
non justice-related privilege, 102
possessive investment in Whiteness, 101–102
privilege, 101–102
social groups, 100
"spared injustice" privilege, 102
US demographics, 103–104
"Soul wound", 182
Spirituality. *See also* Religion
Catholicism, 194
emotional meaning, 28
identification variables, 16
leader, 8
Navajo people, 190
nondominant religions, 68
traditional assumptions, 30

T
Therapeutic relationship, 57–59
Therapist characteristics
competencies and recommendations, 113
counseling and psychotherapy, 113
counselor–client relationship, 112
cultural and social competence, 114
individual and group interventions, 112
power dimension, 112
social justice challenges, 114
Traditional worldview (TWV)
nature subscale, 63
philosophers, 63
process and goals, 64
social relations, 62
tradition and authority, 63
Transgender client (case study)
acculturation index, 220
behavioral observations, 221
childhood and adolescence, 218
clinical interview, 221
counselor biases, 222
cultural identity assessment, 219
DSM-5, 221–222
gender dysphoria disorder, 223
intervention plan, 222–223
posttraumatic stress disorder, 223
psychodynamic treatment, 224
psychosocial history, 219
risk assessment, 221
sexual dysfunction, 223
sexual performance issues, 218
trauma history, 220
worldview, 220
Transgender identity, 23–24
Trauma
emotional abuse and stress, 23
and posttraumatic effects, 164
race-related, 6
refugees, 28
resolution, 159, 163
trauma-informed treatment, 162
Treatment modalities, 162–163
TWV. *See* Traditional worldview (TWV)

U
U-curve, 82
United Nations High Commission for Refugees (UNHCR), 147
Urban refugees, 147

W
Worldview. *See also* Counseling; Cultural identity
acculturation, 185
beliefs and assumptions, 52
bicultural native American client (case study), 195
collectivistic/individualistic cultural systems, 4
Colombian immigrant client (case study), 206–207
cross-cultural counseling, 3
cross-racial African American adoptee (case study), 189
cultural heritage, 135
cultural identity, 156
culture-specific aspects, 52
decision-making and problem solving, 51
definition, 4, 51
EI, 80
Iranian immigrant client (case study), 227
Kluckhohn's existential value, 53
lesbian Latina client (case study), 206, 212–213
native American client (case study), 178
research, 67–69
SAWV, 178
socialization process, 52
transgender client (case study), 220

The manufacturer's authorised representative in the EU is Springer
Nature Customer Service Centre GmbH, Europaplatz 3, 69115 Heidelberg,
Germany. If you have any concerns regarding our products, please
contact ProductSafety@springernature.com

Printed and bound by CPI Group (UK) Ltd, Croydon, CR0 4YY
25/09/2026
02222857-0009